Pregnancy
Care book

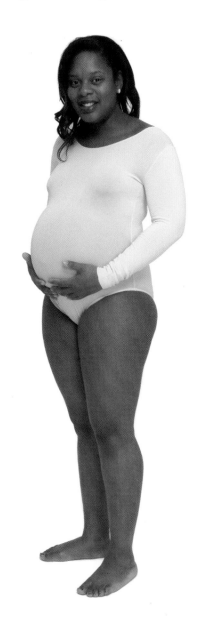

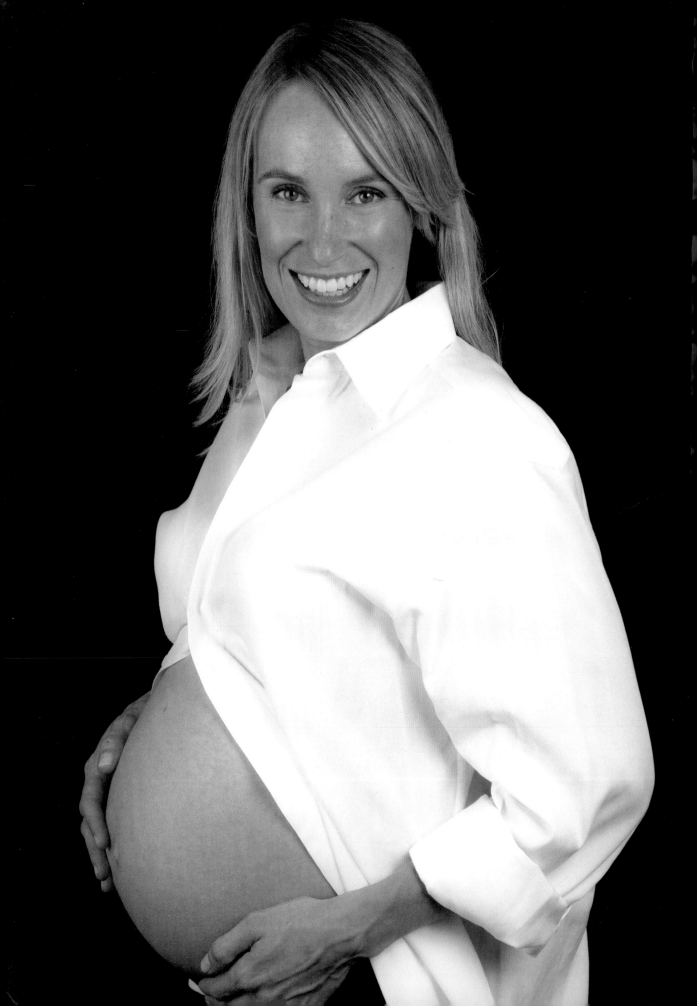

Pregnancy
Care book

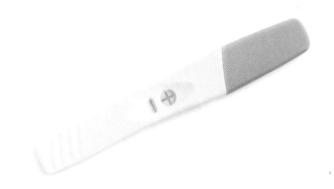

Dr. Michèle Farrugia, MD, FRCS(C)
Dr. Jacqueline Thomas, MD, FRCS(C)
Dr. Paul Bernstein, MD, FRCS(C)

MOUNT SINAI HOSPITAL

Robert
ROSE

For complete cataloguing information, see page 470.

This book is a general guide only and should never be a substitute for the skill, knowledge, and experience of a qualified medical professional dealing with the facts, circumstances, and symptoms of a particular case.

The nutritional, medical, and health information presented in this book is based on the research, training, and professional experience of the authors, and is true and complete to the best of their knowledge. However, this book is intended only as an informative guide for those wishing to know more about health, nutrition, and medicine; it is not intended to replace or countermand the advice given by the reader's personal physician. Because each person and situation is unique, the author and the publisher urge the reader to check with a qualified health-care professional before using any procedure where there is a question as to its appropriateness. A physician should be consulted before beginning any exercise program. The author and the publisher are not responsible for any adverse effects or consequences resulting from the use of the information in this book. It is the responsibility of the reader to consult a physician or other qualified health-care professional regarding his or her personal care.

Editor: Bob Hilderley, Senior Editor, Health
Copy editor: Susan Girvan
Proofreader: Sheila Wawanash
Indexer: Gillian Watts
Design and production: Andrew Smith & Daniella Zanchetta/PageWave Graphics Inc.
Illustrations: Steven Hall/Three in a Box
Front cover photo: © Larry Williams/Corbis
Back cover photo: ©iStockphoto.com/digitalskillet
For a complete list of photo credits, see page 469.

The publisher acknowledges the financial support of the government of Canada through the Book Publishing Industry Development Program (BPIDP).

Published by Robert Rose Inc.,
120 Eglinton Ave. E. Suite 800, Toronto, Ontario, Canada M4P 1E2
Tel: (416) 322-6552 Fax: (416) 322-6396

Printed and bound in Canada

1 2 3 4 5 6 7 8 9 TCP 17 16 15 14 13 12 11 10 09

To all of the women we have cared for and who have
allowed us the privilege and joy of participating
in the birth of their babies

and

To our mentors and colleagues who generously
taught us all that we know and do and who continue
to inspire us to learn, do, and be more.

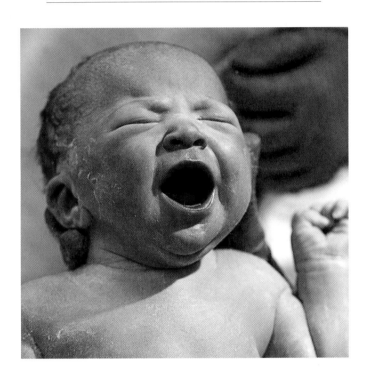

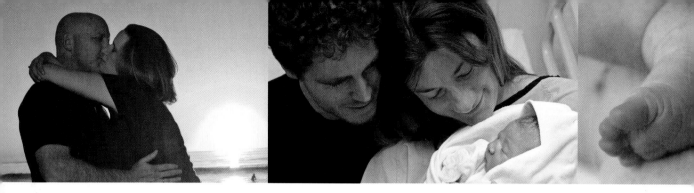

Contents

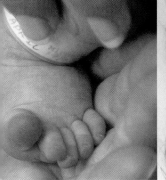
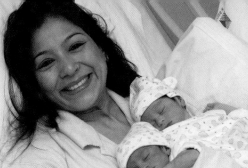
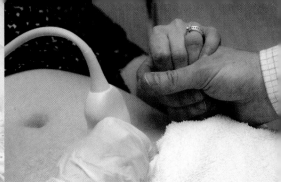

Contributing Editors

Michèle Farrugia, MSc, MD, M.Ed, FRCS(C)
Department of Obstetrics and Gynaecology
Mount Sinai Hospital
Assistant Professor, Faculty of Medicine
University of Toronto

Jacqueline Thomas, MD, MSc, FRCS(C)
Department of Obstetrics and Gynaecology
Mount Sinai Hospital
Assistant Professor, Faculty of Medicine
University of Toronto

Paul Bernstein MD, FRCS(C)
Department of Obstetrics and Gynaecology
Mount Sinai Hospital
Associate Professor, Faculty of Medicine
University of Toronto

Contributing Authors

Yoel Abells, BSc, MHSc, MD, CCFP, FCFP
Lecturer, University of Toronto
Department of Family Medicine
Mount Sinai Hospital

Lisa Allen, MD, FRCSC
Section Head, Pediatric Gynaecology
Division of Endocrinology
Hospital for Sick Children
Head, Gynaecology
Mount Sinai Hospital
Assistant Professor,
Department of Obstetrics and Gynaecology and Paediatrics
University of Toronto

Marshall P. Barkin, MD, FRCS, FACOG, FSOGC
Department of Obstetrics and Gynaecology
Mount Sinai Hospital

Assistant Professor, Faculty of Medicine
University of Toronto

Elizabeth Brandeis, BHSc, RM
Midwives Collective of Toronto
Department of Family Medicine
Mount Sinai Hospital

Laura Crouse, RN, BScN, IBCLC
Mount Sinai Hospital

Ariel Dalfen, MD, FRCP(C)
Perinatal Mental Health Program
Department of Psychiatry
Mount Sinai Hospital
Lecturer, Faculty of Medicine
University of Toronto

Eric Goldszmidt, MD, FRCP(C)
Department of Anaesthesia and Pain Medicine
Mount Sinai Hospital
Assistant Professor, Faculty of Medicine
University of Toronto

Preeti Jain, MD FRCP(C), FAAP
Department of Paediatrics
Mount Sinai Hospital

Elyse S. Levinsky, MD, MHSc, FRCS(C)
Department of Obstetrics and Gynaecology
Mount Sinai Hospital
Assistant Professor, Faculty of Medicine
University of Toronto

Erin Love, BSc, RD
Department of Nutrition and Food Services
Mount Sinai Hospital
Division of Haematology/ Oncology
Department of Paediatrics
The Hospital for Sick Children
Teaching Instructor
Internationally Educated Dietitians Pre-registration Program
Ryerson University

Elliot Lyons, MD, FRCS(C)
Division of General Obstetrics and Gynaecology
Department of Obstetrics and Gynaecology
Mount Sinai Hospital
Assistant Professor, Faculty of Medicine
University of Toronto

Jesseny Rojas
Corrective Exercise Specialist
Holistic Lifestyle Coach

Jodi Shapiro, MD, MHSc, FRCSC
Department of Obstetrics and Gynaecology
Mount Sinai Hospital
Assistant Professor, Faculty of Medicine
University of Toronto

Matthuschka Sheedy, RN, BNSc, ICCE
Coordinator, Prenatal Education Program
Women's and Infants' Ambulatory Health Programs
Mount Sinai Hospital

Dr. Ants Toi, MD, FRCPC
Radiologist, Department of Medical Imaging
Co-director of Center of Excellence in Obstetrical Ultrasound
Mount Sinai Hospital and University Health Network
Associate Professor of Radiology and of Obstetrics and Gynaecology,
Faculty of Medicine
University of Toronto

Beverly Young, MD, FRCPC
Clinical Director, Perinatal Mental Health Program
Department of Psychiatry
Mount Sinai Hospital
Lecturer, Faculty of Medicine
University of Toronto

Introduction

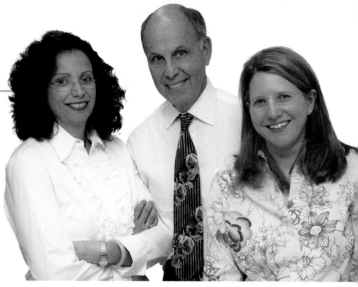

Welcome to the Mount Sinai Hospital *Pregnancy Care Book*! But why another pregnancy book, you might ask? Surely between the plethora of previously published books and the Internet, there is no need for yet another book about pregnancy. At the outset, we asked this question, too. Then we spoke to the people who count — our patients. We soon learned that some books tended to scare women with textbook detail, some were too superficial, and none reflected our approach to pregnancy and childbirth. We set out to write a balanced, practical, and straight-talking guide. We think we've succeeded in clarifying the progress of an uncomplicated pregnancy and have prepared you to handle any complications you might encounter along the road. We're not here to scare you, but rather to prepare you for childbirth.

It is au courant to have a philosophy about pregnancy and birth. We won't be preachy, but we do believe that

- Pregnancy is a condition of health, not a disease
- Pregnancy and birth can be a time of vulnerability to medical problems, and monitoring is wise to ensure continued health
- Birth is a rite of passage but not the most important part of either pregnancy or parenthood
- Safety of mother and child is paramount
- Health-care professionals should support women in their choices

The information in this book is supported by medical research, where it is available. Surprisingly, perhaps, many aspects of obstetric care have not been adequately researched and we can only rely upon expert opinion for guidance. Because opinions can vary, you may find information here that conflicts with information from other sources. We have tried to indicate when a practice is controversial and when the practice is well supported by evidence, but we know that it can be confusing to sort it out. If this is the case, it is probably best to talk with your doctor or midwife.

You can use this book in a number of ways. You may choose to read it cover to cover, following the course of a pregnancy from conception through delivery to care of a newborn. Pregnancy is divided into three trimesters of roughly equal length. We have chapters for each trimester, further divided into month-to-month sections where you will find information about the progress of your pregnancy and the growth of your baby at each stage. Interspersed with these "progress" chapters are "theme" chapters on such subjects as nutrition and exercise in pregnancy.

More likely, you will dip into the book, reading here and there, looking for answers to specific questions that you have. We have designed the book with many DYK (Did you know?) and FAQ (Frequently asked questions) features that should pique your interest. At the beginning of the book, there is a pregnancy diary for you — a space to record medical information and to respond to how you are feeling and what you are thinking. We trust the book is accessible, with many different ports of entry.

Throughout the book, you will find beautiful photographs of "real" pregnant women and their babies. Many are patients and colleagues of ours who deserve more than our thanks.

We are a trio of obstetricians at Mount Sinai Hospital in Toronto, each with a busy obstetric practice caring for pregnant women and delivering their babies. We have been privileged to help women deliver thousands of babies. We are also parents, with eight children among us! We have been on both sides of the examining table and delivery bed. Even with all of our training, the personal experience of pregnancy and birth was special, but sometimes also mystifying. They just don't teach you everything in medical school or residency! We are going to be beside you as you go through your pregnancy, providing you with practical advice every step of the way.

Families come in all shapes and sizes. There are many ways to make a family, and they do not all involve a man and a woman. Sometimes a new baby will have two mothers, sometimes two dads. Sometimes, the woman carrying the pregnancy will not be the same person who will care for the baby after birth. We have been privileged to care for women with all sorts of families and family plans. Sometimes, we simplify the language and refer to a traditional family as a matter of convenience only. Non-traditional families may have some unique issues to face that may not be addressed fully in this book, but there are also many similar concerns we do address. Please bear with us … and forgive us. This book is intended to be welcoming to all families.

We all feel fortunate to be associated with Mount Sinai Hospital. Mount Sinai has become a leader in obstetric care and research, with a worldwide reputation. At Mount Sinai, we deliver more than 6500 babies a year, and while the majority of our mothers have healthy full-term pregnancies, our colleagues care for a significant number of women with very complicated pregnancies. We are fortunate to have a large and well-supported Womens' and Infants' Ambulatory Health Program, with more than 20 obstetricians on staff, half of whom are also subspecialists in maternal-fetal medicine, as well as numerous family doctors and midwives who care for women in our hospital, before, during, and after the birth of their baby. Our neonatal intensive care unit is a leader in its own right. In addition to the obstetric staff, we have a large number and variety of other specialists who help support women and their babies as necessary, including pediatricians, anesthesiologists, radiologists, psychiatrists, internists, and geneticists. We draw upon the expertise of our dietitians, social workers, lactation consultants, and nurses daily as resources for ourselves and our patients. This is the context in which we practice obstetrics, and helps explain how we were able to enlist the support of so many experts to help us write this book. If you look at the contributors page, you will see that we enlisted the help of 15 of our colleagues from many different fields to contribute their expertise so that you have the most relevant and important information on every page.

Our primary goal in this book, and in our practices, is the safe delivery of your baby, and every baby. We have no other agenda.

Michèle Farrugia, MD
Jacqueline Thomas, MD
Paul Bernstein, MD

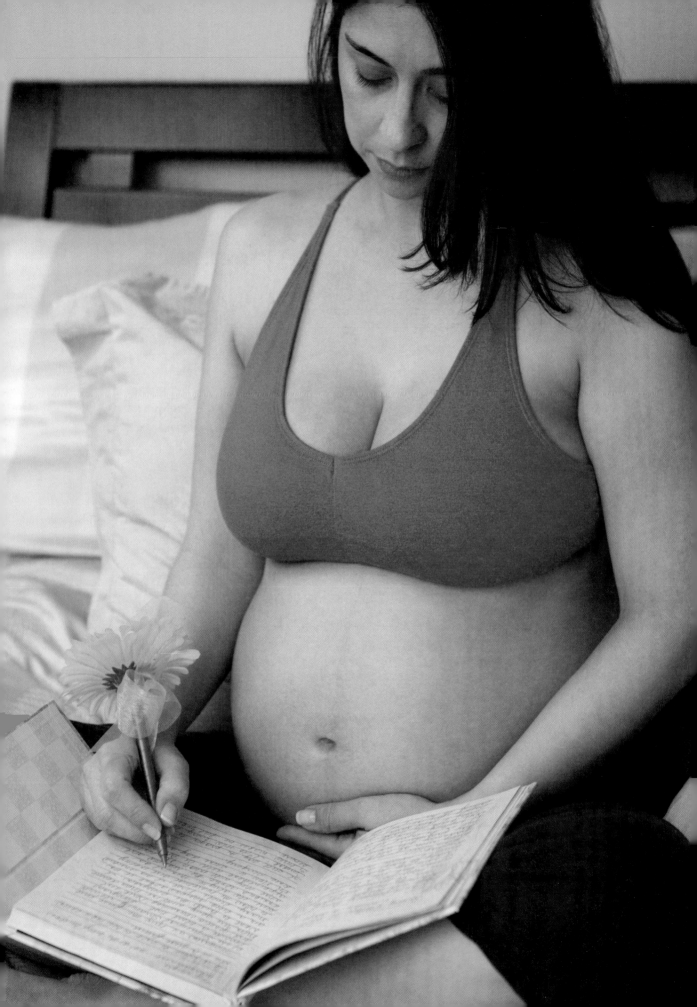

My Pregnancy Diary

Use these pages as a diary of your pregnancy. Information you record here will help your doctor or midwife care for you, and help you trace your progress from conception to delivery and into life with your newborn. Bookmark these pages so you can refer to them quickly. Make lists — they will keep you organized. Jot down your questions — before you forget them. Celebrate your achievements. And write about your experiences and feelings — your child will love to read your pregnancy story one day!

Get started

Sometimes it's hard to get started writing a diary, so we have suggested a few ways to begin. But once started, it is sometimes hard to stop. If you need more room, go ahead and photocopy or scan these diary pages, or tip in other sheets.

Frequently asked questions

As you compose your diary, you are prompted with questions to ask your doctor or midwife. You will have many more than can be listed in this diary. You may want to consult the "Frequently Asked Questions" feature at the end of each chapter. Indeed, the whole book is designed to answer your questions. The diary is just a start.

Contents

Pre-pregnancy (before conception)

Date of my first visit to my doctor to discuss getting pregnant: ....

Date and time of my next scheduled visit: ....

Remarkable firsts at this stage

1. First date we decided to have a baby: ....

2. First date I thought I might be pregnant: ....

Things to do

1. Make an appointment with my doctor.

2. Begin taking vitamins with folic acid, immediately.

3. ....

4. ....

5. ....

6. ....

Questions to ask my doctor or midwife

1. What foods, chemicals, and medications should I avoid?

Answer: ....

2. Where can I sign up for childbirth classes?

Answer: ....

....

3. ....

Answer: ....

....

....

4. ....

Answer: ....

....

5. ....

Answer: ....

....

6. ....

Answer: ....

....

7. ....

Answer: ....

My pregnancy story (part 1)

How do I feel about becoming pregnant? ....

....

....

....

Where can I find support? ....

....

....

....

What will I call my baby? ....

....

First trimester (first 3 months)

Date my baby is due to be born: ....

Date and time of my next visit to my doctor or midwife: ....

Date and time of my first childbirth class: ....

Remarkable firsts at this stage

1. First date I told my partner I was pregnant: ....

2. First date I heard my baby's heartbeat: ....

3. ....

4. ....

5. First ultrasound scan image of my baby

Tape first ultrasound image here

Things to do

1. Consider birth options – home birth or hospital birth, midwife or obstetrician?

2. Talk about genetic screening with my partner and my doctor or midwife.

3. ....

4. ....

5. ....

Questions to ask my doctor or midwife

1. How much weight should I gain during pregnancy?

Answer: ....

....

2. Can I continue to exercise?

Answer: ....

....

3. ....

Answer: ....

....

My pregnancy story (part 2)

How do I feel about becoming pregnant? ....

....

....

What are my hopes and dreams for my baby? ....

....

....

What are my worries and concerns? ....

....

....

Second trimester (second 3 months)

Due date: ....

Dates and times of monthly visits to my doctor or midwife: ....

....

Remarkable firsts at this stage

1. First date I started showing: ....

2. First date I felt my baby kick: ....

3. ....

4. ....

5. Second ultrasound scan image of my baby

Tape second ultrasound image here

Things to do

1. Create a birth plan.

2. Explore the benefits of breastfeeding versus formula-feeding.

3. ....

4. ....

5. ....

Questions to ask my doctor or midwife

1. What can I do to relieve my nausea and vomiting?

Answer: ....

....

2. Is amniocentesis necessary?

Answer: ....

....

3. ....

Answer: ....

....

My pregnancy story (part 3)

How do I feel about becoming pregnant? ....

....

....

How am I feeling physically? ....

....

....

....

What am I concerned about? ....

....

....

....

Third trimester (third 3 months)

Due date: ....

Dates and times of next monthly and weekly visits (4 to 5) to my doctor or midwife:

....

....

Remarkable firsts at this stage

1. First time I couldn't see my feet: ....

2. First time I felt contractions: ....

3. ....

4. Third ultrasound scan image of my baby (if requested)

Tape third ultrasound image here

Things to do

1. Pack my hospital bag.

2. Find a family doctor or pediatrician to care for my baby after I give birth.

3. ....

4. ....

5. ....

Questions to ask my doctor or midwife

1. What kinds of pain relief are safe and effective?

Answer: ....

....

2. How can I prepare for labor and delivery?

Answer: ....

....

3. ....

Answer: ....

....

4. ....

Answer: ....

....

My pregnancy story (part 4)

How do I feel now? ....

....

....

What am I looking forward to? ....

....

....

Who do I imagine my baby will look like? ....

....

....

Labor and Delivery

Projected due date: .... Actual birth date: .... Time: ....

Contractions began: .... Labor lasted: ....

My baby's weight: .... Length: ....

Delivery team members: ....

Remarkable firsts at this stage

1. First sight of my baby: ....

2. First time I held my baby: ....

3. ....

4. ....

5. First photograph of my newborn baby after delivery

Tape newborn picture here

Things to do

1. Review what my doctor or midwife told me about labor.

2. Rehearse with my partner pushing and breathing strategies.

3. ....

4. ....

Questions to ask my doctor or midwife

1. When should I go to the hospital?

Answer: ....

....

2. What happens if I need assistance with the delivery?

Answer: ....

....

3. ....

Answer: ....

....

4. ....

Answer: ....

....

My pregnancy story (part 5)

How did I feel during labor and delivery? ....

....

....

....

How did I feel when I first saw my baby? ....

....

....

....

Postpartum (6 weeks after birth)

Apgar score at 1 minute: .... *At 5 minutes:* ....

Newborn examination results: ....

Next visit to my doctor or midwife: ....

Remarkable firsts in my baby's life

1. First time my baby breastfed or formula-fed with me: ....

2. First time I gave my baby a bath: ....

3. ....

4. ....

5. Photograph of the first time my baby came home

Tape first picture at home here

Things to do

1. Master my breastfeeding technique.

2. Review arrangements for help with household chores and baby care.

3. ....

4. ....

5. ....

Questions to ask my doctor or midwife

1. How long do I have to stay in the hospital?

Answer: ....

....

2. What conditions are being screened for in the newborn examination?

Answer: ....

....

3. ....

Answer: ....

....

4. ....

Answer: ....

....

My pregnancy story (part 6)

How do I feel about being a mother? ....

....

....

....

How do I feel about my baby? ....

....

....

....

....

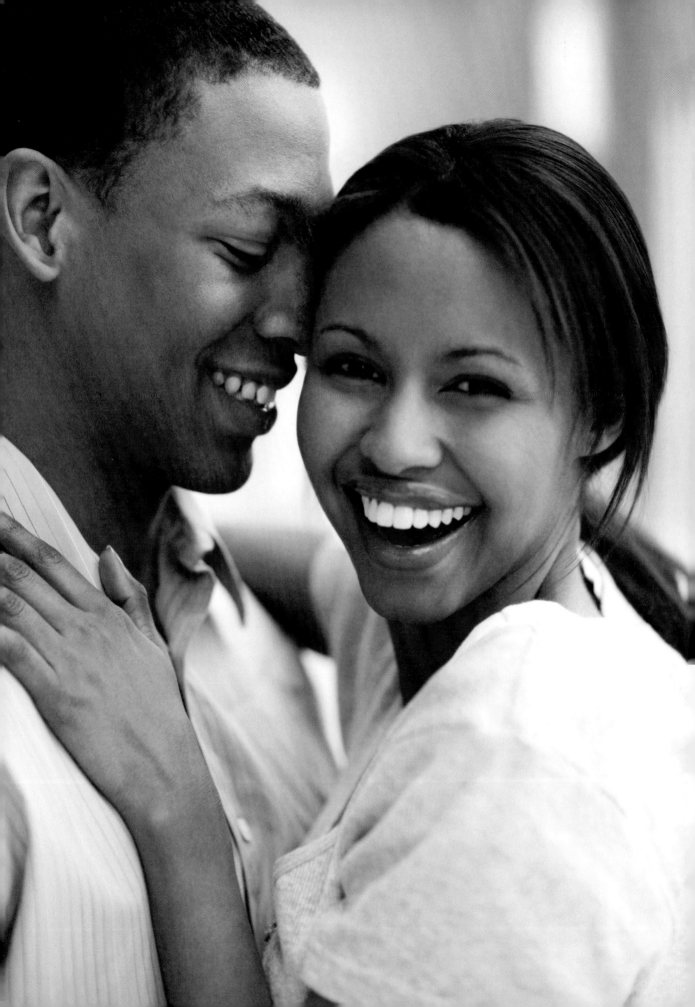

Part 1

Planning Your Pregnancy

Are you ready…

Congratulations! You are about to become a parent. This is a most exciting time as you imagine the changes ahead. But you may have some concerns about the best way to prepare yourself for a pregnancy. Although not every woman plans her pregnancy, many do. If you find yourself unexpectedly pregnant, don't worry. Just catch up by reading on — and seeing your doctor as soon as possible. We're here to help you as best we can.

Language of pregnancy

Amniocentesis, autosomal dominant, beta subunit of human chorionic gonadotropin, Braxton Hicks, chorionic villi, doptone, endometrium, epidural, episiotomy, genetic screening, gestation, hydrops, Kegels, neural tube, oligohydramnios, pica, placenta previa, pre-eclampsia, postpartum, spina bifida, teratogens, thalassemia, trimester, vacuum extraction … you could write a whole dictionary of specialized terms related to pregnancy, with a host of related acronyms to decode — ßHCG, IVF, AMA, Rh+, and VBAC, to name a few. Often these technical terms are needed to be medically precise, but we'll try to keep the language plain, defining terms in their context as we go along. We all will be speaking the same language soon.

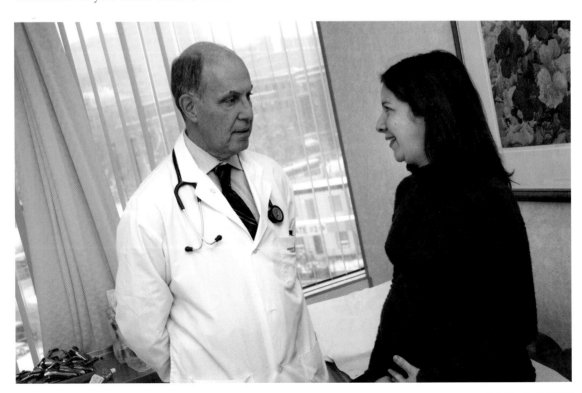

Anatomy of Fertilization

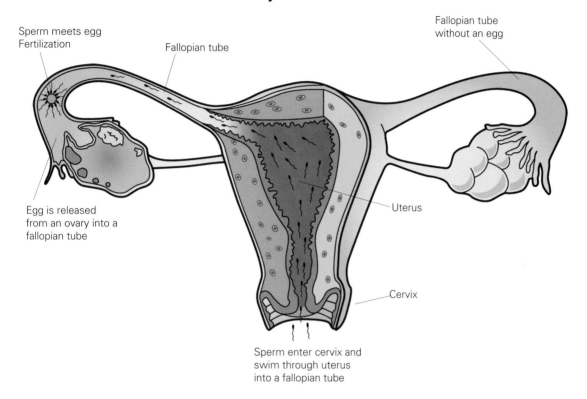

Sperm meets egg
Fertilization

Fallopian tube

Fallopian tube
without an egg

Egg is released
from an ovary into a
fallopian tube

Uterus

Cervix

Sperm enter cervix and
swim through uterus
into a fallopian tube

Ten tips to help you achieve a healthy pregnancy

1. Start taking folic acid, ideally at least 3 months before you plan to conceive, to reduce the risk of serious brain and spine defects in the fetus. For most women, 1 mg daily is adequate.

2. Stop drinking alcohol to reduce the risk of fetal alcohol spectrum disorder. There is no safe level of alcohol ingestion in pregnancy. Say it again, out loud …

3. If you smoke, quit now. Quit yesterday.

4. Don't use recreational drugs or drugs of abuse, such as marijuana, cocaine, or heroin.

5. Arrange for a general medical check-up to address any problems you may have prior to pregnancy.

6. Have a blood test to check your immunity to rubella (German measles) and varicella (chicken pox). If you are not immune, get vaccinated before pregnancy.

7. Stop taking any acne medications with "retin" in their name, such as isotretinoin (brand name Accutane), 1 month before trying to become pregnant.

8. Keep track of your menstrual cycle so you can determine when you may be ovulating.

9. Buy your partner some boxer shorts (instead of briefs) to keep his testicles cooler and his sperm healthier.

10. Have sex often. But not too often. Every 2 days is fine.

Fertility refresher

Most of us learned about fertility and conception — at least, the scientific facts — in high-school health and biology classes. And yet many of us — even those who got an A in biology — would be hard-pressed to describe accurately where sperm and eggs come from or how they find each other and create a new life.

Sounds simple

"Fertility" simply refers to a couple's chances of becoming pregnant. A fertile woman produces an egg during her monthly menstrual cycle. A fertile man produces strong and healthy sperm that can penetrate and fertilize an egg.

Sounds simple, right? Well, of course, it's not. Fertility is determined by the many factors that affect the viability of an egg and the health of sperm, including diet, exercise, timing, sexual behaviors, age, and even emotions. If you are trying to conceive, you might want to start by remembering how female and male reproductive systems interact in conception. Here's a refresher course.

Egg and sperm

Each prospective parent contributes to the baby. You provide the egg (and the incubator), while your partner sends the sperm to the conception party.

Ovulation

Each month, your body undergoes a cycle of physical changes that result in the release of an egg by your ovaries. This process is part of your menstrual cycle. During the cycle (which can range in length from 21 to 40 days, with an average of 28 days), female sex hormones also prepare the uterus to support a pregnancy should the egg be fertilized or to shed the uterine lining (the endometrium) through menstruation if it is not.

Ovulation is your most fertile time. This is when you are most likely to get pregnant. Each month, an egg reaches maturity in one of your two ovaries. Fourteen days before menstruation, rising levels of certain hormones cause the mature egg to be released through the ovary wall. That is, by definition, ovulation.

Few women are aware of ovulation when it happens, so how can you pinpoint the release? By tradition (and because it's the most obvious sign), day 1 of your cycle is considered to be the first day of your period, when your body begins to shed the uterine lining prepared for the last egg. In a 28-day cycle, ovulation occurs about day 14, but if your cycle is longer or shorter, it may happen a day or two later or earlier.

After it's released, the egg travels into the nearest fallopian tube (you have two — they're like small pipes that lead from the ovaries to the uterus). The conception of a baby depends on whether or not your egg is penetrated by a healthy sperm while on its way to the uterus.

Did You Know?

Life of an egg

Like all women, you were born with about 1 million eggs in your two ovaries. You will release about 400 (yes — only 400) of them in your lifetime, beginning with your first period and ending with menopause (age 45 to 55). The average egg lives from 12 to 24 hours after release and must be fertilized during that period if a baby is to be conceived.

Ejaculation

A man's body is constantly producing millions of microscopic sperm, whose sole purpose is to penetrate an egg. Men aren't born with ready-made sperm — they make them. The average sperm lives only a few weeks in a man's body, and around 30 million to 300 million are released each time he ejaculates. Although millions of sperm are produced and released in each ejaculation, only one is needed to fertilize an egg.

Sperm production starts in the testicles, the two glands housed in the scrotal sac beneath the penis. The testicles hang outside of the body because they are sensitive to heat. To produce healthy sperm, they have to stay slightly cooler than normal body temperature. (This is why boxer shorts are recommended for aspiring fathers.) Once the sperm are created, they're stored in the testicles until they get mixed with semen just prior to ejaculation. In men, orgasm propels sperm-rich semen into the vagina at roughly 10 miles per hour.

Fertilization

Fertilization, if it is going to happen, is a matter of timing. The average egg has a lifespan of about 12 hours, while post-ejaculation sperm have a lifespan of up to 72 hours. The sperm either immediately find an egg on its travels through the fallopian tube, or the sperm must hang around waiting for an egg to be released in the hours or days after ejaculation.

Of the millions of sperm ejaculated, only a few hundred of the strongest swimmers will make it into the fallopian tube, where fertilization takes place. Fertilized or not, the egg continues to travel down through the fallopian tube to the uterus.

Did You Know?

Sperm challenges

In their life-or-death swim to find an egg to fertilize, sperm face many challenges, including high acid levels in the vagina and thick, gooey cervical mucus. Sperm travel at a rate of about 1 inch (2.5 cm) every 15 minutes, and the fastest may find the egg in as little as 45 minutes. Their slower brethren can take up to 12 hours. If sperm don't find an egg in the fallopian tubes at the time of intercourse, they can wait there for up to 72 hours. Out of all those millions of sperm released in ejaculation, only a few dozen ever make it to the egg. The rest get trapped, lost, or die along the way. The ones who do get through still have to work very hard to penetrate the egg's outer shell and get inside. When a sperm gets in, the egg changes instantaneously so that no others can enter.

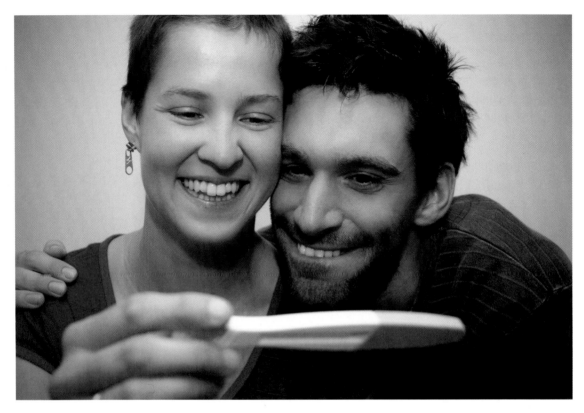

Conception

Once fertilization has taken place, the genetic material in the sperm combines with the genetic material in the egg to create a new cell that starts dividing rapidly. This group of new cells travels the rest of the way down the fallopian tube and usually implants in the wall of the uterus (endometrium) about 2 weeks after the egg has been fertilized. At this stage, conception is considered to be complete. These implanted cells are known as the embryo and will continue to divide to become the fetus in about 8 weeks.

Did You Know?

Timing is everything (almost)

If a sperm defies the odds and arrives at the fallopian tube, an egg must be there, waiting to be fertilized, if conception is to take place. That's why having sex during your fertile time of the month — just before or after ovulation — is the way to conceive a baby. While there are other factors at play as well, if your timing is off, nothing else matters.

Implantation

Once the fertilized egg is implanted, the release of a hormone called human chorionic gonadotropin (HCG) helps ensure the endometrium does not disintegrate and leave the uterus during your menstrual period. Often simply called the "pregnancy hormone," a portion of the HCG hormone, called the beta subunit (ßHCG), is detected in a pregnancy test.

Fertility do's and don'ts

Do — eat a balanced diet. It helps to regulate hormones and nourish the reproductive system. A good diet also helps to maintain a healthy weight. Women who are underweight or overweight may have a harder time becoming pregnant because body fat levels affect the production of sex hormones.

Do — be sure you're getting enough vitamins and minerals. A pregnancy multivitamin with at least 1 mg of folic acid is advised.

Don't — drink alcohol. Some studies have suggested that a woman who consumes three or more drinks a week is more likely to have trouble conceiving. Furthermore, if you become pregnant, it is definitely advisable not to drink at all for the safety of your growing baby. Heavy drinking (14 or more drinks a week) in a male partner can reduce his fertility by altering testosterone levels and sperm production. It can decrease sperm count, increase the production of abnormal sperm, and reduce fertility levels by up to 50%. More moderate drinking (less than 14 drinks per week) in a man probably does not affect his fertility.

Don't — smoke. Smoking impairs both female and male fertility. These effects are likely reversed about a year after you quit smoking. So quit smoking — not just so you can become pregnant, but also for the health of your baby and for your own short- and long-term health.

Don't — drink too much caffeine. Too much caffeine (in coffee, tea, colas, chocolate) can reduce your fertility, but there is no evidence that you need to cut it out altogether. One to two cups a day of coffee or the equivalent dose of caffeine will not impair your fertility. Men can drink as much as they like without impairing their fertility.

Some women have a small amount of bleeding at this time (called an implantation bleed). Not to worry. You may even mistake an implantation bleed for a normal period or maybe a slightly unusual period. Most women have no bleeding and may now begin to suspect they are pregnant because their period is late. It's time to test to see if, in fact, you are pregnant. For more information on pregnancy tests, see Part 2, Early Pregnancy Progress (page 60).

Infertility

If you've been having unprotected sex for a couple of months and are not yet pregnant, you've probably started worrying that it might never happen. Well-meaning friends and family are likely offering advice along the lines of "Don't worry. Just relax." This is one of those times when perfectly good advice is quite useless. You will worry, but you don't need to panic.

Odds are…

Consider the odds. On average, among couples having regular intercourse, 20% of women will conceive within 1 month, 60% within 6 months, and 90% within 18 months. Put another way, even if you do everything "right," you still have only a 20% chance of conceiving in any given cycle.

The point here is that conception doesn't always happen right away. And more often than not, there's nothing seriously wrong — what's preventing success could be something as simple as bad timing!

HOW TO...
Enhance your fertility

If you are having trouble getting pregnant, you might want to take a deep breath and consider some simple things that could improve your chances of success.

1. Have sex frequently

Having sexual intercourse during your fertile period is the key to your success. A simple rule to follow is to have sex every 2 days between day 10 and day 20 of your cycle, if you have a 28-day cycle.

Some people will ask, "Why so much sex?" Well, predicting the time of ovulation is educated guesswork and just counting days may not be good enough. We know that an egg survives only about 12 hours after it is released, so if you are off a day or two with your counting and only have sex on day 14, the sperm will miss the egg altogether. We know that sperm are a little hardier, and some can survive up to 72 hours in the female reproductive system. This means that if you are having sex every 2 days in the mid-point of your cycle, sperm will be hanging around in your uterus and tubes, waiting for the egg to pass by.

Some people will ask, "Why so little sex?" Why not have sex every day, even multiple times a day? Surely that will put more sperm where they need to be... Actually, it won't. Volume of semen and sperm counts will actually be a bit lower if your partner is ejaculating more frequently. So every 2 days is plenty.

2. Monitor ovulation

There are a number of ways that you can monitor your fertility and predict the timing of ovulation more effectively than just by counting days.

- **Basal body temperature (BBT):** Your basal body temperature is your temperature measured more precisely than, for example, when you have a fever associated with a cold or illness. Consistent use of a basal body thermometer will tell you when you have ovulated, because basal body temperature increases *after* an egg is released. Measuring your basal body temperature can help you understand your cycle a bit better, but if you didn't have sex before the temperature rises, you have missed the fertile time.

  You must buy a special basal body thermometer (not just a regular thermometer) from the drugstore in order to measure this temperature precisely. Take your temperature as soon as you wake up in the morning, before you even get out of bed, for the greatest accuracy. You can then graph your temperature on the graph paper supplied with the thermometer. After a few cycles, you can look back at the graphs, and often you will see what is called a "biphasic" curve. The BBT is lower in the first half of the cycle and higher in the second half — on average. For women who have a very regular cycle, this can be a useful method of predicting ovulation. For most women, it is too finicky to be of much use.

- **Ovulation predictor kit:** A more useful way of predicting when ovulation will occur is to use an ovulation predictor kit, available at most drugstores. It will contain several sticks that look like a home pregnancy test. The stick will measure the amount of a hormone called LH (luteinizing hormone) in your urine. The levels of LH in your blood and urine rise sharply just *before* ovulation,

Basal Body Temperature Chart

Cycle Date:																																	
Cycle Day	1	2	3	4	5	6	7	8	9	10	11	12	13	14	15	16	17	18	19	20	21	22	23	24	25	26	27	28	29	30	31	32	33	34
Day of week																																		
37.3/99.4																																		
37.2/99.2																																		
37.1/99.0																																		
37.0/98.8																																		
36.9/98.6																																		
36.8/98.4																																		
36.7/98.2																																		
36.6/98.0																																		
36.5/97.8																																		
36.4/97.6																																		
36.3/97.4																																		
36.2/97.2																																		
36.1/97.0																																		
36.0/96.8																																		

Temperature °C / °F

so if you have a positive test, that means your ovary will release an egg in the next 24 hours … and by now you know what that means … call your partner and make plans. You can begin testing a few days before you anticipate releasing an egg, just to make sure. Most kits will advise you to start testing on day 11 if you have a 28-day cycle.

3. Adjust sexual positions

You and your partner may want to experiment with different positions during intercourse. For a woman to become pregnant, the sperm must be deposited as close as possible to the cervix. Certain positions — missionary and rear-entry intercourse — are better for this than others. Avoid standing, sitting, or the woman-on-top positions — these work against gravity.

4. Don't rise immediately after intercourse

Lie on your back for 15 minutes or so after intercourse. This helps the semen stay close to the cervix and prevents leakage. If you run to the bathroom immediately after intercourse, you will lose some of the semen in the toilet.

5. Boxers, not briefs, for men

If your partner wears boxer shorts, he will reduce the risk of his testicles overheating, which can result in sperm damage.

6. Make sure the vaginal environment is sperm-friendly

Don't douche after sexual intercourse and avoid using vaginal sprays, scented tampons, and artificial lubricants. Don't use any lubricants with intercourse, not even water-based lubricants.

7. Exercise in moderation

Excess body fat can increase the amount of estrogen in a woman's body, throwing the fertility cycle out of balance. Exercise helps to burn off this excess body fat, allowing hormone levels to return to normal. But don't overdo it! Too much exercise can actually impair fertility. Some studies suggest that 7 hours a week of vigorous exercise is associated with reduced fertility. If your periods are very irregular, infrequent, or very light, discuss with your doctor the possible effect of exercise on fertility.

Fertility tests and treatments

Suppose the failure to conceive continues. Doctors recommend fertility testing for women who have been unable to conceive for more than 12 months, perhaps sooner if you are over 35. There may be a time when you'll want to consider these options. Your age and cycle pattern will play a part in helping you and your health-care provider determine when that time has come.

There are male-specific and female-specific fertility tests. The good news is that even a diagnosis of infertility is not the end of the road when it comes to conception, thanks to the medical interventions that are now possible. Roughly two out of three couples who seek such interventions do conceive a baby. Methods used include fertility medication, in vitro fertilization, and surgery.

Fertility drugs

If it turns out that you are having a fertility problem, your health-care provider will probably suggest fertility medication for you, either on its own or combined with assisted reproductive techniques or artificial insemination, as a first step in treatment. Medications can be given either in pill form or as injections. Injectable fertility drugs can be expensive — the final cost will depend on the dosage used. Your health-care provider will help you decide the drug type and dosage best for you.

Intrauterine insemination

During this procedure, sperm are introduced directly into the uterus at the time of ovulation, using a special syringe to increase the chances of fertilization.

Did You Know?

Twin (and more) possibilities

Although you are not likely to plan to have twins, triplets, or more babies, you should be prepared for the possibility. The birth of twins and other multiple gestations have become more common in recent years because of the use of fertility drugs and IVF. While a "multiples" pregnancy has some similarities to a "singleton," there are significant differences. These similarities and differences are highlighted in this book at each stage of pregnancy.

In vitro fertilization

In vitro fertilization (IVF) allows infertile couples to have a child who is biologically related to them. The technique begins when eggs produced using fertility drugs are removed from a woman's ovary, fertilized by her partner's sperm in a laboratory, and allowed to divide for a few days. Resulting embryos are then placed in the woman's uterus to implant and develop naturally. If the first IVF attempt does not achieve a pregnancy, the procedure may be repeated.

IVF is usually the treatment of choice for severe male infertility, blocked fallopian tubes, and poor ovarian function, or when other infertility treatments have not worked. Its success depends on many factors, including the age and reproductive health of both prospective parents. With this procedure, there is an increased chance of multiple births.

Surgery

In recent years, the success of IVF has reduced the number of infertility surgeries performed. Surgery is, however, still used

Guide to...

In vitro fertilization procedures

The IVF procedure is complex, requiring careful timing and coordination of several steps.

- The woman takes fertility drugs so that her ovaries will produce several eggs.
- The surgeon inserts a needle through the vagina into one of the woman's ovaries and removes the eggs.
- The man provides a semen sample, and sperm are separated from the semen in a laboratory.
- The active sperm are combined in the laboratory dish with the eggs.

- About 18 hours later, it is possible to determine whether an egg or eggs have been fertilized and have begun to develop into embryos.
- Two or 3 days later, embryos are transferred into the woman's uterus through the cervix, using a long tube. The woman remains in a resting position for the next hour or so.
- For the next 2 weeks, the woman takes hormones that promote embryo development and enable the uterus to support a pregnancy.
- If the egg or eggs attach to the uterine wall and grow, the woman is pregnant.

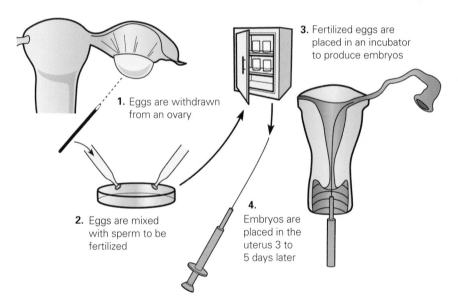

1. Eggs are withdrawn from an ovary

2. Eggs are mixed with sperm to be fertilized

3. Fertilized eggs are placed in an incubator to produce embryos

4. Embryos are placed in the uterus 3 to 5 days later

to treat female fertility–related conditions, such as fibroids (benign tumors in the wall of the uterus), tubal disease, and endometriosis (abnormal tissue growing around the reproductive organs and interfering with reproductive function), or to reverse previous surgery that sterilized the patient.

Fertility surgery on men is used to repair a varicocele (a varicose vein in the testicle, causing reduced sperm count), remove obstructions in the ductal system, reverse vasectomies, and treat performance problems, such as erectile dysfunction. Your health-care provider will discuss these procedures at length with you should they be required.

Genetics primer

Genetics holds the answer to age-old questions: Will we have a boy or a girl? What will "he" look like? Will "she" be tall like your partner or short like your mother? Will "he" have your blond hair and blue eyes or your partner's dark hair and brown eyes? More importantly, genetics can also help predict possible genetic disease conditions — and help us to prevent these conditions as part of planning a pregnancy.

Gene make-up

If remembering the basics of fertility and conception from our high-school health and biology classes is challenging, anything we recall about genetics is often more foggy — and perhaps incorrect, given the recent advances in genetics research. Here are the basics involved in pregnancy.

Heredity

Most living organisms are made up of cells that contain a substance called deoxyribonucleic acid (DNA). DNA is wrapped together to form structures called chromosomes. These are microscopic, rod-shaped bodies that carry hereditary information via genes. Genes are segments of DNA that are carried on the chromosomes and determine specific human characteristics, such as height or hair color. A chromosome can carry thousands of genes.

There are over 30,000 genes in each cell of your body, and each gene carries information involved in determining inherited traits. The passage of traits from one generation to the next is called heredity. Heredity helps to make us who we are: short or tall, with black hair or blond, dark skin or light. Which traits are passed on depends on the genes we inherited.

Chromosomes

Most cells in the human body have 23 pairs of chromosomes, making a total of 46. There are 22 pairs of autosomes (those not involved in determining gender) plus one pair of sex chromosomes. Normal males have 23 pairs of chromosomes, including an X and Y chromosome pair. (It is the Y chromosome that makes them male.) Normal females have 23 pairs of chromosomes, including a pair of X chromosomes.

At the moment of conception, 23 chromosomes from the egg and 23 chromosomes from the sperm cell

Did You Know?

Girl or boy?

Of the 23 pairs of chromosomes, only one pair — sex chromosomes X and Y — determines whether your baby will be a girl or a boy. That determination is actually dependent on which of the father's sperm fertilized the egg. That's because eggs contain only the X sex chromosome, while sperm may contain either the X or the Y. If a sperm cell containing an X chromosome fertilizes an egg, the resulting embryo will be XX (female). If the sperm cell contains a Y chromosome, the resulting embryo will be XY (male).

make up the 23 pairs. Because each parent contributes one chromosome to each pair, each of us has two of every gene on the chromosome. Some characteristics are determined by a single gene; others come from gene combinations.

Dominant and recessive genes

If half of your genes are from your mother and half are from your father, why do you resemble one more than the other? It's because of the way genes combine in your chromosome pairs, and because a gene can be either dominant or recessive. Dominant genes show their effect even if there is only one copy of that gene in the pair. For you to have a recessive characteristic, the recessive gene must be on both chromosomes of the pair. Although eye and hair color are often discussed as traits determined by

simple genetics, multiple genes inherited in a complex way probably determine these physical traits.

- Physical traits determined by dominant genes include freckles, a cleft in the chin, dimples, freely hanging earlobes, and a widow's peak. Thus, if one parent has the gene for dimples, there is a 50/50 chance the child will inherit the same gene and have dimples!

- Physical traits determined by recessive genes include albinism and hitchhiker's thumb. If one parent has a hitchhiker's thumb, that parent has two copies of the responsible gene, one on each chromosome. The child will inherit one of those genes for sure, but the only way that the child will have a hitchhiker's thumb is if the other parent also carries the gene and passes it on.

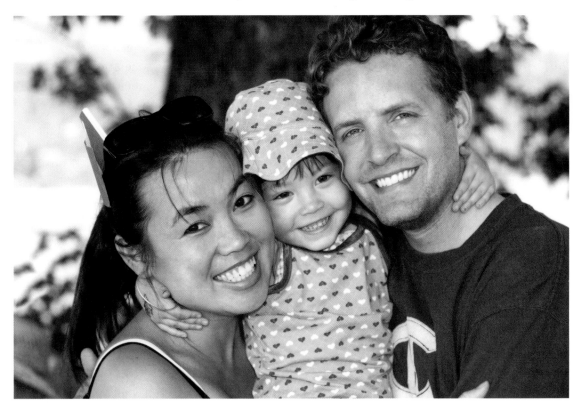

Twin Differences

One egg and
one sperm

Fertilized
egg splits

Identical twins
(in two sacs)

Two eggs and
two sperm

Fraternal twins

Twin genetics

Twins are two offspring resulting from the same pregnancy and occur in about 1 in 80 pregnancies. Twins can either result from the splitting of one fertilized egg during the first 2 weeks (known as "identical"), or they can be the result of the fertilization of two eggs at the same time ("fraternal"). Statistically, about 10% to 20% of twins will be identical and 80% to 90% fraternal. The incidence of identical twins is about the same worldwide, about 3 to 5 per 1000 births, but the incidence of fraternal twins varies with different ethnic groups and with use of assisted reproductive technologies. Fraternal twins are more common for older mothers, with twinning rates doubling in mothers over the age of 35. Many couples don't know they are expecting twins until the first ultrasound scan, normally at 11 to 12 weeks.

Identical twins

Identical twins are genetically identical, and they are always the same sex. The degree of separation in development depends on when the egg splits. If the fertilized egg splits during the first 3 days after fertilization, each embryo will develop with its own placenta and its own amniotic sac. If the embryo splits between days 4 and 8, the two embryos will have a shared placenta, but two separate sacs. In about 1% of identical twinning, the split occurs late, between days 8 and 12, resulting in both a shared placenta and a shared sac. And in rare cases, the embryo splits extremely late (after 13 days), resulting in conjoined twins. The later the split, the higher the risk of losing one or both of the fetuses during the pregnancy.

Fraternal twins

The two fertilized eggs for fraternal twins develop separate placentas and amniotic sacs. Fraternal twins can be of opposite sexes and will look no more alike than any other siblings.

Genetic diseases

Our genes dictate our physical and personality traits — and sometimes what illnesses we may develop as our inheritance. There are many, many genetic diseases, more than 15,000. Some are understood right down to the molecular level, and some are not understood at all. Some occur infrequently, while others are more common. Many can have a serious impact on your child's health as a child and an adult, but some can be prevented with conscientious genetic screening and planning. For more information on genetic diseases, see Part 13, Managing Medical and Environmental Risks (page 429).

Gene mutations

Sometimes it happens that genes are not exact copies of the original — they have changed (mutated). While cells usually recognize and repair gene mutations, sometimes they don't. (The failure to repair cell and gene damage increases as our bodies age.) Having a genetic mutation that may cause disease does not, however, mean that a person will definitely get that disease. Because we inherit a gene from each parent, having one abnormal gene does not cause problems unless it is a dominant condition. However, if both genes in the pair are abnormal, it can result in diseases, such as cystic fibrosis, which is inherited recessively. Other abnormal genes are carried on the X chromosome and only affect boys.

Did You Know?

Abnormal genes vs. abnormal chromosomes

When discussing genetic disease, it is important to differentiate between diseases caused by an abnormal gene and diseases caused by abnormal chromosomes. Cystic fibrosis is an example of a genetic disorder — there are two abnormal genes. Down syndrome is an example of a chromosomal disorder — there is an extra copy of chromosome 21. Disorders of genes are discussed here, while chromosomal disorders are discussed more thoroughly in the section on prenatal screening in Part 4, First Trimester Progress (page 148).

Common genetic diseases

Although considered common relative to other genetic diseases, even these conditions are quite rare, as statistics for incidence in the population indicate.

- Cystic fibrosis (0.4 in 1000 births)
- Hemophilia (0.1 in 1000 births)
- Huntington's disease (0.5 in 1000 births)
- Muscular dystrophy (0.3 in 1000 births)
- Sickle cell disease (0.1 in 1000 births)
- Thalassemia (0.5 in 1000 births)

Genetic inheritance tables for recessive diseases

A traditional way of looking at genetic inheritance is to make a table like the one shown here. The specific genes of one parent are shown across the top; the related specific genes of the other parent are shown down the side. The non-bolded letters represent the possible combinations of the two pairs of genes in their offspring:

	C	**c**
C	CC	Cc
c	Cc	cc

In this table, upper case C represents a normal copy of the gene. Lower case c represents an abnormal copy of the same gene. Therefore, across the top, one parent has one normal and one abnormal copy of the gene. Down the side, the other parent has the same gene arrangement.

Both parents would be considered carriers of the abnormal gene (Cc), which could be a mutation that's associated with cystic fibrosis or some other recessive genetic disease. They carry the mutation but are healthy and do not have the disease.

When these parents have children, there is a 50% chance of having a child with Cc (a carrier of the mutation), a 25% chance of having a child with CC (two normal copies of the gene, not a carrier), and a 25% chance of having a child with cc (two abnormal copies of the gene, which will likely lead to development of the disease).

Alternatively, if one parent was a carrier and one parent was not, the table would look like this:

	C	**c**
C	CC	Cc
C	CC	Cc

In this case, 50% of their offspring would be carriers (Cc), and 50% would not be carriers (CC). None of their children would be expected to develop the disease.

Genetic screening

Parents can be screened with blood tests for their carrier status for many of these common genetic diseases but not so easily for diseases more influenced by lifestyle factors, such as congenital heart disease, diabetes, and hypertension. Carrier screening should be considered when people of your and your partner's ethnic origin have an elevated risk of a particular genetic disease or your family has a history of genetic disease. Carrier screening allows potential parents to make decisions about inheritance risks prior to pregnancy or early in pregnancy. In these cases, consultation with a geneticist or genetic counselor is advised prior to pregnancy.

Populations at higher risk

Certain populations have a higher risk of certain genetic diseases than others. If you are a member of these higher-risk populations, you may want to be screened for these genetic diseases.

- Cystic fibrosis is more common in people of Northern European descent.
- Sickle cell anemia is more common in people of African descent.
- Thalassemia is more common in people of Mediterranean, Asian, and African descent.
- Tay-Sachs disease is more common in people of Ashkenazi Jewish descent and in people of French Canadian descent.

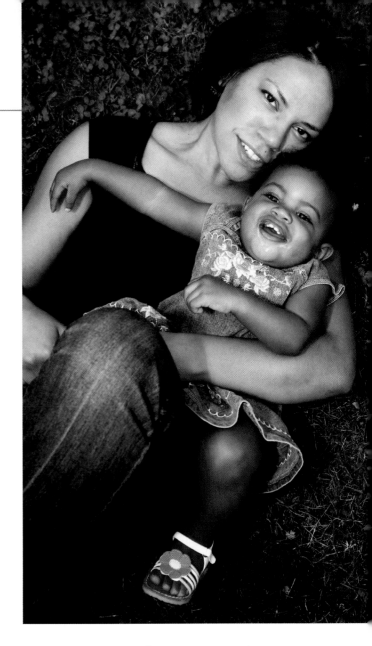

Guide to...

Genetic Disease Management

What do you do if you find that both you and your partner are carriers of a genetic disease? This is a tough question. Don't let these questions scare you — use them to prepare for any problems that may come your way. With the help of your family physician or a genetic counselor, you can consider your options.

- You may wish to proceed with a pregnancy and accept the risk of having a child with a genetic disease.

- You may wish to proceed with a pregnancy and undergo genetic testing of the fetus early in the pregnancy.

- If the fetus is affected, you may then choose to carry on with the pregnancy or terminate the pregnancy.

- If the risk seems too great, you may choose to achieve pregnancy by undergoing in vitro fertilization. The embryo can then be tested in the lab to see if it carries the gene mutation before it is returned to your body to continue with the pregnancy. This procedure may not be available for all genetic diseases.

Pre-pregnancy medical check-up

Besides the possible need for fertility testing and genetic screening, you should visit your doctor while planning your pregnancy to discuss any chronic medical conditions and environmental risks in pregnancy. Your doctor will help you manage these conditions and avoid or reduce your exposure to these risks. The aim is to optimize your health prior to and during pregnancy. The key principle that guides doctors looking after pregnant women is simple — the best thing for the baby is a healthy mother.

If you are 35 years or older, this would be a good time to evaluate your pregnancy plans with your doctor, because there are some additional challenges for women of "advanced maternal age," which are, by no means, insurmountable.

Topics for discussion

When you visit your doctor, time will usually be made to discuss health concerns specific to pregnancy. You should also raise your own questions. Use the "My Pregnancy Diary" inserted in this book to record any questions you may have. These are some of the pregnancy-related concerns your doctor may discuss:

Did You Know?

Poor health in pregnancy

It is important to be as healthy as possible in pregnancy. If you are very ill with an acute or chronic disease at the time you become pregnant or if you are very ill in the first trimester, there is an increased chance of miscarriage. If you are very ill in the second or third trimesters, the risk of stillbirth increases. The rate of preterm labor and delivery also increases. Take the time to take care of your health.

- General health and well-being
- Fertility basics and, if a problem, infertility treatments
- Genetic disease screening and counseling, especially if you are from a population at risk
- Chronic medical conditions and drug treatment options, if applicable
- Most important environmental risks to avoid or minimize now
- Folic acid supplementation
- Treatment of sexually transmitted diseases, if applicable
- Pregnancy after 35, if applicable

Tests

Your doctor may suggest blood tests to determine if you carry a risk of any genetic disease and if you are immune to a few viral and bacterial infections, most importantly, at this stage, rubella (German measles) and varicella (chicken pox). If not immune, you should be vaccinated now.

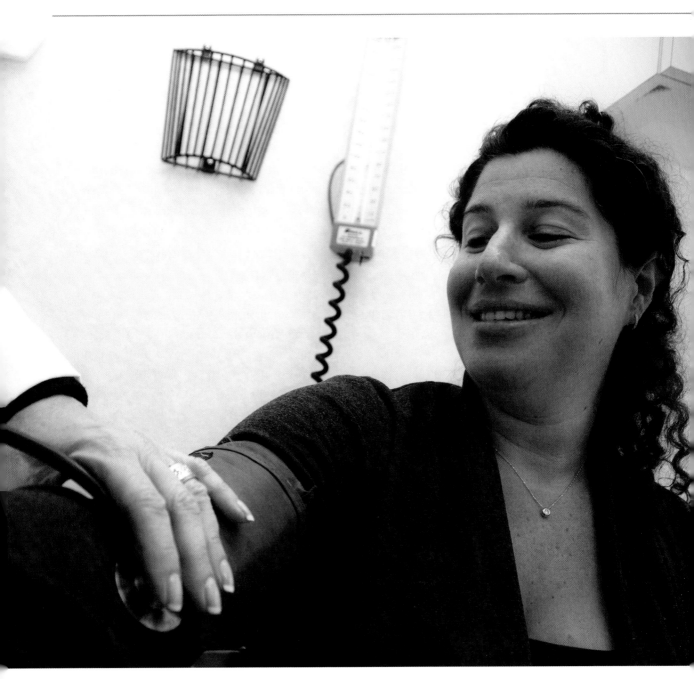

Optimizing your health

If you are a healthy person, there is little else you need to do to optimize your own health prior to pregnancy other than to take care of any chronic conditions, minimize exposure to environmental risk factors, and get vaccinated against specific infectious diseases. Focus on eating a healthy, balanced diet and exercising moderately. Maintain a healthy body weight, neither underweight nor overweight. Don't smoke. Follow a healthy lifestyle ... and your body should take care of the rest.

Chronic medical conditions

If you have any chronic medical problems, let your doctor know that you are planning to get pregnant and discuss how your condition will affect a pregnancy — and how a pregnancy will affect your condition. These effects can be maternal or fetal or both.

Complicated by pregnancy

Conditions that are complicated by a pregnancy can be rheumatological (rheumatoid arthritis and lupus), gastrointestinal (Crohn's disease and ulcerative colitis), cardiovascular (heart disease and hypertension), neurological (multiple sclerosis and epilepsy), or psychological (depression and anxiety). This list is not exhaustive, and the impact of these conditions on each person and each pregnancy varies widely.

Did You Know?

Rule of thirds

A good way to think about how chronic diseases respond to pregnancy is called the "rule of thirds." That is, in one third of patients, the disease will remain stable; in one third, the symptoms will get better; and in one third, symptoms will get worse. The most important predictor of this is the symptoms you are experiencing at the time you get pregnant. If symptoms are "quiet" at the time you get pregnant, it will be more likely that you will not have a flare-up during pregnancy. If symptoms are active when you get pregnant, it is more likely that symptoms will remain active during your pregnancy.

Higher-risk chronic conditions

Some chronic medical conditions have a higher risk than others of affecting a pregnancy. If you have one of these conditions, your doctor will help you in limiting any risk to you and your baby.

- Asthma
- Diabetes mellitus
- Heart disease
- Hypertension
- Mood disorders
- Obesity
- Hypothyroidism
- Hyperthyroidism

For more information on these higher-risk conditions, see Part 13, Managing Medical and Environmental Risks (page 431).

Surgery

If you have a medical condition that requires surgery, you may want to have the surgery done prior to a pregnancy. In general, health-care providers try to avoid operations on pregnant women unless they are absolutely necessary. If surgery is necessary, the operation will likely go ahead regardless of the pregnancy, remembering the principle that what is best for the baby is a healthy mother.

Positive outcomes

Because chronic conditions can have a significant impact upon your ability to conceive and carry a pregnancy to term successfully, be sure to consult your doctor to create a care plan, ideally before becoming pregnant. Not every pregnancy is planned, so if you find yourself pregnant and you have a chronic medical condition, see your health-care providers immediately.

The decision to undergo a pregnancy if you have a chronic medical problem should not be taken lightly, but rest assured that with proper medical care, most women enjoy a healthy pregnancy in spite of any medical challenges they might face.

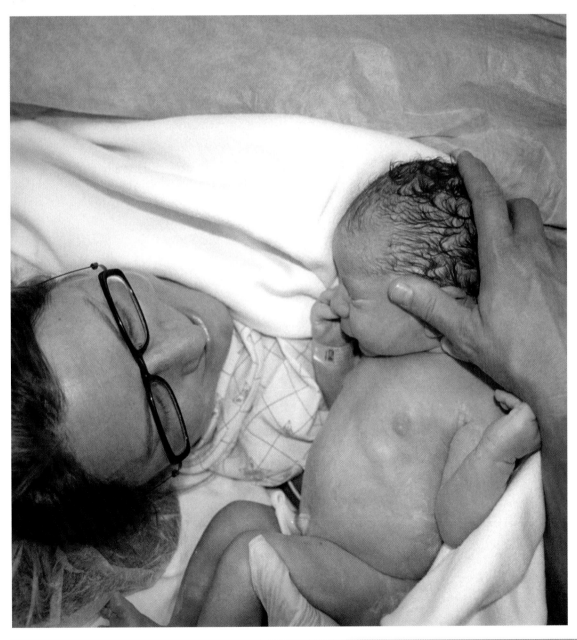

Environmental exposures

Much of prenatal care is directed toward avoiding or reducing the risk of serious complications, caused not only by genetic diseases and chronic conditions, but also by environmental factors, including infectious diseases and medications. Exposure to alcohol, cigarette smoke, chemical pollutants, bacteria, viruses, parasites, and certain drugs can potentially harm a developing fetus in utero or the newborn baby at birth.

Teratogens

Teratogens are environmental agents that can cause structural or functional abnormalities in a developing fetus following exposure in pregnancy. One of the most well-publicized teratogens is thalidomide, a drug once prescribed in Europe and Canada for morning sickness. However, thalidomide was found to cause some exposed babies to be born without limbs.

Crossing the placenta

Teratogens often reach the fetus via the placenta, which is the point of interaction between the mother and the fetus. All that is good for the fetus passes from the mother through the placenta. So, too, does the bad. Anything that is consumed, inhaled, or touched by a pregnant woman has the potential to reach the placenta through the bloodstream, cross it, and enter the fetus. Some substances do cross the placenta, and others do not. Some are safe; some are not. Teratogens are not.

Neural tube defects

During embryonic development, the brain and spinal cord are enclosed in the neural tube, covered over with skin, between week 5 and 6 of pregnancy. If this does not happen normally and the spine and brain are not covered, then, in the presence of a teratogen, a neural tube defect can result. An open neural tube defect can lead to destruction of the brain and nerve tissue.

Anatomy of the Placenta

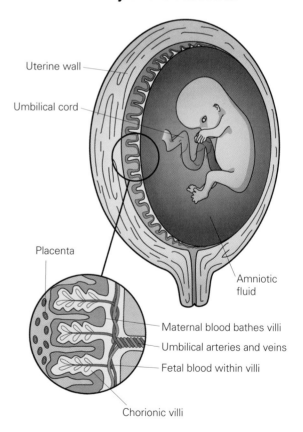

Uterine wall

Umbilical cord

Placenta

Amniotic fluid

Maternal blood bathes villi

Umbilical arteries and veins

Fetal blood within villi

Chorionic villi

Ten key teratogens to avoid in pregnancy

Teratogen	Fetal and newborn effects
1. Alcohol consumption	Can lead to fetal alcohol spectrum disorder involving developmental delay, low birth weight, poor growth, abnormal facial features, lifelong impaired cognitive development, and behavioral problems.
2. Rubella (German measles) infection	Can result in deafness, vision problems, heart problems, mental retardation, and possible fetal death.
3. Varicella (chicken pox) infection	Can result in scarring of the skin, abnormal limb development, mental retardation, and eye problems.
4. Parvovirus (fifth disease) infection	Can attack developing blood cells, leading to anemia and hydrops, which is sometimes associated with fetal death.
5. Toxoplasma parasite	Can have serious consequences for the brain and eyes, leading to deafness, seizures, mental retardation, cerebral palsy, and blindness.
6. Listeria bacterium	Can cause listeriosis, leading to miscarriage, premature delivery, stillbirth, and neonatal death.
7. Mercury ingestion	Can contribute to cerebral palsy, poor physical and mental development, blindness, and deafness.
8. Lead ingestion or inhalation	Can contribute to miscarriage, preterm delivery, low birth weight, and developmental delays.
9. Isotretinoin (Accutane) acne drugs	Can cause severe birth defects, including deformed or absent ears, mental retardation, and hearing and heart abnormalities.
10. ACE inhibitor hypertension drugs	Can damage the kidneys of the fetus and lead to miscarriage when taken during the second and third trimester.

For more information on common teratogens, see *The Complete Guide to Everyday Risks in Pregnancy & Breastfeeding from the Motherisk Program at the Hospital for Sick Children* (Toronto, ON: Robert Rose, 2004).

Neural tube defects are not usually inherited (genetic), but they can be detected in prenatal screening during pregnancy. The best way to reduce the risk of neural tube defects is to avoid or limit exposure to teratogens and supplement your diet with folic acid for at least 3 months prior to conception.

Anencephaly and spina bifida
Neural tube defects can result in a wide range of abnormalities, depending upon where the abnormality lies along the spinal column. If the brain is involved, a condition called anencephaly can result and cause death. If the spine is involved, the condition is called spina bifida. A variety of problems can result,

Did You Know?

Neural tube defect prevalence

Neural tube defects are rare disorders and, fortunately, becoming more rare as we find ways to prevent them. The incidence in the United Kingdom decreased from 4 per 1000 births in the 1970s to 1 per 10,000 births in the late 1990s. Some of this decrease can be attributed to folic acid supplementation. Consuming adequate amounts of folate (folic acid) before and during pregnancy has been shown to reduce the risk of neural tube defects by 50%. Because many pregnancies are unplanned (up to 50%), all women of childbearing age are strongly advised to take a daily multivitamin with adequate folic acid.

including breathing problems, paralysis, hydrocephalus, urinary and fecal incontinence, and sometimes intellectual impairment.

Folate sources

Folate is a water-soluble B vitamin. In dietary form, it is called folate, but in supplemental or fortified form, it is known as folic acid. Some folate is available from food sources, but folic acid supplements are needed to reach and maintain the correct dosage. In Canada, since 1998, folic acid has been added to white flour and pasta, making these fortified grain products a good source of folate. For more information on folate, including a list of common food sources, see Part 3, Eating Well for a Healthy Pregnancy (page 112).

Folic acid dose

- All women contemplating pregnancy should take 1 mg of folic acid daily for 3 months prior to conception and continue until 6 to 8 weeks after birth or until breastfeeding is finished. Some groups of women require additional folic acid.
- Women with a family history of neural tube defects, a previous child with spina bifida, or a history of Type 1 diabetes or epilepsy should take as much as 5 mg of folic acid daily for 3 months prior to conception and continue until 6 to 8 weeks after birth or until breastfeeding is finished.
- Most multivitamins and prenatal vitamins contain 0.4 mg folic acid, so you will need to take an additional supplement to reach a 1 mg dose. You can buy a specific 1 mg folic acid supplement.
- If you have been advised to take more folic acid, don't just take more multivitamins, because this could give you too much of some vitamins, such as vitamin A, that can be harmful to the fetus at high doses. Instead, take 1 multivitamin and then 3 to 4 tablets of 1 mg folic acid.

Neural Tube

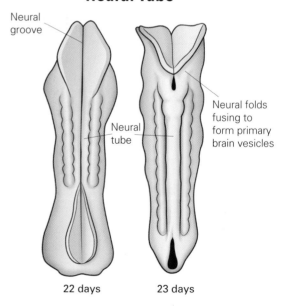

Between day 22 and 23 of embryo development, the neural tube closes, covering spinal nerve tissue.

Environmental exposures in pregnancy

Viral and bacterial infections	Bacterial vaginosis Hepatitis C Influenza Parvovirus Rubella (German measles) Varicella (chicken pox) Yeast infections
Sexually transmitted diseases	Chlamydia Genital warts Gonorrhea Hepatitis B Herpes Human immunodeficiency virus (HIV) Syphilis Trichomonas
Over-the-counter and prescription medications	Unsafe drugs
Complementary and alternative remedies	Vitamin A (more than 10,000 IU) Herbs that induce uterine contractions
Lifestyle risks	Alcohol Cigarette smoke Hot tubs and saunas Recreational drugs and drugs of abuse
Food-borne bacteria and parasites	Listeriosis Toxoplasmosis
Food contaminants and additives	Artificial sweeteners Caffeine Herbal teas Mercury in fish Polychlorinated biphenyls (PCBs)
Chemical pollutants	Air pollution Carbon monoxide Heavy metals (lead, mercury, arsenic) Household risks Organic solvents Pesticides Trihalomethane (byproduct of chlorination)
Occupational hazards	Agricultural fertilizers and pesticides Radiation exposure Refinery precipitants and contaminants

For more information on these risks in pregnancy, see Part 13, Managing Medical and Environmental Risks (page 428).

Infectious diseases

Some infectious diseases can also seriously affect the health of the fetus and your newborn child. An infection occurs when your body is invaded by a bacterium, virus, fungus, or parasite. Some infections, like the common cold, the flu, or stomach flu, will make you miserable for a short while but have no long-lasting impact upon your health or your baby. Other infections, such as hepatitis B or HIV, may have few initial symptoms but be long-lasting and have life-threatening implications for both you and your baby. However, with some preparations and precautions, you can reduce, even avoid, your exposure to infections.

Immunization

Unfortunately, pregnancy does not make you immune to the many bugs lurking in the environment, and you will come into contact with some of them. Fortunately, you may already be immune to some of these diseases due to previous exposure or immunization. In many cases, immunity can be screened for with a blood test. If you are not immune, it is advisable to be vaccinated prior to pregnancy, particularly against rubella (German measles) and varicella (chicken pox). It is also advisable to receive the flu shot annually, especially if you are pregnant or thinking about becoming pregnant.

STDs

Some infectious diseases are transmitted sexually. During delivery, the fetus can be exposed to any sexually transmitted diseases (STDs) the mother may have. Some can be treated immediately, but others, like human immunodeficiency virus (HIV), can have long-term consequences for the newborn child. For more information about infections in pregnancy, see Part 13, Managing Medical and Environmental Risks (page 439).

Did You Know?

Fetal and maternal risk

When you have an infection during pregnancy, consider its impact on you and the fetus. Sometimes, you will be just fine, maybe even barely notice the infection, but the microorganism can cause serious harm to the fetus. Sometimes health-care providers screen for a particular infection because identification and treatment will significantly reduce fetal risk. For example, medical treatment of HIV-infected mothers can significantly reduce the risk that the baby will develop HIV.

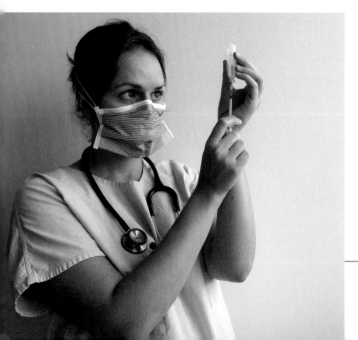

Medications

Many women are concerned about the possible effects of drugs on the fetus and newborn child. Women commonly use over-the-counter and prescribed medications in pregnancy, either to treat pre-existing chronic medical problems or to help cope with some pregnancy symptoms. Even if you don't have a chronic health problem, you might need to use prescription medications for just a few days or weeks of your pregnancy to treat something like a bladder or throat infection. Be sure to check with your doctor before stopping any medication or reducing the dose.

Drug safety

Fortunately, most drugs are considered to be safe for the mother and do not adversely affect the growing fetus. Do not assume you will need to stop your medications. In many cases, it is better to have your underlying medical condition well treated by medication than to stop your medication suddenly and become ill at the beginning of a pregnancy.

Unfortunately, a few drugs are not safe or their safety is not known. Some medications are known to be harmful to the fetus when taken in pregnancy, particularly in the early weeks. Some of these drugs may be damaging even if taken up to 3 years before you become pregnant. These drugs should be avoided or substituted with a safe alternative, if possible.

But if the medication is needed, it may be more harmful to you and to your baby if you stop taking the medication. For more information on medications unsafe and safe in pregnancy, see Part 13, Managing Medical and Environmental Risks (page 448).

Common safe medications in pregnancy

- Acetaminophen (pain)
- Diclectin (nausea)
- Gravol (nausea)
- Tums (heartburn)
- Benadryl (antihistamine)

Guide to...

Taking medications in pregnancy

Here are a few general guidelines for taking prescription medications during pregnancy:

- Always, always discuss any medications you are taking with your health-care provider, preferably before you get pregnant.

- Never, never take someone else's prescription drugs.

- Take only medications prescribed to you or recommended by a health-care provider who is aware that you are pregnant.

- Don't stop taking or change the dosage of a prescribed drug you are taking without discussing it first with your health-care provider. Before taking any new medication or changing the dose, consult your doctor and pharmacist.

Pregnancy after 35

You may not look or feel old at age 35 or 40, but from a reproductive point of view, you are aging rapidly ... women classified as being at an advanced maternal age (AMA) — 35 or older on her due date — face some special risks. Pre-planning your AMA pregnancy can help ensure a healthy outcome.

Complications

Although, in general, pregnancy in older women is successful, the risk of complications is approximately twice that for women giving birth under the age of 30. Part of planning a pregnancy in advanced maternal age is evaluating these risks against the benefits — and consulting with your health-care providers.

Fertility and conception

Advanced maternal age is associated with a decline in fertility, an increase in the incidence of miscarriage, and the risk of ectopic pregnancy. The chances of pregnancy involving multiples and problems related to the placenta are also increased in AMA.

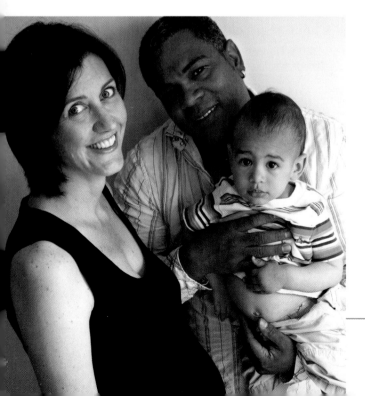

Fetal abnormalities

Advanced maternal age increases the incidence of trisomy 21 (Down syndrome). The risk of giving birth to a baby with trisomy 21 at 35 years of age is 1 in 385, at 40 it is 1 in 100, and at 44 it is 1 in 40. The risk of structural and functional abnormalities, such as heart defects, is also increased with AMA.

Chronic medical conditions

The incidence of many medical conditions, such as hypertension, diabetes, and other chronic illnesses, is higher in older mothers. Maternal diabetes increases the risk of chromosomal and other structural abnormalities in the fetus.

Preterm labor and delivery

Incidences of low birth weight and perinatal death are more likely with increasing maternal age.

Good news

In spite of these increased risks, the chance of having a healthy baby and a healthy mother are still excellent. There are many studies suggesting that although the risk for these complications is increased in AMA, the actual risk of a poor outcome is minimally increased in women over 30 years of age.

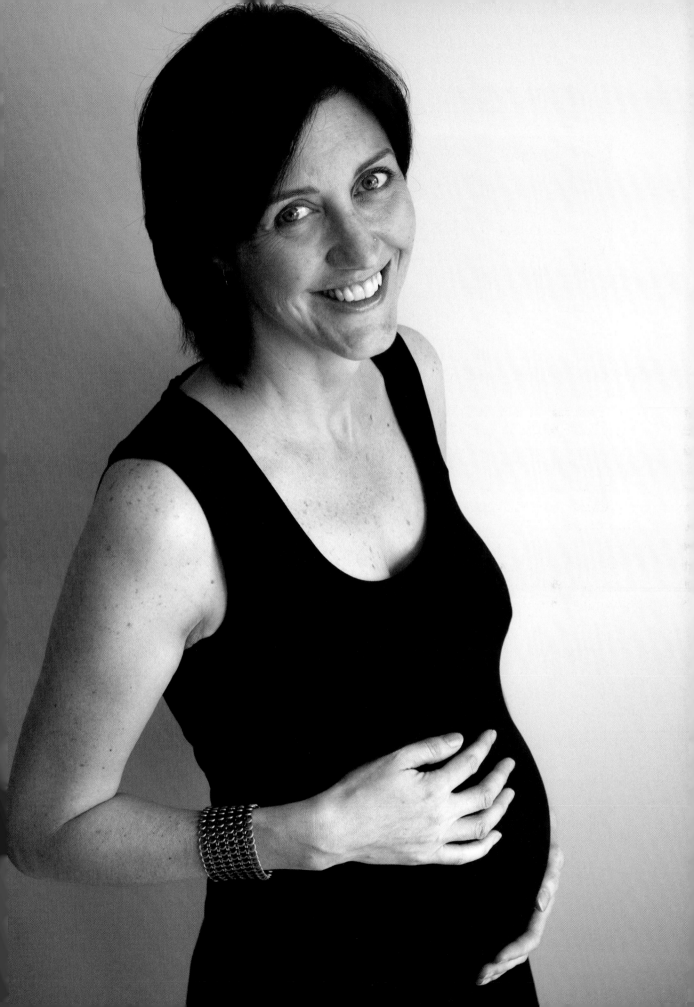

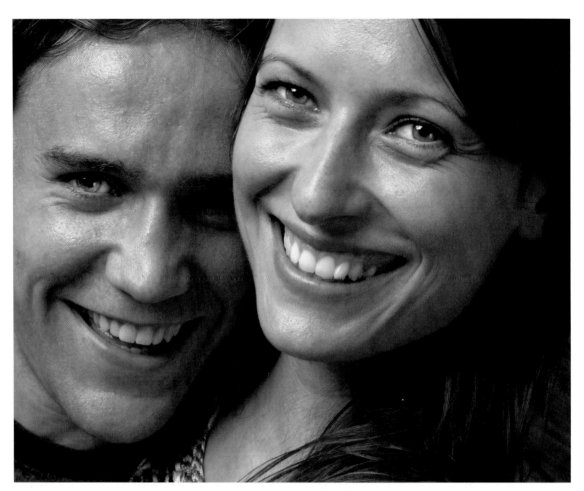

F.A.Q.

We answer many questions from pregnant women and their partners. Here are some of the most frequently asked questions. Be sure to ask your health-care providers any other questions that may arise. If they don't have the answers, they will refer you to a colleague who does.

Q: Do I need to see a doctor before I get pregnant?

A: While not absolutely essential, it's a good idea. This way, you can discuss any health issues and medications you may be taking with your doctor to determine if anything should be done prior to conception. Your genetic risk factors can be evaluated and investigated if necessary. Your immunity to rubella (German measles) can be checked, and if necessary, you can be vaccinated prior to pregnancy. You can also review the appropriate amount of folic acid you should be taking, and review your menstrual cycle and ways to plan conception in your most fertile time.

Q: *What if I had a few drinks before I even realized I was pregnant?*

A: This is a very common concern. Don't dwell on it; there is nothing you can do now to change it and there is likely no significant harm done. Resolve to stop drinking as soon as you hear the pregnancy test is positive.

Q: *Do I need to get rid of my cat?*

A: No! While cat feces can carry a parasite called toxoplasmosis, you will not be exposed unless you are the person changing the kitty litter. Start delegating now (a good parenting skill to learn) and have someone else take care of that job. You can still enjoy your cat and cuddle with it.

Q: *Why do neural tube defects occur?*

A: We don't always know, but it is believed that neural tube defects may be caused by a combination of multiple factors, including genetic and environmental factors. Some of the big environmental factors include folate deficiency in mothers and anti-seizure medications.

Q: *How is sickle cell disease inherited?*

A: Sickle cell disease is an inherited condition most often found in people of African descent. In order to inherit sickle cell disease, a baby has to inherit one sickle cell gene from each parent. That is — there are two sickle cell genes present. If only one sickle cell gene is present, then it is called sickle cell trait. If the mother has sickle cell trait or disease, and if the father of the child is also affected, there is a chance that their child will be affected by sickle cell disease. If both parents have the sickle cell gene, prenatal testing can be done to see if the fetus has sickle cell disease. A person with sickle cell *trait* may have anemia but is otherwise healthy. A person with sickle cell *disease* may have anemia and other serious problems, such as bone pain, increased susceptibility to infections, and even trouble breathing in enough oxygen to supply the body. These symptoms tend to occur during "crises" that can be precipitated by illness, stress, surgery, and other events, including pregnancy.

Q: *I have a family history of babies being born with abnormalities and I am very concerned about this happening to me. What should I do?*

A: You need to discuss this with your doctor, and maybe even with a genetic counselor. Try and find out as much information as you can about the medical problems of each baby so that the risk of similar problems recurring in your pregnancy can be estimated.

What's next

Pregnancy! Do you feel ready now to take the trip from conception to birth during the next 9 months? That's not long to wait to see your new baby. Meanwhile, there's lots of things to do and hurdles to jump, but with everyone's support, you can do it. But first... how do you know you're pregnant? Read on.

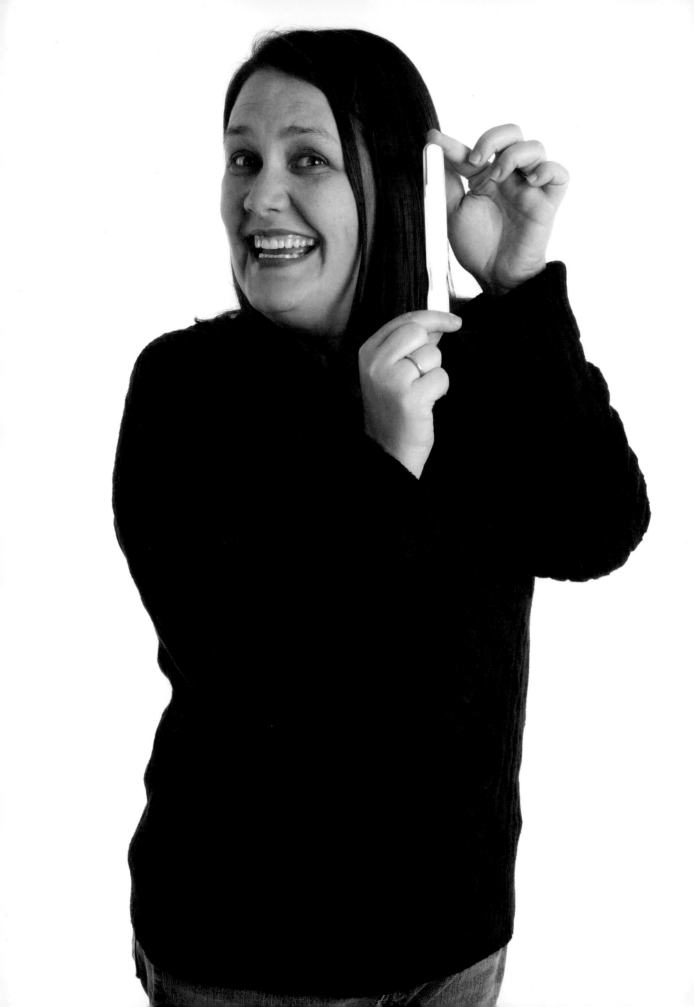

Part 2

Early Pregnancy Progress

Month 1 (Week 1 to 4)

So you think you are pregnant…

But how do you know for sure? Most women are anxious to know the answer to this question. There are some simple tests that determine if you are pregnant, and once you have estimated the date of conception, you can estimate the date your child is due to be born and begin planning the coming months of pregnancy. Your pregnancy journey can take many different roads … Bon voyage!

Pregnancy tests

For many women, especially those with regular periods, the first sign of pregnancy will be a missed period. You may have some bleeding at the regular time, but it may be lighter or just a bit different. This blood is shed as the embryo implants in the wall of the uterus 2 weeks after conception. Either a blood or a urine pregnancy test can be used to confirm a pregnancy at this early stage by determining the presence of the hormone known as the beta subunit of human chorionic gonadotropin (ßHCG). Just remember it as the pregnancy hormone!

Feeling pregnant

If you are not having regular periods for any reason, it may be harder to tell if you are pregnant. For some women, the earliest sign is how they are feeling — perhaps slightly nauseous, very tired, with sore breasts and the urge to urinate frequently. In this case, blood and urine tests can make the diagnosis

of pregnancy, but an ultrasound may also be used. An ultrasound scan can also help to date a pregnancy, especially if the date of the last period is uncertain.

Did You Know?

Home pregnancy tests

Are home pregnancy tests reliable? Yes — if you follow the instructions on the packaging carefully. Most tests will detect very low amounts of the pregnancy hormone ßHCG in urine, generally at levels present by the first day of your missed period. Using first morning urine ensures that the ßHCG concentrations in your urine are highest and, therefore, more easily detectable, but this is not always necessary — check the packaging on the test. False negative tests can occur if the hormone concentration in the urine is too low for the test to detect — perhaps because you are testing too soon in your pregnancy or too late in the day.

Anatomy of Cell Division and Conception

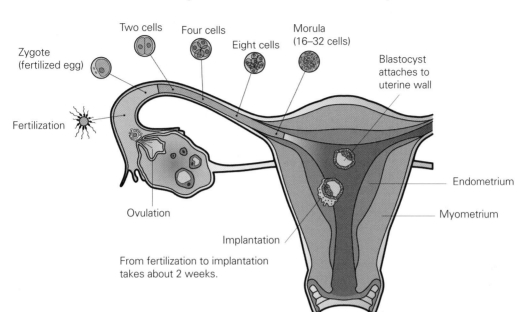

From fertilization to implantation takes about 2 weeks.

Twin possibilities

Consider the possibility of twins (or more) if symptoms of pregnancy are exaggerated. Often there is more fatigue and more morning sickness, while the uterus gets bigger much sooner, making the expectant mother with multiples show earlier than the mother carrying a singleton. Multiples are typically confirmed with an ultrasound scan.

Ten tips for a healthy early pregnancy

1. Confirm you are pregnant! A home urine test should do the job.
2. Calculate your due date. Mark it on the calendar.
3. Don't drink alcohol. To say it again … there is no safe level of alcohol ingestion in pregnancy.
4. Continue taking 1 mg of folic acid to prevent neural tube defects in the highly vulnerable period of week 4 to 6 of gestation.
5. Meet with your doctor to assemble your pregnancy-care team and schedule visits for the next 9 months.
6. Research the various maternal-care models and birthing philosophies. Take your time making a choice. It's important to be happy with these decisions.
7. Explore childbirth classes available in your community and sign up for an early pregnancy class.
8. Watch for signs of trouble and seek medical advice if you have bleeding or pain.
9. Eat a healthy diet.
10. Take a deep breath … life will never be the same.

Calculating your due date

Once you know you are pregnant, you can calculate your due date. There are several reliable ways of *estimating* your due date based on gestational age, but don't expect your baby to arrive on precisely that day! Consider your due date as more of a due week … most babies arrive plus or minus 1 week of their due date.

Gestational age

The age of a fetus is referred to as its gestational age. While 9 months is considered to be the conventional gestational term, health-care providers use weeks to measure the progress of a pregnancy. There are actually 40 weeks in the average full-term pregnancy, which works out to about 10 months, not 9. Confused?

Did You Know?

Due date values

You need to have your best estimate of your due date, or birth date, for a number of valuable reasons, besides settling your own curiosity:

- First, it will help you plan your personal life.
- Second, it will help your health-care providers conduct routine tests at appropriate times.
- Third, if you are at risk of delivering your baby early, your doctor can use your due date to help determine your baby's stage of development and the safety of preterm delivery.
- Fourth, if you have not delivered by 10 days after your due date, your doctor will rely upon it while considering when to induce post-term labor.

This confusion in measuring gestational age can be explained by the fact that, conventionally, a pregnancy is deemed to begin officially on the first day of the last menstrual period (LMP), even though it doesn't really begin until conception, about 2 weeks later. So 40 weeks – 2 weeks = 38 weeks, which is a little more like 9 months. To be more precise, an average pregnancy is 282 days from conception.

Still confused? You'll get the hang of it soon enough.

Naegele's rule

How long have you been pregnant? A human pregnancy averages 9 months or 40 weeks or 282 days from the date of conception. To estimate your due date, you can use Naegele's rule: subtract 3 months from the first day of your last menstrual period, then add 7 days. For example, if the first day of your last period was June 14, subtract 3 months … March … and add 7 days … March 21 is your due date! If your menstrual cycle is normally shorter or longer than 28 days, this will need to be adjusted a little. Your health-care provider may use a "pregnancy wheel" to help calculate the due date. A "dating" ultrasound is sometimes used in the first 3 months to confirm or adjust your due date.

Pregnancy wheel

In order to determine a due date, the two wheels are spun around until the last menstrual period is aligned with the actual calendar day. Then, you can look at the wheel and read the calendar date that matches up to 40 weeks. Here, the first date of the last period was April 22 and the due date is January 29.

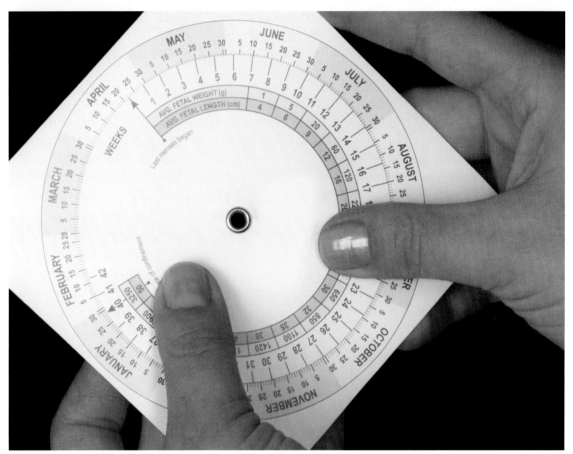

Pregnancy time periods

The 40 weeks of pregnancy are commonly divided into trimesters:

● First trimester: month 0 to 3 or week 0 to 12 (some people say 0 to 14)

● Second trimester: month 4 to 6 or week 13 to 27

● Third trimester: month 7 to 9 or week 28 to 40

The first few weeks after conception are sometimes called early pregnancy. Some people call the first 3 months (12 weeks) of a baby's life the fourth trimester, mainly because the baby's growth and development continue as quickly in these 3 months as they did during pregnancy. But strictly speaking, the period of time after birth is referred to as the postpartum period, and it lasts 6 weeks.

Fetal growth and development

In the 4 weeks since you missed your last menstrual period, you have been pregnant only for the 2 weeks since conception. In that short 2-week period, the fertilized egg has been active.

Pregnancy milestones

At 2 to 4 weeks gestation

- The fertilized egg has implanted in your uterus and started to grow by cell division into a ball-shaped, fluid-filled blastocyst.
- The blastocyst has divided into two, with one half being inside the other. The outer half will become the placenta, while the inner half becomes the embryo and eventually your baby.

- In turn, this inner half has divided into three layers:
  Inner layer: forms the internal organs, thyroid gland, and gastrointestinal tract lining
  Middle layer: forms the muscle, bone, cartilage, and blood vessels
  Outer layer: forms the brain, nervous system, skin, and hair
- At this early stage, the embryo measures $\frac{1}{70}$ to $\frac{1}{2}$ inch (0.36 to 1 mm).

Embryo at 4 Weeks

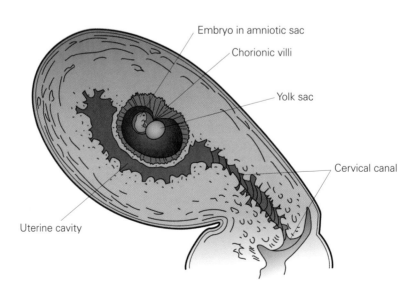

Embryo in amniotic sac

Chorionic villi

Yolk sac

Cervical canal

Uterine cavity

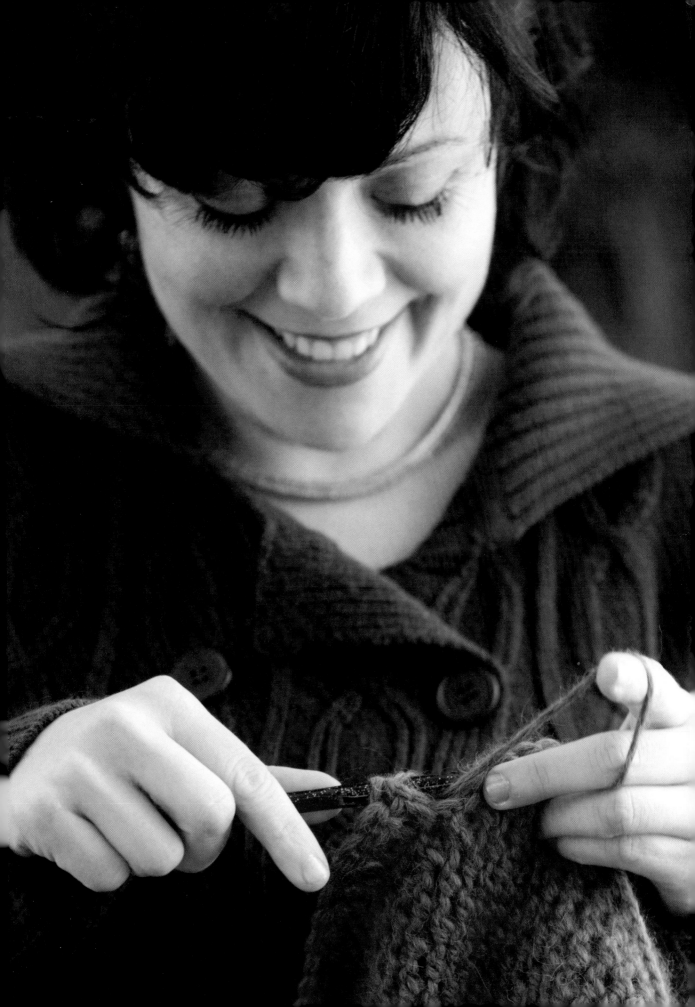

Looking and feeling pregnant

Now that you are pregnant, there are many changes going on inside your body. Some of these physiological changes are obvious to you, but others may not be. These changes are occurring so that your body can support the growing fetus and prepare you for the delivery of your newborn baby.

Weight gain

Most women will gain weight in pregnancy. The majority of weight gain is related to the uterus and its contents (fetus, placenta, and amniotic fluid), while other weight gain occurs in the breasts. The rest is attributable to normal fluid gain of approximately 7.4 quarts (7 liters). Half of this fluid comes from the fetus, placenta, and amniotic fluid, while the rest is the result of increased blood volume during pregnancy. Blood volume increases by approximately 50%! The majority of this increased blood volume is water, but the number of red blood cells also increases. For more information on weight gain in pregnancy, see Part 3 (page 106).

Cardiovascular system

In pregnancy, your resting heart rate will increase by about 10 to 15 beats per minute, and your cardiac volume (the volume of blood in your heart at any one time) will increase by about 10%. With so much more blood flowing through your heart, your doctor may notice a new murmur, which, in most cases, is normal. Your resting blood pressure will decrease in the early part of pregnancy and plateau in the beginning of the third trimester before

gradually increasing to your pre-pregnancy reading by the end of your pregnancy. When pregnant, you will experience vasodilation (or widening of the blood vessels). Standing still for long periods of time may cause you to feel faint or lead to the development of varicose veins.

Hair and skin

High levels of estrogen and progesterone stimulate more hair growth on your scalp, face, and body. This cycle reverses itself after delivery, when this hair will start to

Did You Know?

Hormones of pregnancy

Levels of the pregnancy hormone increase rapidly in early pregnancy, doubling approximately every 48 hours, and then gradually declining by about 16 weeks of gestation. This is why many women feel less morning sickness after the first trimester. The two other major hormones involved in pregnancy, estrogen and progesterone, increase greatly in pregnancy. Initially produced by the ovaries, their production is largely taken over by the placenta as it develops.

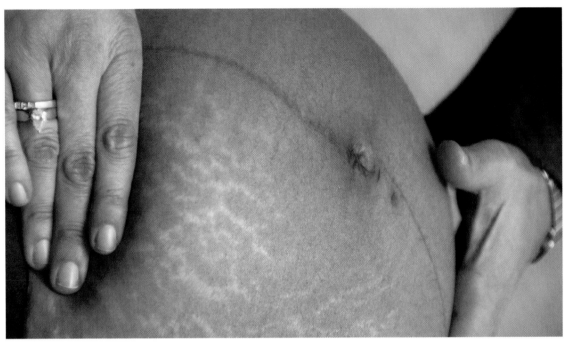

■ Linea nigra

fall out. You will also notice darkening around your nipples and a dark, vertical line from your belly button down to the pubic area, called the linea nigra, a result of the hormone stimulation in pregnancy. It will fade after delivery. You may also notice dark spots, called chloasma, on your skin, particularly on your face. They, too, will fade when hormone levels return to normal after pregnancy.

Breasts

Your breasts change greatly in pregnancy as your body prepares them for lactation. In addition to the increasing size of the breast, the size of the areola increases and darkens. By the second trimester, the first milk, called colostrum, can be expressed. The breasts also become more sensitive to the touch as your pregnancy progresses.

Gastrointestinal effects

As a result of higher progesterone levels and the increasing weight of your uterus, gut motility is slowed down and constipation is common. Hemorrhoids are also common as the weight of your pregnancy causes the veins of the pelvis to become engorged. Another common complaint is heartburn as stomach acid reflux burns the lower part of the esophagus due to the lower esophageal sphincter losing its closing capacity.

Did You Know?

Kidney function

The clearing capacity of the kidneys (the glomerular filtration rate) increases by about 40% during pregnancy. If you have a pre-existing kidney disease, this extra strain on your kidneys may be a problem. Be sure to discuss this with your doctor prior to pregnancy, if possible.

Choosing your health-care providers

While the first thing you should do after discovering you are pregnant is to celebrate, next in order is to make an appointment with your health-care provider, who will help assemble a team to guide you through pregnancy, labor and delivery and into life with your newborn baby.

Maternity-care models

There are many different models of maternity care in North America. You will need to decide which model best suits you — your personality, your expectations, your desires, and your location. Be sure your caregivers are knowledgeable, competent, and well-trained people you like and trust. They're going to guide you through one of the richest experiences of your life.

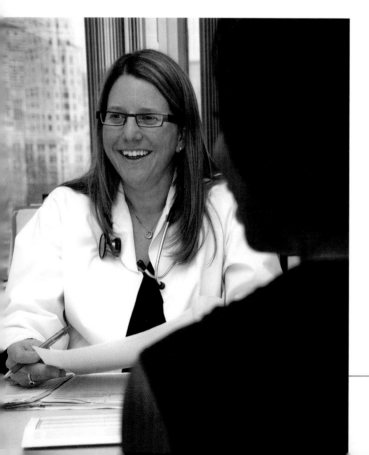

Primary caregivers

If your pregnancy is going well, you will probably not need to see anyone else other than a primary caregiver — obstetrician, family doctor, or midwife. If you develop any problems in your pregnancy that fall outside their scope of practice, they will refer you to a specialist.

Obstetricians

Obstetricians have specialized training in caring for pregnant women from pre-conception to the postpartum period, providing maternity care to women with both complicated and uncomplicated pregnancies. They are skilled at performing all types of vaginal delivery and Caesarean sections. In some smaller communities, obstetricians provide ongoing pregnancy care to women with more complicated pregnancies and act as a back-up to family doctors and midwives. All obstetricians will expect you to deliver your baby in the hospital.

An obstetrician does not provide newborn care, so you will need to have a different doctor examine your newborn baby and provide ongoing pediatric care. Your obstetrician may not continue to see you regularly after your postpartum visit, and if

Did You Know?

On-call doctors and call groups

Not all babies are born between 9 a.m. and 5 p.m. In fact, most are not. To address this need for off-hours care, doctors have formed "call" groups for evenings and weekends. All doctors in the group take turns being your "on-call" doctor. While not all patients will be cared for by their own doctor, it does ensure continuity of care within the group — and no doctor is up for several nights in a row, sleepless, before attending you in labor. Some hospitals have moved to 24-hour call systems so that, even during the daytime, the on-call doctor is responsible for caring for all maternity patients in the hospital (for labor, delivery, and specific problems). Ask your doctor how the call group works, and how to reach the on-call doctor.

she does, it will not be to provide general medical care, so you will need a family doctor for your ongoing care.

Family doctors

Many, but not all, family doctors provide prenatal care and deliver babies. Family doctors generally provide care to healthy women with relatively uncomplicated pregnancies. They are skilled at vaginal deliveries, and, in some places, usually rural, are trained in how to do Caesarean sections. Almost all family doctors will expect you to deliver your baby in the hospital. They will look after both you and your baby after birth, and continue to provide care to your family as the baby grows. This is the "family" aspect of family medicine.

While some family doctors continue to offer prenatal care and attend the deliveries of their patients' babies, others will follow their patients only during the prenatal period, usually until 28 weeks, and then refer the patient to either another family physician who delivers or an obstetrician. Following delivery, they will tend to the postpartum needs of the mother and the baby.

Referrals and consultations

Although family physicians treat many complications of pregnancy, you may be referred to an obstetrician for a consultation and shared care. If your pregnancy is particularly high-risk, the obstetrician may assume full care, although it is important to involve yourself in the decision-making process. You may still want your family doctor to participate in some aspects of your ongoing obstetrical care, and your doctor may wish to be present at, or assist in, your labor and delivery. Although family physicians in smaller communities might perform Caesarean sections, in most centers this is done by an obstetrician or general surgeon, assisted by the family doctor.

Midwives

The word "midwife" comes from the Old English "with woman." In many countries, midwifery care is the norm for expectant mothers. In fact, four out of five babies worldwide are born into the hands of midwives. In North America, a growing number of midwives are creating more care options for healthy, low-risk childbearing women. In many places, midwives have been integrated into health-care systems as fully funded primary caregivers. Many midwives have hospital privileges.

Midwives look after healthy women with healthy pregnancies. They are skilled

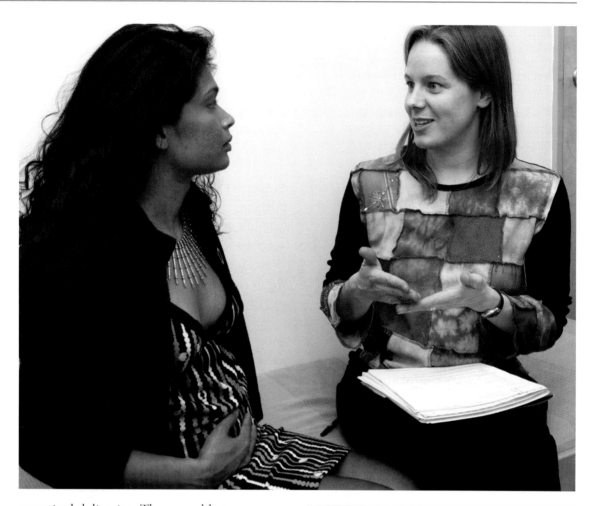

at vaginal deliveries. They are able to order standard lab tests and ultrasound scans. Midwives are typically part of an interdisciplinary team, able to work in collaboration with physicians if certain complications arise. In cases that become high-risk, care is transferred to an obstetrician. Midwives cannot perform Caesarean sections or instrumental deliveries (forceps or vacuum). If you have a pre-existing medical condition, such as diabetes or epilepsy, that makes your pregnancy high-risk, care by a midwife is not an option.

Midwives offer the option of birth at home, in the hospital, and, in some jurisdictions, in birth centers, and provide

Did You Know?

Midwife qualifications

Qualified midwives have graduated from a duly recognized midwifery educational program, successfully completing the prescribed course of studies, and have acquired the requisite qualifications to be registered or legally licensed to practice midwifery in a specific jurisdiction. Midwifery has been recognized as a health-care profession by the International Confederation of Midwives, the International Confederation of Gynecologists and Obstetricians, and the World Health Organization.

postpartum care of mother and baby, including breastfeeding support. This makes midwifery care an appealing option for women seeking personalized, holistic health care, as well as for healthy women with little social support or complex social needs.

Specialists

If you already have or develop a medical problem in pregnancy, you may be referred to a specialist. For example, if you have bad asthma, your doctor may want to get the advice of a respirologist. If you have diabetes or thyroid disease, you may need to see an endocrinologist. Some communities have access to a wider number of specialists than others. Some specialists, like geneticists, are often limited to major or special hospitals, and you may need to travel to meet with them.

Other specialists are less visible but equally important to the team caring for you during your pregnancy and delivery. You may not know them ahead of time, or indeed ever meet them, but they will be there if and when you need them.

Perinatologists

Perinatologists are obstetricians with further training in looking after complicated pregnancies. They are sometimes called maternal-fetal medicine (MFM) specialists. If it's suspected that your fetus has a significant problem, or if you have a significant medical problem, you may be referred to a perinatologist, either to look after your pregnancy or to provide advice to the referring midwife or doctor. Perinatologists always work out of a hospital, often only out of large or special-care hospitals in larger cities.

Did You Know?

Pain managers

Anesthesiologists are highly trained doctors who not only provide anesthetics in the operating room but are also trained in pain management. You may first meet an anesthesiologist when you arrive at the hospital in labor, or you may meet earlier in your pregnancy to discuss any concerns you have about pain management. Anesthesiologists give epidurals for pain relief in labor, and if you need a Caesarean section, they will give you the anesthetic for that operation. In many cases, anesthesiologists also help with postpartum pain relief. While the obstetrician is attending the delivery, the anesthesiologist is responsible for monitoring and stabilizing your vital signs, and administering IV fluids, medications, and blood products as necessary.

Pediatricians

In some places you may have the choice of having a family doctor or a pediatrician provide general well-baby care to your child after delivery. If you wish to have a pediatrician provide medical care to your baby, or if your baby is expected to have medical problems, meet ahead of time so that you can get to know each other — you may see your pediatrician quite a lot in the first year of your baby's life!

Neonatologists

A neonatologist is a pediatrician specializing in looking after newborn babies, generally in the neonatal intensive care unit. Neonatologists are responsible for the medical needs of the tiniest and sickest newborn babies.

Respiratory therapists

These health-care professionals are trained to manage all aspects of respiratory function. You may encounter a respiratory therapist assisting the anesthesiologist in ensuring your baby has successfully begun to breathe on his own.

Radiologists

Radiologists are doctors who specialize in reading X-rays, ultrasounds, and other medical images. Usually an ultrasonographer does your ultrasounds, so you may not meet a radiologist directly, but the ultrasound images collected by the ultrasonographer will be read by radiologists, who prepare the final report for your doctor or midwife.

Psychiatrists

If you or your doctor is concerned that you might have a significant mental health problem, you may be referred to a psychiatrist. A psychiatrist will diagnose and treat these problems. One of the more common, but by no means the only, reason for referral in pregnancy or the postpartum period is for depression.

Geneticists and genetic counselors

If you or your health-care providers are concerned about your risk of genetic disease, you may see a geneticist or a genetic counselor. A geneticist is a medical doctor who specializes in genetic diseases, while a genetic counselor is not a doctor but has highly specialized training in genetics.

If your medical history, medical issues in your family, or experiences in a previous pregnancy suggest an increased risk of genetic disease, it is often a good idea to discuss this ahead of time with a genetics counselor or geneticist. You can review

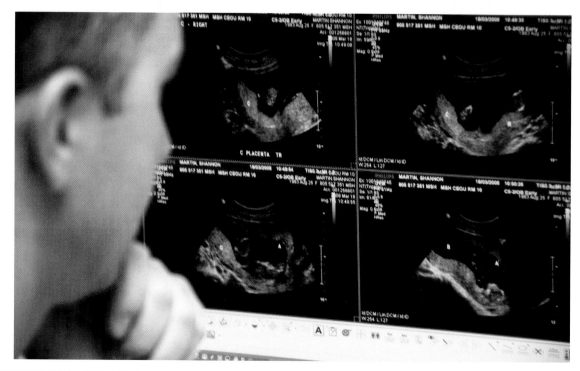

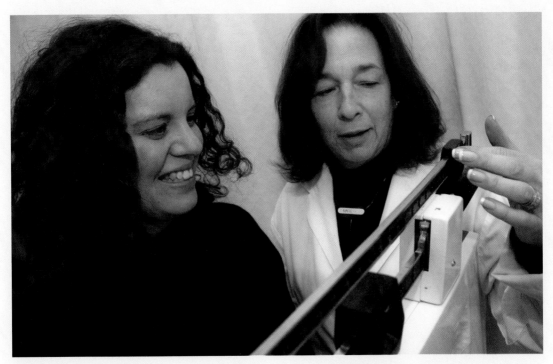

Did You Know?

Nursing care... and more

Prenatal nurses, labor and delivery nurses, and postpartum nurses will be on the front line of your pregnancy, helping your primary care giver at every stage, checking your blood pressure, listening to the baby's heart rate, monitoring your contractions, administering medications, checking your progress in labor, and communicating with your doctor or midwife to advise her of your progress. At the time of delivery, nurses will often do the initial care of your baby and help you with breastfeeding, if needed. Clinical nurse specialists have extra training in a particular obstetric field and may work in a collaborative fashion with your doctor.

your family history and discuss your risks. Sometimes it is advisable for you and your partner to undergo specific testing.

You will often see a geneticist if there are any abnormalities suspected or detected in your fetus after genetic screening tests. The geneticist will help you understand what the specific problem is, what the consequences might be for the baby, and the options for next steps. A geneticist can also help you understand recurrence risk and how to prepare for your next pregnancy.

Lactation consultants

Lactation consultants (LCs) are there to help you breastfeed as successfully as possible. Many, but not all, are nurses. LCs have extra training to help you overcome any problems you or your baby may have with breastfeeding. In some larger hospitals, LCs may run a breastfeeding clinic or center where you can go for advice in the postpartum period, even after you have been discharged. Many LCs also work privately in the community.

Nutritionists and dietitians

A nutritionist or dietitian with special knowledge about pregnancy can be a valuable resource if you are concerned about your diet or if you have a history of eating disorders, such as anorexia nervosa or bulimia. They can also be very helpful if you are heavy to begin with and are concerned about how to control your weight gain in pregnancy. Women diagnosed with gestational diabetes also benefit from meeting a nutritionist to learn how to manage their diet. Your doctor or midwife can refer you to a nutritionist if needed.

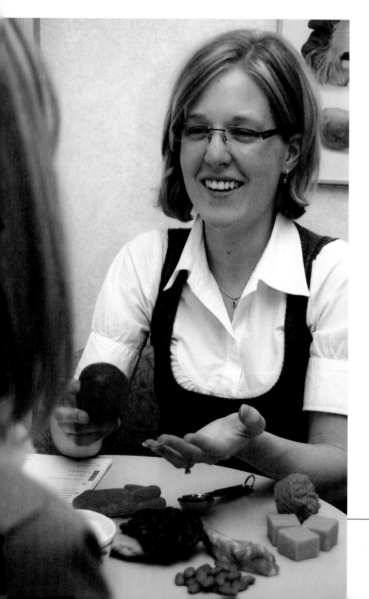

Did You Know?

Doulas

Doulas are private, non-medical labor support coaches. Unlike midwives, doulas are not trained or licensed to provide clinical care. However, the acceptance of doulas in maternity care is growing rapidly with the recognition of their important contribution to improved physical outcomes and emotional well-being of mothers and infants.

Doulas assist you in preparing and carrying out your birth plan by:

- Staying by your side throughout labor
- Providing emotional support and physical comfort measures
- Facilitating communication between you, your partner, and clinical-care providers
- Visiting you and your child after delivery

Social workers

Social workers provide a wide range of services to women during pregnancy. They can provide counseling for all sorts of personal problems, including (but not limited to) relationship problems such as abusive relationships, grief, depression, and substance abuse. If you are having trouble figuring out what employment or government benefits you are entitled to or how to negotiate with your employer, a social worker can help you. A social worker can also assist if you need help with housing or need to know where to go to solve immigration issues.

Guide to...

Medical trainees

You may or may not choose to have medical trainees involved in your care. Consider this decision carefully. The health-care practitioners of tomorrow need the opportunity to practice what they have learned. Remember that trainees are always closely supervised.

Medical students

Medical students are training to be doctors. Most medical students you encounter will be in their last 1 to 2 years of a 4-year program. They are very closely supervised, and while they may speak with you and perform a general physical examination on their own, they will not perform any pelvic exams without the presence of their supervising doctor. You are most likely to encounter medical students in large teaching hospitals, but they may also travel to various parts of the country for training in smaller towns and hospitals.

Interns

Interns are first-year resident doctors. They are closely supervised by a fully qualified doctor but may work a little more independently than a medical student. For example, the intern or resident doctor may examine you and then report back to the supervising doctor over the telephone. Interns are most likely to be found in large teaching hospitals.

Resident doctors

Residents are doctors undergoing further training in their chosen field. You will most commonly encounter residents specializing in family medicine or obstetrics and gynecology. If you need medical care from another specialty, you may also encounter residents in those specialties. Residents may be at various levels of training. For example, obstetrics and gynecology is a 5-year training program (following medical school), so someone who is a senior resident has delivered hundreds and hundreds of babies and has lots of experience already. Nevertheless, residents are still under the supervision of a fully qualified doctor.

Fellows

Fellows are doctors who have completed a residency in their chosen specialty and are pursuing further training in an even more specific field in order to be sub-specialists. For example, a fellow in maternal-fetal medicine (MFM) is a fully qualified obstetrician undergoing 2 to 3 years of further training in MFM.

Nursing students

Nursing students you may encounter are usually in their last year of training. They work under the direct supervision of a fully qualified nurse.

Midwifery students

Midwifery students will be closely supervised by a fully qualified midwife or doctor.

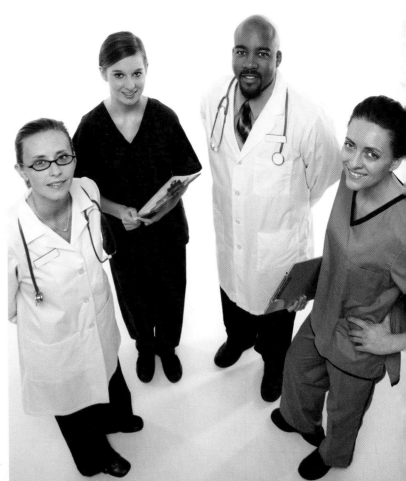

Early pregnancy medical check-up

Once your pregnancy has been confirmed, your primary care giver will schedule a series of appointments with you that run from week 12 (or earlier) through to 6 weeks postpartum. Most women in uncomplicated pregnancies are seen once a month between week 12 and 32 , then every 2 weeks until week 36, and then weekly until delivery.

Most health-care providers schedule your first prenatal appointment toward the end of the first trimester. You may like to be seen earlier if you are not wholly confident about the progress of your pregnancy — and most women aren't. Rest assured that as long as you are not having any bleeding, your pregnancy is probably progressing quite well.

Plan of medical check-ups in uncomplicated pregnancy

Visit	Trimester Month Week gestation	Topics for discussion	Examinations, tests, and measurements
Pre-pregnancy		• Fertility • Genetics • Chronic conditions • Infectious diseases • Environmental risks • Drug safety	• Fertility tests (if necessary) • Genetic screening • Immunization (rubella and varicella)
Early pregnancy	First trimester Month 1 Week 3–	• Schedule of visits • Calculation of due date	• Confirm pregnancy
1	First trimester Month 1 Week 12 or less	• Fetal progress • Maternal symptoms • Medical history • Physical and internal exam • Genetic screening • Pregnancy-care plan	• Routine blood and urine labs: hemoglobin (anemia), Rh factor, rubella, varicella, hepatitis B, syphilis, sickle cell anemia, thalassemia • Doptone (fetal heartbeat) • Screening for trisomy 13, 18, 21 (Down syndrome)

1 (continued)			• Diagnostic genetic tests: chorionic villi sampling (if desired) • Dating ultrasound • Pap smear and vaginal swabs
2	Second trimester Month 4 Week 15–17	• Fetal progress • Maternal symptoms • Blood test results • Follow-up genetic screening and diagnostic tests	• Routine weight, BP, urine protein measurements • Diagnostic genetic tests: amniocentesis (if desired)
3	Second trimester Month 5 Week 20	• Fetal movement • Maternal symptoms • Screening results	• Routine weight, BP, urine protein measurements • Anatomical scan (Level II ultrasound) for fetal health and development, gender
4	Second trimester Month 6 Week 24	• Fetal progress • Maternal symptoms • Signs of preterm labor	• Routine weight, BP, urine protein measurements • Gestational diabetes mellitus screening with oral glucose challenge test • Hemoglobin levels for anemia
5	Third trimester Month 7 Week 28	• Fetal progress • Maternal symptoms • Signs of preterm labor • Prenatal classes • Gestational diabetes mellitus screening follow-up	• Routine weight, BP, urine protein measurements • Uterine height • Rh negative factor testing and treatment
6	Third trimester Month 8 Week 32	• Fetal progress • Maternal symptoms	• Routine weight, BP, urine protein measurements • Uterine height
7	Trimester 3 Month 8 Week 34	• Fetal progress • Maternal symptoms	• Routine weight, BP, urine protein measurements • Uterine height • Ultrasound if at risk

Visit	Trimester Month Week gestation	Topics for discussion	Examinations, tests, and measurements
8	Trimester 3 Month 9 Week 36	• Fetal progress • Maternal symptoms • Preparation for labor • Plans for breastfeeding	• Routine weight, BP, urine protein measurements • Uterine height • Group B streptococcus swab • Ultrasound scan if at risk
9	Third trimester Month 9 Week 37	• Fetal progress • Maternal symptoms • Signs of labor • Group B streptococcus swab results • Ultrasound results	• Routine weight, BP, urine protein measurements • Uterine height • Ultrasound if at risk
10	Third trimester Month 9 Week 38	• Maternal symptoms • Signs of labor • Ultrasound results	• Routine weight, BP, urine protein measurements • Uterine height • Ultrasound if at risk • Vaginal exam to check cervix (optional)
11	Third trimester Month 9 Week 39	• Fetal progress • Maternal symptoms • Signs of labor	• Routine weight, BP, urine protein measurements • Uterine height • Ultrasound if at risk • Vaginal exam to check cervix (optional)
12	Third trimester Month 9 Week 40	• Due!	• Apgar test for newborn • If not born, ultrasound for fetal well-being and vaginal exam to check cervix
13	Third trimester Month 9 Week 41	• Overdue! • If not born, plans for monitoring baby in next week • Plans for inducing labor • Fetal health • Maternal symptoms	• Ultrasound for fetal well-being • Biophysical profile • Vaginal exam to check cervix
Postpartum	Week 6	• Labor and delivery review • Baby care • Breastfeeding • Mother care • Coping • Sleep • Mood • Contraception • Next pregnancy	• Physical exam • Check perineum and uterus • PAP smear if required • Test for diabetes mellitus at 3 months (if required)

Birthing philosophies

There is a large amount of conflicting information available about the best way to have a baby. While the information presented here will not resolve the conflicts, it may give you some insight into the origins of the different philosophies. It is probably safe to suggest that many practitioners and women are influenced by one or more of these different approaches, often picking and choosing the elements they like best from among them.

Birth as an illness

Early in the 20th century in Western cultures, pregnancy was "pathologized" as an illness, and doctors thought a successful pregnancy, labor, and birth required medical intervention. Women often knew little about labor and delivery ahead of time, only that it was a painful, dangerous, and terrifying event. A woman in labor was typically drugged until semi-conscious for pain relief and positioned flat on her back with her legs in stirrups for delivery. Because she was semi-conscious, she was not able to push, so most babies were delivered with the assistance of forceps and a wide episiotomy (incision at the opening of the vagina). The baby was whisked away to be looked after in a nursery. Breastfeeding was considered inferior to formula feeding.

New attitudes

Fortunately, some forward thinkers thought that labor and birth could be a better experience for women and babies and became advocates of a different style of birth. If you are interested in any one of these methods, you will need to seek out specific prenatal education guided by the particular philosophy. Some methods, such as hypno-birthing, involve very specific, focused prenatal education. Elements of these methods are incorporated into prenatal education classes. For example, most modern prenatal educators will advise you to be as active as possible in labor, to use breathing and distraction techniques to help you relax and manage pain, to ensure you have a good labor-support team in place, and to gather information in an effort to dispel your fears.

Dr. Grantly Dick-Read

Dr. Dick-Read, an English obstetrician, pioneered the natural childbirth movement in the 1930s. The story goes that he offered a woman chloroform for pain relief in labor, and she refused it. Afterwards, when he asked her why she refused it, she responded, "Because it didn't hurt. It wasn't supposed to, was it?" This made Dr. Dick-Read question all his training and experience, which told him that pain was an inevitable part of childbirth.

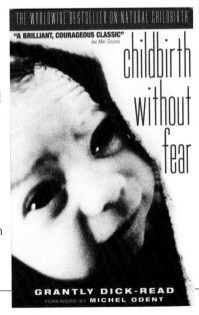

THE WORLDWIDE BESTSELLER ON NATURAL CHILDBIRTH

"A BRILLIANT, COURAGEOUS CLASSIC"
INA MAY GASKIN

childbirth without fear

GRANTLY DICK-READ
FOREWORD BY MICHEL ODENT

From that point on, he came to believe that fear was a major contributor to the pain of childbirth. He described a fear-tension-pain syndrome and believed that if fear and tension could be lessened, pain would be reduced. In 1933, he published a book entitled *Childbirth without Fear* and founded the National Childbirth Trust, an organization dedicated to providing education about pregnancy and birth to women — a radical concept in those days. He was one of the first to encourage fathers to be present in the labor and delivery rooms.

Dr. Ferdinand Lamaze

Dr. Lamaze was a French obstetrician working in the 1950s. He visited Russia and observed women using a birthing method called "psychoprophylaxis,"

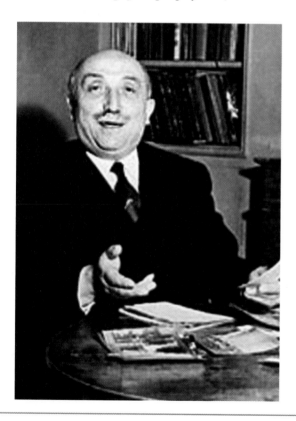

Did You Know?
Hypno-Birthing
Marie Mongan first wrote about hypno-birthing in her 1989 book, entitled *HypnoBirthing: The Mongan Method: A Breakthrough, Natural Approach to Safer, Easier, More Comfortable Birthing*. In hypno-birthing, hypnosis techniques are used to achieve the relaxation, freedom from tension, and diminished pain in natural childbirth described by Dr. Dick-Reed.

in which women were trained to use breathing and distraction techniques to distract their minds from the pain of labor. The Lamaze method combines teaching breathing techniques — different patterns for each stage of labor — with education about labor, as well as visualization, relaxation, and communication strategies. Partners are a crucial part of the Lamaze process, coaching women through the different breathing techniques.

Dr. Frederick Leboyer

Dr. Leboyer, another French physician, published his seminal book, *Birth without Violence*, in 1974, arguing that the trauma of the standard medical birth influences the behavior of the child later in life. In his method, babies are born into calm, gentle surroundings among dim lights and soft voices. Babies are handled gently, avoiding sudden and startling movements — no more slapping the bottom to stimulate breathing! He advised placing the baby on the mother's chest immediately after birth and delaying cutting the cord until it had stopped pulsating. Babies might be placed in a warm bath shortly after birth to simulate the warm, watery intrauterine environment.

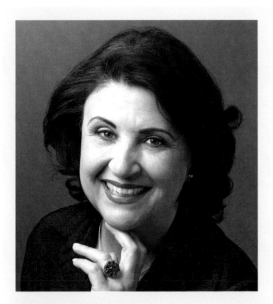

Did You Know?

Active Birth Movement

Another English childbirth educator, Janet Balaskas, published a book called *Active Birth* in 1982. The basic premise of her work is that birth is easier and more successful when women are in an upright position during labor and birth, either standing, kneeling, squatting, or on all fours. The Active Birth Movement she founded incorporates movement and breathing techniques found in Hatha yoga.

Dr. Michel Odent

Dr. Odent, a French surgeon, was asked to perform many Caesarean sections early in his career but began to question why so many interventions were necessary. His work led him to conclude that women instinctively knew how to labor and that they merely needed to be supported and protected during labor. He created a *salle sauvage* in his hospital, a room comfortable enough that a couple might want to make love there, in a bed with a low platform and lots of pillows. Women were free to walk around the room during labor and assume whatever position they wished for delivery. In such a comfortable environment, women could shed their inhibitions, contributing to the release of endorphins, natural painkillers circulated from the brain. Dr. Odent was one of the first to provide water births. He became well known for having low rates of complications and providing effective pain relief for his patients. He did not support prenatal education, since he believed that women knew instinctively how to give birth.

Sheila Kitzinger

Sheila Kitzinger, an English anthropologist, published one of the first natural childbirth education books available in the 1960s. Influenced by Dick-Read and Lamaze, she advocated natural childbirth and encouraged the use of a number of different relaxation and visualization techniques. She remains a strong advocate for the empowering effect of natural birth.

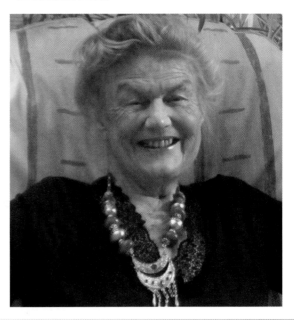

Delivery options

Although most births — 99% by some estimates — in North America now take place in a hospital setting, a very small but growing number of couples are choosing alternatives to hospital birth, including giving birth at home or in special hospital birthing rooms.

Hospital or home birth?

The irony is that hospital birth is actually the new kid on the block. Up until the 1920s, most North American births took place at home, with women attended by midwives, doctors, or even experienced neighbors or family members. In many other countries and cultures, giving birth at home is still the norm, with birth viewed not as a medical experience but as an integral part of family life.

There are many reasons for the North American shift away from home births to hospitals. Some had to do with efficiency — physicians can attend to several patients if they are all in a single place. But part of the shift was also due to negative attitudes toward midwives. From the 1930s through the 1960s, midwifery practice in North

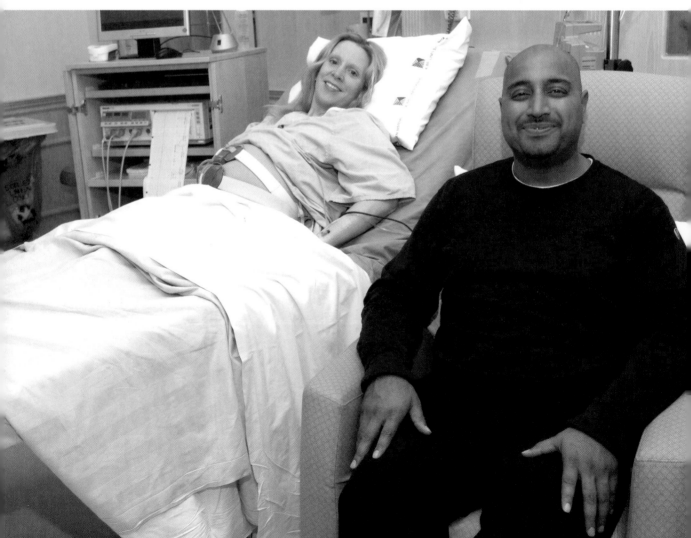

Guide to...

Pros and cons of hospital birth and home birth

Doctor's perspective

- **Hospital birth:** Doctors support hospital birth, almost exclusively. The principle concern is safety. Doctors feel it is the safest place for both mother and baby because of the access to additional doctors and nurses, as well as specialized equipment in case of an emergency.

- **Home birth:** Most doctors acknowledge that the risk of any significant and serious negative outcome is low in appropriately selected women planning a home birth, but fear of that one poor, potentially devastating outcome is enough for many to advise against the practice.

Midwife's perspective

- **Hospital birth:** Like doctors, midwives acknowledge that the majority of women choose a hospital as the place to give birth because it offers ready access to a wide range of health-care professionals and equipment. For that reason, it is an ideal choice when there are known health risks for the baby or mother. It also makes sense for couples more comfortable with a conventional childbirth.

- **Home birth:** For a woman who has been screened to make sure she is at low risk for complications, a carefully monitored home birth has proven to be a safe and successful alternative. The familiar home environment may contribute to the mother's sense of comfort and control.

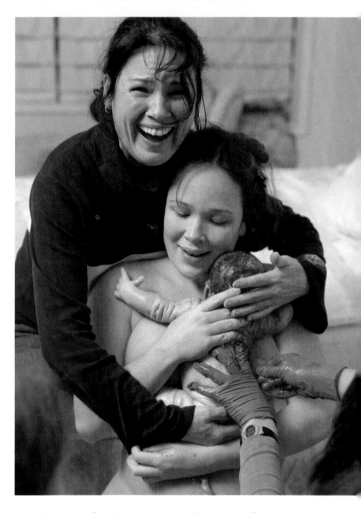

America was either systematically restricted or done away with entirely, and birth became the realm of medical professionals. By the 1950s, most births in North America were taking place in hospitals, but with the women's movement in the 1960s and 1970s came renewed interest in home birth.

Today, medical doctors advocate hospital birth for the safety of the mother and her baby, while midwives feel home birth is a good choice for the overall well-being of mother and child. The choice is yours, but take the time to review the pros and cons of both birth locations.

HOW TO...
Evaluate hospital care

Not all hospitals are alike. Before you decide on one for your labor and delivery, here are a few questions to ask:

1. What is the hospital's rate of using tests, intervention procedures (such as Caesarean sections), and drugs?

2. Does the hospital have one or more birthing rooms, and what are the rules concerning their use?

3. What are the hospital's overall childbirth policies and restrictions (for example, limitations on having children with you)?

4. Will the hospital allow you to have a midwife with you during labor and delivery?

5. After birth, are you encouraged to keep your baby with you all the time?

6. Should you want to breastfeed, are lactation specialists available to help if you need it?

7. Is the hospital a "Level 3" (tertiary care) facility with specialized care for very sick newborns?

Birthing rooms

Couples trying to decide between a hospital delivery and a home birth might want to consider a third option — a birthing room within a hospital. This is often a perfect compromise.

The hospital birthing room resembles a cozy bedroom or hotel room with a special birthing bed or chair designed so you can assume a variety of positions throughout your labor.

Although birthing rooms are meant for standard, complication-free deliveries, easy access to medical interventions in case of unexpected complications make birthing rooms within hospitals appealing to those who don't want an institutional setting but who are concerned about possible emergencies during a home birth.

Water births

Women in labor often find pain relief and comfort when in a tub of warm water. Water baths have been introduced into some hospitals, and some women delivering at home set up baths for a water birth.

Using the birthing philosophies of Dr. Leboyer and Dr. Odent, some midwives advocate a water birth as a gentle transition from in utero amniotic fluid into the world. In a water birth, the baby is born into the water and lifted out of it as the umbilical cord stops pulsating. At that point, the baby will take a first breath.

In labor, the calming effects of warm water in a birthing pool can aid relaxation. The water's buoyancy also makes is easier for you to move around and get comfortable without expending too much energy, and being immersed in water may make contractions more bearable.

Some women use the water baths as a way to relax in labor and then deliver the baby "on land."

Water birth safety

Currently, there is virtually no scientific evidence looking at the risks or benefits of water birth to the baby. At minimum, there is a potential for water inhalation and infections; both have been reported to cause significant problems for some babies. The frequency of this occurrence is not known. Advocates of water birth believe it is safe and report good outcomes for both mother and baby, based upon anecdotal evidence. Check with your doctor or midwife to see if this option for delivery is available in your community.

HOW TO...

Choose a midwife for home birth

1. Ask about her training and her certifications or licenses, as well as about her experience attending other births.

2. Make sure you discuss her childbirth philosophy and find out whether it's in line with your own thinking.

3. Ask about her contingency plans. How does the midwife handle problems or complications if they develop during labor? What standard and emergency equipment does she carry? What are her plans for transportation to a hospital in case of an emergency? What kind of relationship does she have with the obstetricians at the hospital?

4. Establish her fees and find out exactly what they cover.

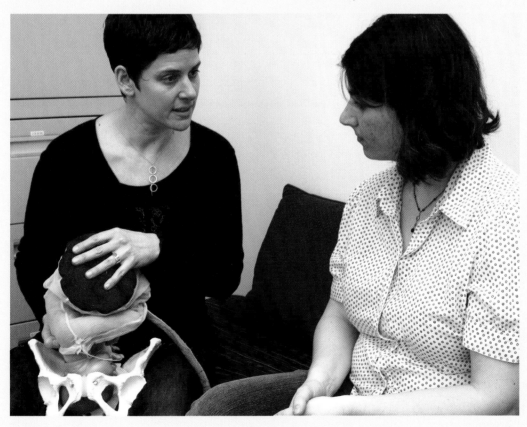

Childbirth classes

Childbirth classes (also called prenatal classes) are designed to help prepare you for labor, birth, and early parenthood. They provide a forum for asking questions, gathering information, and socializing with other expectant couples. By attending classes, you and your partner can acquire the skills and confidence needed to make birth a positive experience. For many people, these classes are a rite of passage, something they know they are supposed to take part in prior to the arrival of their first child. For others, they are a foreign concept because the knowledge needed to birth a child is either passed down from generation to generation, or it is something that women just experience without any preparatory guidance from others. Remember that these classes are only the beginning of your learning journey as a parent, and that you will continue to search for answers as your new bundle of joy grows up!

Types of childbirth classes

There are many different types of classes delivered in prenatal education programs. The type of class you choose will depend on what your needs are and how effective your support network is. It may depend on your schedule, but it also depends on your learning style. For some, group classes provide an opportunity to share ideas and to connect with others going through similar experiences. For others, the idea of sitting in a classroom with other expectant mothers and couples is not appealing, and they would prefer to meet one-on-one with an educator to have their individual learning needs met.

Some women absorb things quickly and may prefer to learn as much as possible in one shot at a weekend series of classes. Some need time to digest the information received, so an evening series might be a better choice. Remember also that the longer the series, the greater the likelihood that plenty of time will be spent on each topic, and the more time the educator will have to answer your questions. There are also drop-in classes and online classes.

Early pregnancy classes

Early pregnancy classes cover basic prenatal-care guidelines, available screening tests and their impact, anatomy and physiology associated with early pregnancy (including typical physical discomforts and possible remedies), and risk factors (including the impact of the environment, stress, smoking, alcohol, and drugs on the baby). There is often a focus on nutrition and physical activity for the mother.

Later pregnancy classes

The classes most people associate with prenatal education focus on physical and emotional preparation for childbirth and the postpartum experience. Anatomy and physiology associated with the later stages of pregnancy, warning signs of preterm labor, recognition of labor, and the stages of labor common to all women are covered in these classes. Non-medical and medical interventions to support the laboring woman are discussed, including self-help comfort measures, mainstream and alternative techniques for relaxation and labor support, and common medical pain management techniques. Common interventions, such as fetal monitoring, inductions, and Caesarean sections, are usually explained in terms of risk vs. benefit to the mother and baby, and parents are often taught how to be part of the decision-making team when they find themselves in unexpected situations.

Did You Know?
Breastfeeding classes
Breastfeeding classes, whether stand-alone or as part of a series, tend to cover a variety of topics, such as the benefits of breastfeeding, the risks of formula feeding and supplementation, anatomy and physiology of the breast, strategies to promote successful breastfeeding, and tips on how to recognize and prevent complications. Advice on how and where to find breastfeeding support play an integral role in these classes.

Postpartum classes
These classes focus on your adjustment to parenthood, with information and advice on hospital postpartum routines, physical and emotional changes you can expect during the postpartum period, and how to deal with these changes. Detailed explanation of newborn care, behavior, and breastfeeding are usually offered.

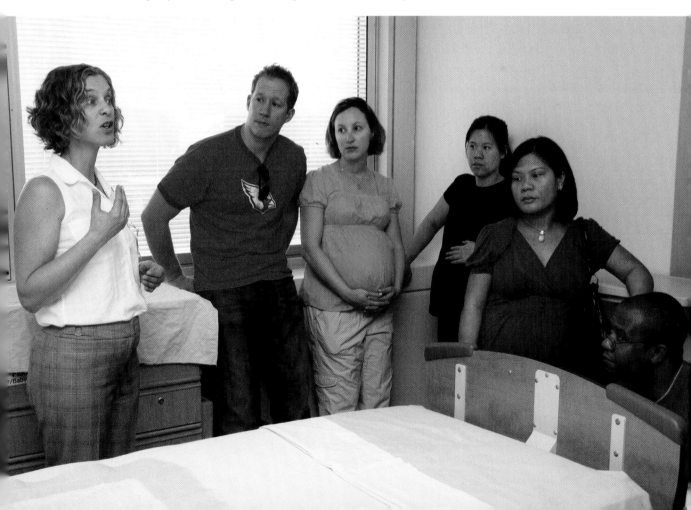

Guide to...
Childbirth class content

Although childbirth classes may vary in their learning style and birthing philosophy, most provide the following basic information, support, and guidance:

- Explanation of the pregnancy's progress in each trimester and postpartum
- Description of physical and emotional changes you may experience
- Details of medical procedures and interventions you may require
- Demonstrations of the different birth positions
- Guidance in choosing pain relief options
- Hands-on learning of massage skills, relaxation strategies, and breathing techniques
- List of community pregnancy-support groups and breastfeeding resources
- Advice on involving your partner and family in your pregnancy and birth
- Insight into relationship changes in the family during pregnancy and after delivery
- Guidance in initiating breastfeeding and tips for ensuring success
- Preparations for unexpected outcomes

Specialized classes

Most classes are designed for first-time parents and help both partners get involved in the preparations for labor and birth. These generic classes usually cover a variety of topics, including prenatal issues, labor and delivery, role of

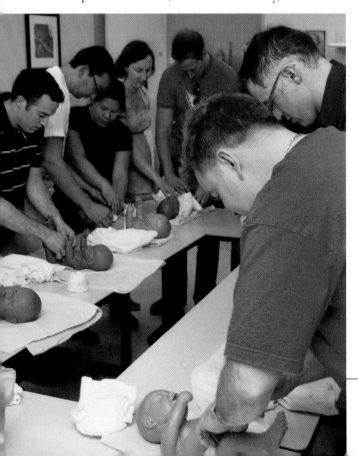

support persons, breastfeeding, postpartum care of the newborn and mother, and adjustment to parenting. They are the most common type of classes offered. However, specialized classes may be found. The availability of these classes is largely determined by where you live, with larger cities generally having more options.

- **Refresher classes:** These classes are aimed at women who have already had children and tend to focus on only those issues of interest to them. For example, second-time mothers often want to talk about their previous birth experiences and be updated on research and changes in birth practices but may not need information on feeding their babies.
- **Group-specific classes:** Classes may be offered to certain clientele, such as adolescents, those expecting multiples, single parents, cultural groups, parents from diverse family structures, or bereaved parents.
- **Women-only classes:** Single women, gay women, and those whose partners are away may find these classes particularly useful.

• **Childbirth philosophy classes:** A few of the most common childbirth philosophies are the Lamaze, Leboyer, or Odent. Many of these ideas are incorporated into general childbirth education classes. If you are interested in exclusive education on any one of these methods, you will need to find a class that is guided by that philosophy.

Sponsors and teachers

Public health units, hospitals, community health centers, non-profit organizations, private businesses, and independent educators all offer prenatal classes. They can be taught by registered nurses, physiotherapists, social workers, or psychologists, as well as by lay persons with an interest in childbirth, such as doulas. In addition, classes focused on breastfeeding may be taught by certified lactation consultants or by individuals who have taken a course in lactation support.

Ideally, the educator is either certified or is working toward certification. There are a number of organizations that provide certification in childbirth education, and some will provide certification for prenatal education separately from postpartum education.

Signing up

Your health-care provider may be able to provide a list of childbirth classes in your area. If not, phone your local public health department or hospital, ask your friends, search via the Internet, or look in the Yellow Pages under prenatal classes. Book early, and if you're planning to attend a class that's not run by a local hospital or health center, make sure that the instructor has been properly trained.

Guide to...
Questions to ask before you sign up

• Who sponsors the classes and is there a cost?
• Is there financial assistance available if the cost is prohibitive?
• Where will the classes be given?
• When are the classes offered (daytime, evening series, weekend programs)?
• How many classes are there in a series?
• Can you visit a class before you decide?
• How long is each class?
• How many couples are in each class?
• Are private classes offered?
• Can you bring more than one support person or come alone?
• What types of classes are offered — generic all-inclusive, early pregnancy, labor and birth preparation only, postpartum experience, or breastfeeding?
• What types of learning techniques are used?
• What birth philosophies and methodologies are covered?
• What do you need to bring?
• Is the instructor certified or affiliated with any organization?
• Can the instructor provide references?

Pregnancy support

Pregnancy is an exciting time, but it's not unusual for pregnant women to sometimes feel tired and stressed. Fatigue is normal, especially in the early months. Activities that you used to breeze through — going to work, taking care of your other children — can suddenly seem overwhelming. You might feel stressed about all that you have to do regarding work, taking care of the house, and getting ready for your baby.

Don't try to push through it all alone. Your partner, parents, friends, and family — even your other children — are great sources of strength and support. Asking for help and accepting it can make your pregnancy more relaxing and enjoyable. Sharing the work can make everyone involved feel part of the experience.

Partners

In most cases, your partner is the first person you look to for help and support during your pregnancy. It's important to involve your partner as early as possible in the experience of pregnancy, engaging him or her in open discussions about what you are experiencing and feeling — both your concerns and your excitement. Psychologically and emotionally, if not physically, your partner is also going through pregnancy. If they are actively involved, many partners will develop a strong bond with their unborn child. It may be a good idea to join a pregnancy support group together.

Parents and in-laws

Your partner isn't the only person you can lean on during pregnancy. Your parents and in-laws may be eager to assist but might be worried about overstepping boundaries. In fact, it might take a while to find the balance between maintaining your privacy and independence and allowing the whole family to enjoy the pregnancy together.

Your parents and in-laws might be able to help by babysitting your other children, running errands, cooking meals, grocery shopping, and stocking up on useful items, such as diapers, baby clothes, nursery furniture, and bedding. After your baby is born, you might want to involve grandparents in the baby's care, which will make them feel needed and useful, and will take some of the pressure off you. Two-way, open communication about needs and expectations is the key to making it all work, during pregnancy and beyond.

Did You Know?

Ongoing support

Drawing strength from others during pregnancy depends on your ability to ask for and accept help — and your willingness to let the important people in your life get involved. After the baby is born, your helpers will want to continue assisting in large and small ways. Open communication and flexible expectations will help you discover the best ways for this to happen.

Siblings and friends

Siblings can be a great source of support. They may be particularly excited and eager to help if you are the first in your generation to have a baby. Prospective aunts and uncles can be very keen. If they've already had a baby, they can be a good source of information regardless of their distance from you. If they live in the area, siblings could be a source of baby gear as well as assistance. Friends can play the same role as relatives, helping with everyday chores, such as cleaning and cooking, and baby preparations, such as painting the nursery or shopping for clothes.

Children

If you have one or more older children at home, they can help as well. You've probably spent some time preparing them for the birth of a new sibling, talking about how the baby will be cared for, what things the baby will need, and where the baby will sleep. You may have discussed how your child can help once the new baby arrives. Why not start even earlier?

Did You Know?

Singles support groups

Support groups for single pregnant women and single parents in your community are good places to find other people who share your situation. Talking with them may help you to feel less isolated. Alternatively, if you have a computer with Internet access, you might want to join one of the many online communities of single parents.

Single parenthood can be rewarding and joyful. Just remember to let yourself lean on others and to ask for help when you need it.

Getting your baby's siblings to help while you are pregnant will get them used to participating, and might even relieve some of your own work. Let them do small household chores, such as helping fold the laundry, and baby-specific tasks, such as helping pack your suitcase for the hospital. After a long day on your feet, a foot massage from your little one can be a great way to relax and share some private time.

Guide to...

Being a great partner

Partners can participate and help in many ways during pregnancy. Not only does this lift some of the weight off your shoulders, it can contribute to developing a new bond called parenthood between you and your partner. Here are just a few suggestions:

- Participate in prenatal classes to learn what to expect during pregnancy and labor
- Attend prenatal medical check-ups
- Take over many of the household chores, such as cleaning, cooking, and grocery shopping
- Offer foot and body massages (they're relaxing and can contribute to the developing bond of parenthood)
- Help create a birth plan
- Exercise and eat healthy meals together
- If applicable, cut down on or quit smoking and reduce alcohol intake

F.A.Q.

We answer many questions from pregnant women and their partners. Here are some of the most frequently asked questions. Be sure to ask your health-care providers any other questions that may arise. If they don't have the answers, they will refer you to a colleague who does

Q: Can I have a midwife and a doctor?

A: Not usually. Both doctors and midwives provide primary care. Midwives and doctors work together if you are in midwifery care and complications arise in your pregnancy or labor, but in most cases, your midwife is still your primary care giver. If your complications become quite complex, your care will need to be transferred to a doctor, and then your midwife may choose to stay involved in a supportive role. If you are under a physician's care and are looking for someone to provide added emotional and physical support, you should consider hiring a doula.

Q: What's the difference between a midwife and a doula?

A: Midwives are regulated health professionals who provide comprehensive prenatal, intrapartum, and postpartum care. Midwives are trained to attend to all of your normal pregnancy-, birth-, and postpartum-related health-care needs. While midwives provide emotional support and physical comfort measures in labor, they are also responsible for all of your clinical-care needs. A doula is solely responsible for providing information and emotional and physical support. She has training and expertise in helping a woman and her family through the pregnancy and birth process, and often provides postpartum support and breastfeeding assistance. A doula plays no medical role in your care and cannot provide medical advice.

Q: Why do I feel so short of breath?

A: Perceived breathlessness, or dyspnea, can happen in 70% of pregnancies. There is no change in physical activity level associated with this breathlessness. In pregnancy, there is a slight increase in respiratory rate, but a large increase in tidal volume (the amount of air with each breath). This compensates for the increasing size of the uterus and its effects on respiration.

Q: What is natural childbirth?

A: "Natural childbirth" usually refers to those births in which no interventions were used. There were no medications to stimulate labor or control pain, and the child was born vaginally without the aid of forceps or vacuum.

Q: Why are medical doctors opposed to natural childbirth?

A: This is a widely held misconception! Doctors are not opposed to natural childbirth. If a woman is able to cope well with the birthing process, in whatever way she can, then most doctors will support her decision, assist her as much as they can, and, indeed, salute her for her courage and fortitude! However, doctors are also willing to provide medications as indicated, including pain medication, should the laboring woman choose to have it. Some doctors are concerned that the current emphasis and high value placed upon natural childbirth can lead women to feel disappointed with themselves and unhappy with their experience if they do choose to use medications in labor and require a forceps delivery, or even a Caesarean section.

Q: I'm spotting! What should I do?

A: Do not panic. There are many potential causes of bleeding in early pregnancy. Often there is a bit of bleeding as the embryo implants into the wall of the uterus — called an implantation bleed. There can also be a bit of bleeding behind the developing placenta — called a subchorionic hemorrhage. In these cases, the pregnancy outcome is often just fine.

Other causes include miscarriage and ectopic pregnancy. The best way to differentiate between these causes is by having an ultrasound.

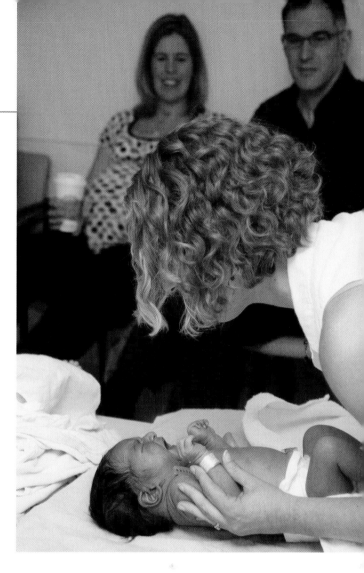

You are undoubtedly anxious, but if the bleeding is quite light, your doctor can arrange for an ultrasound to be done during office hours, saving you a long wait in an emergency room. Of course, if the bleeding is heavy (two pads/hour for more than 2 hours), then you should seek emergency care.

What's next

Hungry? Many pregnant women crave to eat for two. While that's overdoing it a bit, you do need to consume some more calories and other nutrients to keep yourself and the fetus healthy.

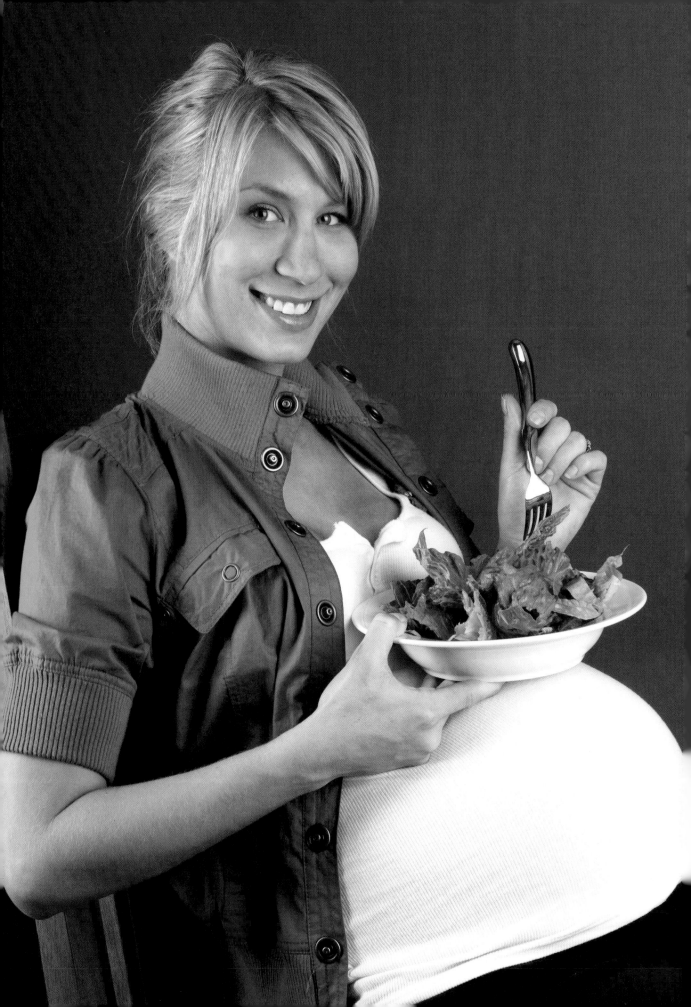

Part 3

Eating Well for a Healthy Pregnancy

Eating for two (or more)

There is some truth in the old wives' tale that you need to eat for two when you are pregnant. Additional food energy is needed to nourish both you and the fetus, and some common nutrients should be taken as supplements to make up for any pregnancy-related deficiencies. Maintaining a diet that meets these needs is a tall order, but eating can still be fun. There are very few foods that you should avoid during your pregnancy.

Special nutrient needs

Food provides the body with the energy it needs for all daily activities. Energy comes from the macronutrients you consume — carbohydrate, protein, and fat. The energy from food is measured in calories, and you may hear the terms "energy" and "calories" used interchangeably. The body converts macronutrients into energy to use for daily living with the help of micronutrients:

vitamins, minerals, amino acids, and essential fatty acids.

During pregnancy, higher amounts of specific nutrients are required to help support the 50% increase in blood volume; the development of the placenta, which aids in the transfer of nutrients from you to the fetus; your increase in body weight, including breast growth for lactation; and the growth and development of the

Nutrient needs in pregnancy

Nutrients (per day)	DRI before pregnancy	DRI during pregnancy	UL during pregnancy
Macronutrients			
Carbohydrate (g)	130	175	N/A
Fiber (g)	25	28	N/A
Protein (g)	46	71	N/A
Micronutrients			
Calcium (mg)	1000	1000	2500
Vitamin D (IU)	200	200	2000
Iron (mg)	18	27	45
Folic acid (mcg)	400	600	1000
Zinc (mg)	8	11	40
Omega-3 fatty acid (g)	1.1	1.4	Avoid supplements
Vitamin B_{12} (mcg)	2.4	2.6	Not determinable
Vitamin A (IU)	700	770	1000

Guide to...

Dietary definitions

DRI: The Dietary Reference Intakes (DRIs) have been developed by the U.S. Institute of Medicine to determine the amount of macronutrients and micronutrients required daily. The DRIs provide recommended intakes for healthy persons living in North America, based on the most recent scientific data. The DRIs consider specific life stages, including pregnancy and lactation. The needs of the fetus during pregnancy and the need for optimal production of breast milk during lactation are considered when determining the nutrient needs of pregnant and lactating women.

RDA: The Recommended Dietary Allowance is the average daily dietary intake level required to meet the nutrient needs of almost all (97% to 98%) healthy individuals in a group defined by age, gender, and activity level.

UL: The Tolerable Upper Limit (UL) states the maximum amount of a nutrient that is safe to consume on a daily basis without posing adverse health effects. Regular daily consumption of certain nutrients above the UL can increase the chance of developing a disease or disorder. During pregnancy and breastfeeding, this value is especially important to consider, because some nutrients are considered teratogenic (harmful to the fetus) if consumed in quantities above the UL.

fetus. Ensuring that all macronutrient and micronutrient needs are met throughout pregnancy and that the appropriate amount of weight is gained will promote your health and improve the outcome for your baby.

Trimester energy demands

Determining the energy needs of pregnant women in each trimester is based on individual pre-pregnancy requirements. Your pre-pregnancy energy requirement takes into account your age, height, weight, and level of physical activity.

Calorie calculation

For example, the average recommended intake of calories for a 30-year-old pregnant woman, 5'5" (165 cm) in height, weighing 150 pounds (68 kg) before pregnancy, and at an "active" level of physical activity (60 minutes of moderate intensity activity daily) is 2477 calories each day.

Extra calories: Her extra calorie needs in each trimester are:
- **First trimester:** no difference from pre-pregnancy energy requirements of 2477 calories
- **Second trimester:** 340 calories additional each day, or a total of 2817 calories
- **Third trimester:** 452 calories additional each day, or a total of 2929 calories

Activity level factor: If this woman was not at an active level of physical activity, but less or more active, the requirements would differ for the first trimester, and this new base number would affect the total number of calories required in the other trimesters:
- **Sedentary level:** 1982 calories
- **Light level:** 2202 calories
- **Active level:** 2477 calories
- **Very active level:** 2807 calories

Guide to...

Meeting second and third trimester calorie requirements

To add another 340 healthy calories per day in the second trimester and boost your intake to 452 more calories than your regular daily diet in the third trimester, try adding these food servings:

Food item (standard serving)	Calories per serving
Second trimester (add 340 calories)	
Add a morning snack:	
¾ cup (175 g) vanilla yogurt (1% MF)	185
½ cup (125 mL) blueberries	45
Add an afternoon snack:	
1 cup (250 mL) decaffeinated latte made with 1% MF milk	110
Third trimester (add 452 calories)	
Add a morning snack:	
1 banana	100
Add an afternoon snack	
1 cup (250 mL) carrots	60
2 stalks celery	12
2 tbsp (25 mL) low-fat vegetable dip	80
Add an evening snack	
1 2-oz (60 g) bran muffin (homemade)	200

Calorie content

To determine the calories you normally consume daily, recall what you ate in a average day and add up the calories in each food and beverage consumed. (Don't forget the snacks between meals and any snacking while preparing meals.) To determine your calorie intake in your first trimester, keep track of the food you eat for a few days. Lists of the calorie content of common foods are available on the Internet, as are electronic calorie counters. You can also meet with a dietitian to have your usual calorie intake calculated.

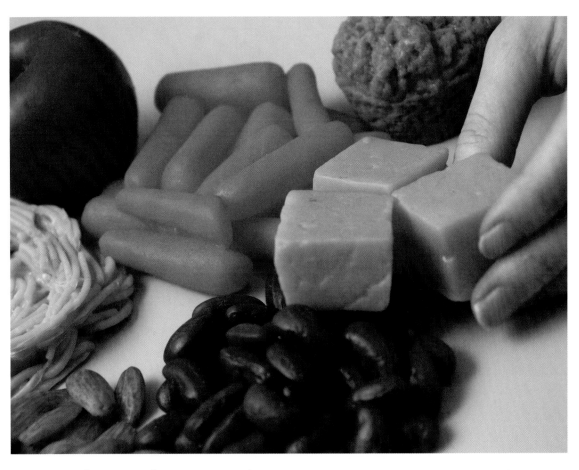

Ten tips for good nutrition during pregnancy

1. Follow the US Department of Agriculture (USDA) MyPyramid food guide or Canada's Food Guide to Healthy Eating for food choices and meal plans.
2. Don't be afraid to eat the recommended amount of calories for each trimester or to gain the recommended amount of weight.
3. Continue taking a prenatal vitamin and mineral supplement each day with at least 1 mg of folic acid and 15 mg of zinc, especially in the first trimester but throughout your pregnancy.
4. Eat a diet rich in fiber so you feel full but don't feel constipated.
5. Consume at least 3 servings of calcium-rich milk products each day.
6. Be sure to drink 12 cups (3 L) of fluids every day to keep well hydrated.
7. Include plenty of omega-3 fatty acids in your diet, especially in the third trimester.
8. Be careful not to consume excess amounts of vitamin A — more than 10,000 IU can contribute to fetal abnormalities.
9. Avoid fad diets.
10. Enjoy your food! Some women find food more flavorful, not at all nauseating in pregnancy.

Macronutrients

You will get the energy you need by eating food rich in the three macronutrients —
carbohydrate, protein, and fat. In pregnancy, these macronutrients need to be eaten
in specific proportions for optimum calorie intake and control of weight gain.

Carbohydrate

Carbohydrate provides energy to all cells in the body. The brain depends on carbohydrate as its sole source of energy. Carbohydrates are made up of starches, sugars, and fiber. Sugars are short-chain, easily digested carbohydrates and include both monosaccharides (glucose, fructose, and galactose) and disaccharides (lactose, sucrose, and maltose). You're probably familiar with these names from reading food labels. Starches are long-chain carbohydrates and include polysaccharides and modified starches. Starches are digested more slowly than sugars. Fiber is a part of carbohydrate that is not digested by the body and does not contribute to energy intake or increases in blood sugar.

Carbohydrates are found in grain products (such as breads, oats, and cereals), vegetables (potatoes and carrots), fruits (apple and banana), and some dairy products (milk).

- DRI for carbohydrate in pregnancy is 175 g per day.

Low-carbohydrate fad diets

Diets that are low or lacking in a specific macronutrient are not safe to follow during your childbearing years. For example, popular low-carbohydrate diets focus on decreasing overall calories by decreasing the amount of carbohydrate consumed.

However, decreasing carbohydrate can lead to an inadequate intake of the essential nutrients that come with carbohydrates, such as iron, folate, some B vitamins, and fiber. Diets low in iron can result in anemia, and diets low in folate can place the fetus at risk of neural tube defects. If your carbohydrate intake is insufficient,

Did You Know?

Acceptable macronutrient distribution ranges (AMDR)

Health agencies have established a range of intakes of energy from carbohydrate, protein, and fat that is associated with the least amount of risk of disease and, at the same time, can provide essential nutrients. Intakes that are below or above the range can increase the risk of chronic disease.

AMDR is expressed as a percentage of total energy and emphasizes the proper (not equal) balance among the three macronutrients. It is based on age, gender, and life stage, including pregnancy and lactation.

AMDR in pregnancy

Carbohydrate: 45% to 65%
Protein: 10% to 35%
Fat: 20% to 35%

Carbohydrate content of common foods

Food item (standard serving)	Carbohydrate (g) per serving DRI: 175 g total
Breakfast	
1 cup (250 mL) multigrain cereal	20
1 cup (250 mL) milk	13
½ cup (125 mL) raspberries	8
Morning snack	
1 apple	20
Lunch	
2 slices whole wheat bread	30
½ cup (125 mL) raw vegetables (mix of cucumber, peppers, celery)	3
1 cup (250 mL) cranberry juice (unsweetened)	30
Snack	
1 cup (250 mL) milk	13
Dinner	
½ sweet potato	15
1 cup (250 mL) green beans	10
1 cup (250 mL) milk 1% MF	13

your body will use the protein stored in your muscles as an energy source. Your "low-carb" diet can lead to a decrease in lean muscle mass.

There is no scientific evidence that low-carbohydrate diets will help you lose weight and maintain the weight loss for a long period of time, except, possibly, for the unhealthy loss of lean muscle mass. Postpartum depression has also been linked to diets that are low in calories and carbohydrates.

Did You Know?

Calories per gram

Contrary to popular belief, carbohydrates are not more "fattening" than protein or fat. Carbohydrates contain 4 calories per gram, which is less than half the number of calories in a gram of fat (9) and the same number found in a gram of dietary protein.

Glycemic index of common carbohydrates

Low-GI foods	Medium-GI foods	High-GI foods
Skim milk	Banana	Dried dates
Plain yogurt	Raisins	Instant mashed potatoes
Sweet potato	Split pea soup	Baked white potatoes
Oat bran bread	Whole wheat bread	White plain bagel
Oatmeal	Brown rice	Soda crackers
Lentils	Couscous	French fries
Kidney beans	Rye bread	Ice cream
Chickpeas		Table sugar

Adapted by permission from Kalnins D and Saab J, *Better Food for Pregnancy: Nutrition Guide Plus More Than 125 Recipes for Healthy Pregnancy and Breastfeeding* (Toronto, ON: Robert Rose, 2006).

Glycemic index

The glycemic index (GI) measures the body's blood glucose response to the consumption of 1 gram of a specific carbohydrate. Foods are classified as being low-GI (for example, oat bran cereal and lentils) or high-GI (for example, white bread and potatoes). A low-GI food is absorbed relatively slowly in the body, accompanied by a lower rise in blood glucose, offering health benefits over high-GI foods, which increase blood glucose rapidly after consumption. Generally speaking, low-GI foods are also higher in fiber and less processed than high-GI foods, making them healthier food choices for most people. You should aim to eat low-GI carbohydrates.

Fiber

Fiber helps to keep bowel movements regular, helps make you feel full, helps normalize blood sugar and blood cholesterol levels, and reduces the risk of cardiovascular disease. There are two types of fiber — soluble and insoluble. It is important to consume a balance of both types.

Soluble fiber is found mainly in legumes, fruit peels, root vegetables, psyllium, and oats. It's the fiber that helps with the regulation of blood sugar and cholesterol levels. Insoluble fiber is found in whole grains, vegetables, nuts, and seeds and helps to keep bowel movements regular.

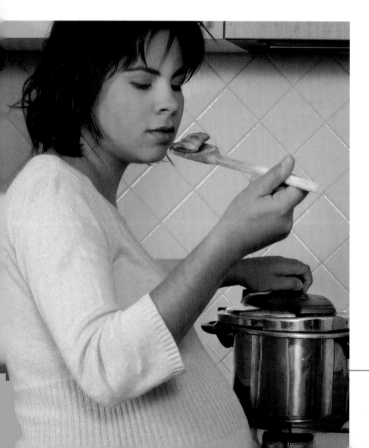

Fiber content of common foods

Food item (standard serving)	Fiber (g per serving) DRI: 28 g
Breakfast	
1 cup (250 mL) raisin bran cereal	6.7
Snack	
½ cup (125 mL) blackberries	4.0
Lunch	
1 whole wheat pita bread	4.7
1 apple with skin	2.6
Snack	
4 tbsp (60 mL) almonds, roasted	4.2
Dinner	
½ cup (125 mL) broccoli, boiled	2.0
1 baked potato with skin	3.8

During pregnancy, women often experience constipation and hemorrhoids — a diet rich in fiber and fluid is the best way to promote normal bowel regularity.

- DRI for fiber in pregnancy is 28 g per day (21–38 g per day recommended for the non-pregnant population).

Protein

Dietary protein is made up of amino acids, the building blocks for cells and tissues. In pregnancy, this protein is used for the growth and development of fetal and maternal tissues, organs, and bones. It supports the mother's breasts, uterus, placenta, and blood volume. Protein also helps to increase satiety (feeling full). Protein should be part of every meal. The food groups that contain the most protein are meat and alternatives (fish, legumes, nuts, seeds, and eggs) and milk and alternatives (milk, yogurt, and cheese).

- DRI for protein during pregnancy is 71 g (including an additional 25 g in the second and third trimester).

Fats

The fats you consume are the most concentrated source of energy, providing 9 calories per gram (versus 4 calories per gram for protein and carbohydrate). Fat in food is needed to transport fat-soluble vitamins (vitamin A, D, E, and K). Dietary fats also provide the essential fatty acids your body requires. Fats are found in milk and milk alternatives, meats and meat alternatives, and some commercially prepared foods. Foods from the vegetables and fruit and grain products groups do not contain significant amounts of fats.

There are a few different types of fats, or fatty acids, found in food. Some are healthy, others are required, and some increase disease risk. Understanding the different fats can help you choose safer foods.

Saturated fats

Saturated fats are found in animal products (meat and dairy products) and commercially prepared foods made with butter and lard (pastries and baked goods). Saturated fats contribute to heart disease by elevating total cholesterol and low-density lipoprotein ("bad") cholesterol levels. Limit your consumption of foods with these dietary fats.

Unsaturated fats

Unsaturated fats are found in plant foods (nuts, seeds, and oils) and include both

Protein content of common foods

Food item (standard serving)	Protein (g per serving) DRI: 71 g
Vegetables and fruit	
½ cup (125 mL) vegetables	1–4
½ cup (125 mL) fruit or 4 tbsp (60 mL) dried fruit	1–2
Grain products	
½–1 cup (125–250 mL) breakfast cereals enriched with iron	1–5
½ cup (125 mL) pasta, rice, barley, couscous, quinoa	2–8
1 slice bread	3
Milk and alternatives	
1 cup (250 mL) milk	8–10
¾ cup (175 g) yogurt	7–10
1.75 oz (50 g) cheese	10–15
Meat and alternatives	
2.5 oz (75 g) meat (beef, chicken, pork, lamb, veal)	15–30
2.5 oz (75 g) fish and seafood (salmon, halibut, sardines, shrimp)	10–25
1 egg	6
¾ cup (175 mL) legumes (white beans, soybeans, lentils, chickpeas, kidney beans)	8–21
5 oz (150 g) tofu	7–21
2 tbsp (25 mL) nuts or seeds (pumpkin seeds, sesame seeds, sunflower seeds, peanuts, walnuts, almonds, cashews)	5–10
2 tbsp (25 mL) peanut butter	15
Second and third trimester additional protein To add the required extra 25 g per day to your diet in the second and third trimester, try eating these foods:	

Food item (standard serving)	Protein (g per serving)
Morning snack	
¾ cup (175 g) 1.5% MF strawberry yogurt	8
Afternoon snack	
1 cup (250 mL) skim milk	9
¼ cup (50 mL) almonds	8

monounsaturated (found in canola and olive oil and almonds) and polyunsaturated fats (found in fish oil, sunflower oil, walnuts, and seeds). These fats are a healthier choice than saturated fats because they do not raise the low-density lipoprotein levels. Rather, they can lead to an increase in high-density lipoprotein ("good") cholesterol levels and help to protect against heart disease. Choose plant-based foods rather than meat-based foods because they are rich in unsaturated fats.

Trans fats

Trans fats are similar to saturated fats in that they raise low-density lipoprotein ("bad") cholesterol levels and lower high-density lipoprotein ("good") cholesterol levels. Similarly, trans fats should be limited in your diet.

Trans fats are found naturally in small amounts in animal products, but most are created commercially by adding hydrogen to liquid fats to make them more solid, a process known as hydrogenation. Fats are hydrogenated to increase shelf life and improve the taste and texture of foods. They are found most often in frozen foods, pastries, convenience snack foods (such as crackers, potato chips, French fries, and cookies), and in products containing hydrolyzed or partially hydrolyzed vegetable shortening.

Trans fat free

Trans fats have been shown to increase the risk of cardiovascular disease, and their consumption should be limited at all times, including during pregnancy. Food companies have made an effort to reduce the amount of trans fat in their foods, and many convenience foods boast "trans fat free"

Fat sources

Monounsaturated fats
Oils (olive, canola, peanut)
Non-hydrogenated margarine
Avocados
Nuts (almonds, cashews, pecans, pistachios, hazelnuts)
Polyunsaturated fats
Fish (salmon, trout, mackerel, sardines)
Oils (canola, safflower, sunflower, corn, soybean, sesame)
Non-hydrogenated margarine
Nuts and seeds (walnuts, almonds, pecans, sunflower seeds, flaxseed)
Eggs fortified with omega-3 fatty acid
Saturated fats
Fatty meats (cold cuts, dark poultry meat, poultry skin, fatty cuts of beef)
Full-fat milk products (homogenized and 2% milk, cheese, full-fat yogurt)
Butter and clarified butter (ghee), lard, hard margarine
Eggs
Oils (coconut, palm)
Trans fats
Found in many commercially prepared convenience foods (crackers, potato chips, baked goods such as cookies, cakes, muffins)
French fries
Partially hydrogenated oil or partially hydrogenated margarine
Vegetable shortening

on the packaging. Look on the label and choose foods with no trans fats, or look at the ingredient list and avoid foods containing hydrolyzed or partially hydrolyzed fats.

Healthy weight gain

No pregnant woman looks forward to gaining more weight than necessary during pregnancy, so let's talk about the numbers right away. A woman who is at a healthy weight at the onset of pregnancy is advised to gain between 25 to 35 pounds during 9 months.

Enough calories

Looking at it another way, growing a healthy baby takes more than 85,000 calories, in addition to the calories you need for your own energy requirements. If you gain about 1 pound per week during the second and third trimesters, it's a good sign that you are getting enough calories.

Of course, if you were underweight at the start of your pregnancy, your health-care provider may recommend that you gain 28 to 40 pounds, and, likewise, if you were overweight before pregnancy, you may be advised to gain only 15 to 25 pounds.

Average weight gain distribution in pregnancy

Source	30 lbs (13.7 kg)
Fetus	7.5 lbs (3.4 kg)
Maternal fat and protein stores	7.0 lbs (3.2 kg)
Retained water	4.0 lbs (1.8 kg)
Breasts	3.0 lbs (1.4 kg)
Increased blood volume	3.0 lbs (1.4 kg)
Uterus (womb)	2.0 lbs (0.9 kg)
Amniotic fluid	2.0 lbs (0.9 kg)
Placenta	1.5 lbs (0.7 kg)

While you may think you know which category you fit into already, it's best if you use the body mass index (BMI) scale to get an accurate picture.

Restriction and restraint

Whatever your BMI and weight gain numbers are, it's important not to restrict your weight gain by dieting or skipping meals. This could have serious effects on the development of the baby. But don't let yourself go either. It's okay to give in to the occasional craving for potato chips or candy bars, as long as you're making healthy choices about the nutrients you consume overall. But while you're at it, why not forgo that candy bar and snack on something sweet and also rich in vitamin C, like an orange or some berries?

Don't worry — with a little extra effort, you'll be able to fit into your regular clothes after your baby is born! Until then, pay careful attention not only to your caloric intake but also to the amounts of folic acid, zinc, protein, iron, and calcium you're getting from all sources (food as well as supplements).

Weight gain imbalance

Weight gained during pregnancy is made up of the weight of the baby, breast tissue, amniotic fluid, placenta, uterus, blood, maternal fat tissue, and other fluids. Not gaining enough weight can increase the risk of a baby being born prematurely or with low birth weight, which can lead to health issues. Gaining too much weight can lead to a high birth weight baby, making the delivery more difficult and also putting the baby's health at risk. It can also increase your risk of developing gestational diabetes.

Did You Know?

High BMI

Research suggests that women with a BMI greater than 35 who remain weight neutral throughout pregnancy are at no greater risk of premature birth or delivery of a low birth weight baby than those with a healthy weight and the recommended weight gain, and may in fact reduce their risk of gestational diabetes.

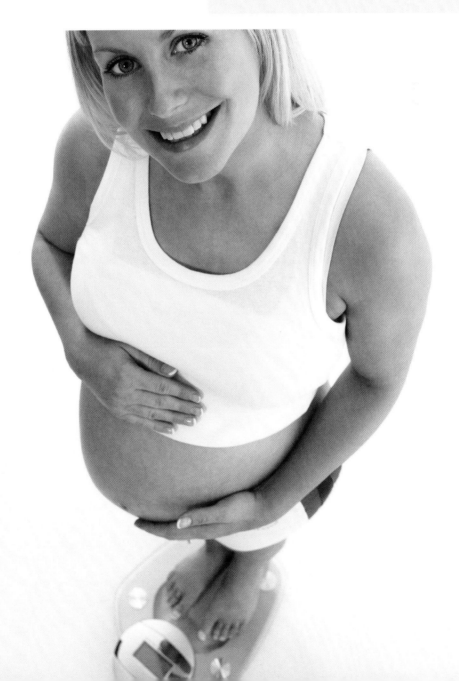

HOW TO...

Calculate and interpret BMI

In order to determine how much weight you should gain, you first need to know your pre-pregnancy body mass index (BMI). The BMI is a number based on your weight and height.

BMI calculation in imperial measure:

(Weight in pounds x 700) ÷ (Height in inches x Height in inches) = BMI
For example: (145 pounds x 700) ÷ (65 inches x 65 inches) = 24

BMI calculation in metric measure:

Weight in kilograms ÷ (Height in meters x Height in meters) = BMI
For example: 65.9 kilograms ÷ (1.65 meters x 1.65 meters) = 24

You may want to use your pregnancy diary to record these calculations. You can also use the BMI electronic calculator or the charts online at the National Center for Health Statistics (www.cdc.gov/nchs) or ask your health-care provider for help.

Interpreting BMI Categories

- **Healthy weight:** If your BMI prior to pregnancy was between 18.5 and 24.9, you are within the healthy weight range before pregnancy.
- **Underweight:** If your BMI was below 18.5, you are underweight.
- **Overweight:** If it was above 24.9, you are overweight.
- **Obesity:** If your BMI was above 30, you are considered to be obese.

Pregnancy weight gain recommendations

- **Healthy weight:** If your BMI is in the healthy range, gaining 25 to 35 lbs (11.5 to 16 kg) is recommended.
- **Underweight:** If your BMI is in the underweight category, gaining 28 to 40 lbs (12.5 to 18 kg) is suggested.
- **Overweight:** If your BMI is in the overweight category, gaining 15 to 25 lbs (7 to 11.5 kg) is recommended.
- **Obese:** If your BMI is in the obese category, gaining 11 to 20 lbs (5 to 9 kg) is recommended.
- In all BMI categories, gaining 2 to 8 lbs (1 to 3.5 kg) in the first trimester is suggested.
- For healthy-weight pregnancies, gaining 1 lb (0.4 kg) each week in the second and third trimester is recommended.

Micronutrient supplements

Micronutrients include vitamins, minerals, essential fatty acids, amino acids, and enzymes. They are required to fuel all metabolic pathways in the body to help produce energy. In addition, many vitamins and minerals have been identified as helping with disease prevention and cellular repair.

Key micronutrients

In pregnancy, some micronutrients are of key importance and, if consumed in the recommended amounts, can help in maintaining your weight and preventing diseases and disorders such as nausea and vomiting and gestational diabetes. If consumed in appropriate amounts, they can also help promote healthy fetal development, ensure an appropriately grown infant born at term, and aid in preventing childhood and adult obesity.

It is suggested that all pregnant women take a prenatal multivitamin supplement. The most important single supplements used during pregnancy are calcium, vitamin D, iron, folic acid, zinc, omega-3 fatty acid, and vitamin B_{12}. Vitamin A should be taken only under the supervision of your health-care providers. Work with them to develop a nutrient supplementation program that ensures your good health and your baby's.

Calcium

Calcium is needed to maintain your teeth and bones and is required for normal function of muscles, nerves, and heart.

In pregnancy, calcium is essential for the growth and development of the fetal skeleton. For calcium to be absorbed effectively, vitamin D and other minerals need to be consumed in adequate amounts. If calcium intake is deficient, your body will pull calcium from your bones, where it is stored, and your bones will gradually become weaker. Dietary sources of calcium include all dairy products, tofu, fish bones found in canned fish, and some vegetables, such as kale and broccoli.

- DRI for calcium in pregnancy is unchanged from pre-pregnancy at 1000 mg per day. Although the requirement for calcium is not increased in pregnancy, it is important that the DRI is met, because calcium is absolutely essential for normal fetal development.

- UL for calcium is 2500 mg per day. The body can only absorb up to 500 mg calcium at one time, so if you are taking supplements that contain 500 mg, be sure to do so in separate doses at different times of the day.

Calcium and vitamin D content of common foods

Food item (standard serving)	Calcium content (mg per serving) DRI: 1000 mg	Vitamin D content (IU per serving) DRI: 200 IU
1 cup (250 mL) calcium-fortified beverages (soy milk, orange juice)	320–370	86–100 (not all soy milks or fortified juices are vitamin D–fortified)
1 cup (250 mL) milk	300–325	100
1.75 oz (50 g) cheese	250–350	
¾ cup (175 g) yogurt	200–320	
2.5 oz (75 g) fish with bones (canned sardines, canned salmon with bones)	185–300	180–225
5 oz (150 g) tofu (if set with calcium sulfate; regular, firm, extra-firm)	234	
1 cup (250 mL) dark leafy vegetables (broccoli, kale, bok choy)	100–250	
¼ cup (50 mL) almonds	90–120	
½ cup (125 mL) cottage cheese	73	
1 orange	52	
6 medium scallops or oysters	40–90	
¼ cup (50 mL) hummus	20	
1 tbsp (15 mL) cod liver oil		1360
1 tbsp (15 mL) fortified margarine		60
¾–1 cup (175–250 mL) breakfast cereals		40 (depending on amount fortified)
1 egg yolk		20
3.5 oz (100 g) beef liver		15

Vitamin D

Vitamin D supports calcium in the prevention of osteoporosis in your body and, in pregnancy, also supports calcium in normal bone and skeleton formation in the fetus.

Vitamin D is a fat-soluble vitamin found in fortified milk, powdered and evaporated milk, fortified soy beverages, margarine, and fatty fish (salmon and trout). It is also made by your skin in large amounts after sunlight exposure. If you live in Canada or the northern United States (where sunlight is minimal in the winter months), it is especially important to obtain vitamin D through dietary or supplementary sources when sunlight is weak. Of course, if you use sunscreen, your body won't manufacture vitamin D during exposure to the sun regardless of the time of year.

- DRI for vitamin D is 200 IU per day. However, recent literature on the prevention of osteoporosis and cancer suggests that this value should in fact be much higher, closer to 2000 IU and perhaps even higher (even greater than the UL for vitamin D), per day for pregnant and lactating women.
- UL for vitamin D is 2000 mg per day and, like calcium, will typically only be reached with dietary supplements.

Iron

Iron is required for the maintenance of blood cells, for cell growth, and for carrying oxygen to body tissues. The majority of iron is found in the hemoglobin of red blood cells. In pregnancy, your iron requirements are almost doubled to support your expanded blood volume, which is needed for fetal tissue development and to compensate for blood loss during delivery. Good dietary sources of iron include meat and poultry, fortified cereals, legumes, and firm tofu.

- DRI for iron in pregnancy is 27 mg per day.
- UL for iron is 45 mg per day.

Iron absorption

Iron absorption is inhibited by calcium (including supplemental calcium and foods rich in calcium), phenolic compounds (found in tea and coffee), and oxalates (found in strawberries, tea, and rhubarb). Iron absorption is enhanced by vitamin C. Eat your iron-rich foods with a vitamin C source during meal times

Iron content of common foods

Food item (standard serving)	Iron content (mg per serving) DRI: 27 mg
Heme iron sources (better absorbed by the body)	
2.5 oz (75 g) meats (beef, chicken, pork, lamb, veal)	0.5–3.5
2.5 oz (75 g) fish (salmon, halibut, sardines)	0.3–1.9
2.5 oz (75 g) seafood (clams, shrimp)	0.3–2.3
1 egg	0.7
Non-heme iron sources	
¾ cup (175 g) legumes (white beans, soybeans, lentils, chickpeas, kidney beans)	1.7–6.5
5 oz (150 g) tofu	1.2–2.4
2 oz (60 g) dried fruit (apricots, raisins, prunes)	1.1–3.7
2 tbsp (60 mL) seeds or nuts (pumpkin, sesame, sunflower seeds; peanuts, walnuts, almonds, cashews)	0.5–5.2
¾ cup (30 g) breakfast cereals enriched with iron	0.5–8.0
1 slice bread, 1 pita bread	1.0–2.0
2 tbsp (25 mL) wheat germ	1.4
1 cup (250 mL) pasta, egg noodles	1.6–2.7

Did You Know?

Anemia risk

Women who are unable to meet their iron needs from dietary sources should speak with their health-care provider about supplemental iron. Some organizations suggest routine iron supplements during pregnancy. If iron intakes are low, the risk of anemia is increased. Anemia during pregnancy can increase the risk of premature birth and low birth weight infants.

and consume your calcium-rich foods during snack time. If taking single supplements, separate your doses of iron and calcium.

Folate

In its dietary form, this B vitamin it is called folate, but in supplemental or fortified form it is known as folic acid. During pregnancy, folate is a key nutrient for both you and fetus. For you, it helps prevent anemia by supporting increases in your blood volume, helps with normal placenta development, and helps support growing maternal tissue. For the fetus, it is crucial in the normal rapid growth and development of all fetal cells, can help ensure the fetus is an appropriate size at birth, and can help prevent neural tube defects. Neural tube defects (spina bifida and anencephaly) can result if there are not adequate amounts of folate in the

Folate content of common foods

Food item (standard serving)	Folate or folic acid (mcg per serving) DRI: 600 mcg
½ cup (125 mL) cooked spinach or asparagus	140
1 cup (250 mL) dark leafy lettuce	60–80
½ cup (125 mL) orange juice	25–60
¼ cup (50 mL) sunflower seeds	77
½ cup (125 mL) cooked broccoli, Brussels sprouts, beets, green beans, corn, carrots, sweet potato, snow peas, turnip, or cabbage	10–90
½ avocado	80
1 serving (1 medium or ½ cup/125 mL) fruit: orange, raspberries, blueberries, strawberries, cantaloupe, honeydew melon, banana, grapefruit	1–40
¾ cup (175 g) cooked legumes (lentils, chickpeas, kidney beans)	70–265
¼ cup (50 mL) nuts (cashews, walnuts, peanuts)	3–40
1 tbsp (15 mL) wheat germ	25
1 slice whole wheat or white bread	45–60
¾ cup (175 mL) breakfast cereal	15–75
1 cup (250 mL) milk	13
1 egg yolk	30

first 4 to 6 weeks of pregnancy, before the neural tube closes. For more information on neural tube defects and folic acid, see Part 1, Planning Your Pregnancy (page 48).

Fortification

Good sources of folate include organ meats, wheat germ, fruit, and vegetables. However, it is difficult to obtain the DRI of 0.6 mg in pregnancy from food alone, which is why it is recommended that women in their childbearing years take a supplement of folic acid prior to becoming pregnant and throughout pregnancy. In Canada, white flour and pasta are fortified with folic acid to help meet requirements.

- DRI for folate during pregnancy is 0.6 mg (600 mcg) per day total (from food and supplemental form), but we recommend 1 mg per day. This is higher than for non-pregnant women. Most multivitamins and prenatal vitamins will contain 0.4 mg folic acid or more. Some groups of women require additional folate: those with a family history or previous history of neural tube defects, women with Type 1 diabetes, or women taking anti-epileptic drugs should speak with their physician prior to pregnancy and may be advised to take as much as 5.0 g (5000 mcg) of folic acid.
- UL for folate is 1.0 mg (1000 mcg), unless otherwise stated for specific populations.

Zinc

Adequate zinc is extremely important during the first trimester, when organs are being formed. Red meat is the best source of zinc, but that presents a problem for vegetarians. In that case, make sure you take a daily

> ### Did You Know?
> #### Zinc absorption
> Iron intake helps with zinc absorption. If supplements of iron are consumed in amounts greater than 30 mg per day, ensure that the supplement you are consuming also contains 15 mg of zinc, or consider speaking with your physician about adding a zinc supplement.

supplement that includes 15 mg of zinc throughout your pregnancy or ensure that your prenatal multivitamin contains 15 mg of zinc. Because it is important in the first trimester, you may want to start taking zinc before you become pregnant.

- DRI for zinc is 11 mg per day.
- UL for zinc is 40 mg per day.

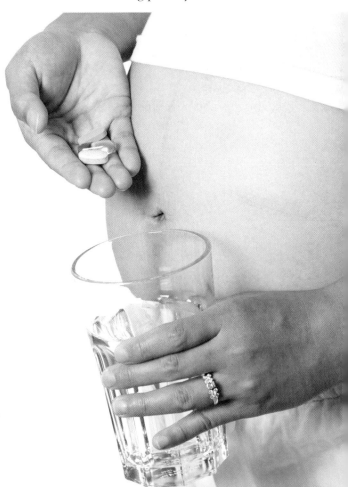

Essential fatty acids

Essential fatty acids (EFAs) must be consumed in food because your body cannot manufacture them. That is why they are called "essential." They are needed for many processes in the body and can promote health by reducing the risk of heart disease and inflammatory diseases, such as arthritis. The two most common types of EFAs are omega 3 (also known as linolenic acid) and omega 6 (also known as linoleic acid). Omega-3 fatty acid is converted to docosahexaenoic acid (DHA) and eicosapentaenoic acid (EPA) during metabolism. Omega-6 fatty acid is converted to arachidonic acid (AA).

Supplement risks

Essential fatty acids supplements are recommended during breastfeeding but not during pregnancy. They have not been adequately tested for their dose-related safety. Taking too much omega-3 fatty acid could have harmful effects on fetal growth and development of bone mass, for example. Another concern is that many omega-3 supplements are derived from fish sources, and high levels of

heavy metals may be a problem. Because the known benefits for the fetus of omega-3 fatty acid during pregnancy have only been studied from omega-3 EFA obtained from food sources, it is recommended that you obtain omega-3 fatty acid from food.

Did You Know?

Essential in pregnancy and infancy

Both DHA and AA are essential for the development of the central nervous system and visual function of the fetus. The fetus obtains omega-3 fatty acid from the maternal diet through the placenta during pregnancy and from the mother's milk during breastfeeding. Women eating diets rich in omega-3 fatty acid will have higher levels of omega-3 fatty acid to pass along to the fetus.

In addition, infants appear to be unable to convert omega-3 fatty acid to DHA in adequate amounts after birth. Your baby will rely on DHA in your breast milk or in commercially prepared infant formulas. The amount of DHA present in your breast milk is directly proportional to the amount you consume.

Omega-3 fatty acid content of common foods

Food item (standard serving)	Omega-3 fatty acid content (g per serving) DRI: 1.4 g
2.5 oz (75 g) fatty fish (salmon, trout, tuna)	0.2–1.4
1 oz (30 g) flaxseed	1.8
1 tbsp (15 mL) flaxseed oil	6.9
1 tbsp (15 mL) canola oil, soy oil	0.9–1.3
1 oz (30 g) walnuts	2.6
1 oz (30 g) other nuts	0.1–0.3

Vitamin B_{12} content of common foods

Food item (standard serving)	Vitamin B_{12} content (mcg per serving) DRI: 2.6 mcg
2.5 oz (75 g) organ meat (liver)	200–420
2.5 oz (75 g) fish and seafood (salmon, trout, crab, sardines, clams)	0.3–74.0
1 egg	0.65
1 cup (250 mL) milk	0.90–1.20
1.75 oz (50 g) cheese (hard)	0.42–1.67
$3/4$ cup (175 mL) yogurt	0.30–1.0
1 cup (250 mL) soy milk (enriched)	1.80–2.85
2.5 oz (75 g) beef	2.0
$1/2$ chicken breast	0.3
$3/4$ cup (175 mL) cereal fortified with vitamin B_{12}	6.0

Foods that contain omega-3 fatty acid include fatty fish (salmon and trout), canola and soy oils, flaxseed and flaxseed oils, walnuts, and eggs or dairy products fortified with omega-3 EFAs. Foods that contain omega-6 fatty acid include meats, egg yolks, and some oils (corn, sunflower, safflower, and peanut oil).

- DRI during pregnancy is 1.4 g per day (0.6% to 1.2% total calories) for omega-3 fatty acid and 13 g per day for omega-6 fatty acid (5% to 10% total calories).

Vitamin B_{12}

Vitamin B_{12} is a water-soluble vitamin found only in animal products, although some non-animal products, such as cereals, are fortified with vitamin B_{12}. It is needed for normal function of the central nervous system and to maintain healthy red blood cells and body tissues. Women with diets low in vitamin B_{12}, such as vegetarians and vegans, and women lacking an intrinsic factor needed for vitamin B_{12} absorption can be at risk of pernicious anemia. Infants are at risk of compromised growth and development if vitamin B_{12} is deficient.

- DRI for vitamin B_{12} is 2.6 mcg per day.
- UL for vitamin B_{12} has not been determined.

Did You Know?

Vitamin B_{12} deficiency signs

If you suffer from nausea and vomiting during the first trimester and have an aversion to animal food, you may have a vitamin B_{12} deficiency. If you suspect your diet is lacking in vitamin B_{12}, speak with your health-care provider and ask to have your blood levels checked. Folic acid consumed in amounts greater than the established UL (1.0 mg, or 1000 mcg, per day) may mask a vitamin B_{12} deficiency in the blood test.

Vitamin A

Vitamin A is a fat-soluble vitamin that aids in the visual function and development of the fetus. However, if consumed in excess amounts, it can be teratogenic (harmful to the fetus), especially if it is consumed in excess during the first trimester. As a fat-soluble vitamin, excess vitamin A is stored in your body, whereas excess amounts of water-soluble vitamins are lost in the urine each day.

Vitamin A consumed from foods is rarely a concern because most foods rich in vitamin A contain amounts well below the UL. The one exception is bovine and porcine liver, which contain stored amounts of vitamin A. During pregnancy, eating liver should be avoided or limited. Be sure to read the label of all supplements you are taking, and if you are taking more than one supplement, add up the amount of vitamin A in all tablets consumed to ensure the total amount is below 10,000 IU per day.

- DRI for vitamin A is 2300 IU (700 mcg) per day.
- UL for vitamin A is set at 10,000 IU (3000 mcg) per day.

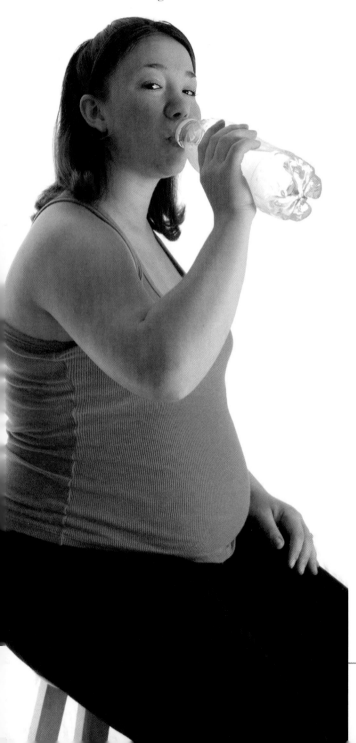

Fluids

In pregnancy, it is very important that you stay well hydrated to support the expansion of blood volume and the growth of both your tissues and fetal tissues. The recommended daily fluid intake is 12 cups (3 L). Fluids include all non-caffeinated beverages and foods with fluids, such as soup. If you enjoy hot beverages, try non-caffeinated teas, hot chocolate made with milk, or hot water with lemon. If you find it difficult to drink 12 cups of fluid each day, try making meals with liquids and keep a glass of your favorite beverage next to you.

- DRI for fluids in pregnancy is 12 cups (3 L) per day.

Food guides

One of the best ways to ensure you are eating a healthy, balanced diet with the appropriate portions (serving sizes) is to follow the nutritional advice in the United States Department of Agriculture (USDA) MyPyramid guidelines or in Canada's Food Guide to Healthy Eating. Planning meals based on these guides will ensure that you meet your growing energy requirements during pregnancy, gain weight appropriately, and receive adequate amounts of key macronutrients and micronutrients. There is also an added benefit — lifelong eating according to these guides helps reduce your risk of chronic diseases, such as diabetes, obesity, heart disease, osteoporosis, and some cancers.

Food groups

MyPyramid divides food into five groups — grains, vegetables, fruits, milk, and meat and beans — while Canada's Food Guide identifies four groups — vegetables and fruit, grain products, milk and alternatives, and meat and alternatives. The recommendations for the number of servings to consume daily from each food group are categorized by gender and age. Recommendations are also given for food group choices and serving sizes during pregnancy and lactation.

Nutrient distribution

Nutrients are distributed differently among the food groups, making it important to eat a varied yet balanced diet.

- Vegetable and fruit group contains fiber, folate, vitamin C, vitamin A, antioxidants
- Grain products group contains carbohydrates, thiamin, riboflavin, niacin, iron (found in fortified grains in Canada), folic acid (found in fortified grains in Canada), and fiber in whole grains

- Milk products and alternatives contain protein, vitamin B_{12}, vitamin D, and calcium
- Meat and alternatives contain protein, iron, zinc, vitamin B_{12}, and essential fatty acids

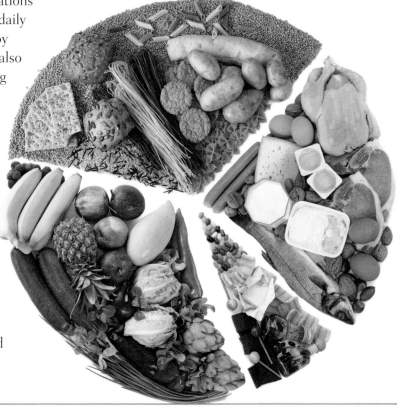

Recommended Number of *Food Guide Servings* per Day

	Children			Teens		Adults			
Age in Years	2-3	4-8	9-13	14-18		19-50		51+	
Sex	Girls and Boys			Females	Males	Females	Males	Females	Males
Vegetables and Fruit	4	5	6	7	8	7-8	8-10	7	7
Grain Products	3	4	6	6	7	6-7	8	6	7
Milk and Alternatives	2	2	3-4	3-4	3-4	2	2	3	3
Meat and Alternatives	1	1	1-2	2	3	2	3	2	3

What is One Food Guide Serving?
Look at the examples below.

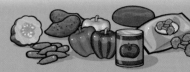

Fresh, frozen or canned vegetables
125 mL (½ cup)

Bread
1 slice (35 g)

Bagel
½ bagel (45 g)

Milk or powdered milk (reconstituted)
250 mL (1 cup)

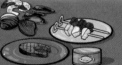

Cooked fish, shellfish, poultry, lean meat
75 g (2 ½ oz.)/125 mL (½ cup)

The chart above shows how many Food Guide Servings you need from each of the four food groups every day.

Having the amount and type of food recommended and following the tips in *Canada's Food Guide* will help:

• Meet your needs for vitamins, minerals and other nutrients.
• Reduce your risk of obesity, type 2 diabetes, heart disease, certain types of cancer and osteoporosis.
• Contribute to your overall health and vitality.

For the full guide, please contact Health Canada or visit their website.

Source: Health Canada. Used with permission.

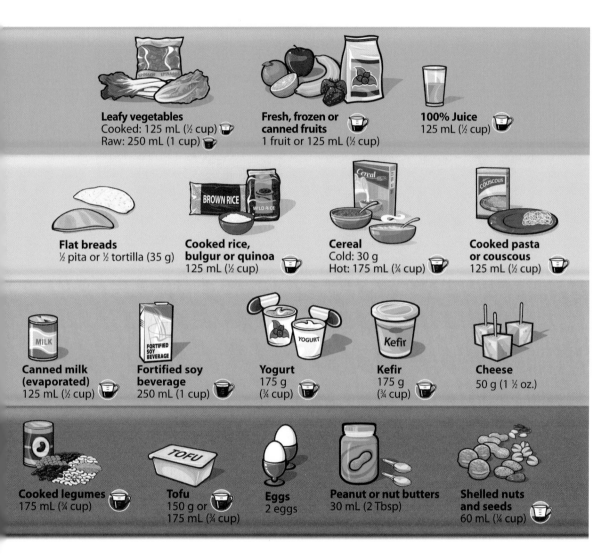

Serving size

When following the food guides, pay attention to both the recommended number of daily servings and the recommended serving size. When serving a portion of these foods, use the following rules of thumb:

- 2 servings of grain products equals 1 cup (250 mL) of rice or pasta, which is about the size of an adult fist

- 1 serving of meat and alternatives equals a chicken breast that is about the size of the palm of your hand, a deck of cards, or a computer mouse

- 1 serving of fruit equals an apple that is about the size of a tennis ball

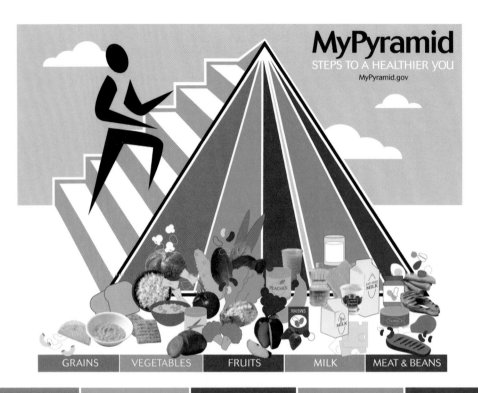

MyPyramid
STEPS TO A HEALTHIER YOU
MyPyramid.gov

GRAINS	VEGETABLES	FRUITS	MILK	MEAT & BEANS

GRAINS	VEGETABLES	FRUITS	MILK	MEAT & BEANS
Make half your grains whole	Vary your veggies	Focus on fruits	Get your calcium-rich foods	Go lean with protein
Eat at least 3 oz. of whole-grain cereals, breads, crackers, rice, or pasta every day 1 oz. is about 1 slice of bread, about 1 cup of breakfast cereal, or ¹/₂ cup of cooked rice, cereal, or pasta	Eat more dark-green veggies like broccoli, spinach, and other dark leafy greens Eat more orange vegetables like carrots and sweetpotatoes Eat more dry beans and peas like pinto beans, kidney beans, and lentils	Eat a variety of fruit Choose fresh, frozen, canned, or dried fruit Go easy on fruit juices	Go low-fat or fat-free when you choose milk, yogurt, and other milk products If you don't or can't consume milk, choose lactose-free products or other calcium sources such as fortified foods and beverages	Choose low-fat or lean meats and poultry Bake it, broil it, or grill it Vary your protein routine — choose more fish, beans, peas, nuts, and seeds

For a 2,000-calorie diet, you need the amounts below from each food group. To find the amounts that are right for you, go to MyPyramid.gov.

Eat 6 oz. every day	Eat 2¹/₂ cups every day	Eat 2 cups every day	Get 3 cups every day; for kids aged 2 to 8, it's 2	Eat 5¹/₂ oz. every day

Find your balance between food and physical activity
- Be sure to stay within your daily calorie needs.
- Be physically active for at least 30 minutes most days of the week.
- About 60 minutes a day of physical activity may be needed to prevent weight gain.
- For sustaining weight loss, at least 60 to 90 minutes a day of physical activity may be required.
- Children and teenagers should be physically active for 60 minutes every day, or most days.

Know the limits on fats, sugars, and salt (sodium)
- Make most of your fat sources from fish, nuts, and vegetable oils.
- Limit solid fats like butter, stick margarine, shortening, and lard, as well as foods that contain these.
- Check the Nutrition Facts label to keep saturated fats, *trans* fats, and sodium low.
- Choose food and beverages low in added sugars. Added sugars contribute calories with few, if any, nutrients.

MyPyramid.gov
STEPS TO A HEALTHIER YOU

U.S. Department of Agriculture
Center for Nutrition Policy and Promotion
April 2005
CNPP-15

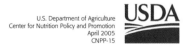

Diets for adolescents in pregnancy

Adolescents need to pay special attention to their nutrition during pregnancy because they require additional energy and protein for their own continuing growth and for the development of the pregnancy. Adolescents who become pregnant within 2 to 3 years after their first menstruation are at especially high risk of compromising their growth potential.

Adolescent requirements

Calcium requirements are higher for adolescents who are pregnant. The DRI is 1300 mg per day, rather than 1000 mg for adult pregnancies. Weight gain should be at the higher end of the range to promote the growth of the adolescent and help reduce the risk of low birth weight infants, which is 6.5% in an adolescent population versus 5.7% in a non-adolescent population.

Did You Know?

Vegetarian diets

Vegetarian diets can be maintained throughout pregnancy, but women following restrictive vegetarian diets may have to consume additional vitamin and mineral supplements. The nutrients that are most insufficient in some vegetarian diets are protein, iron, zinc, vitamin B_{12}, calcium, vitamin D, and omega-3 fatty acid. Ask your health-care provider to set up a consultation with a dietitian to ensure all nutrient requirements are being met and assess whether additional supplements are warranted. Besides dietary intake analysis, nutrient levels can be measured by blood test as another way to determine your nutrient status.

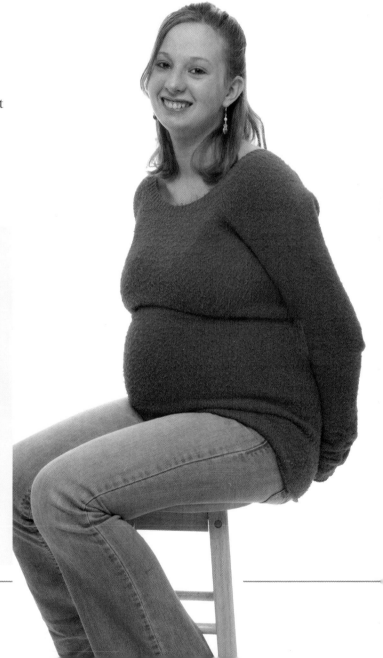

Diets for mothers of multiples

Women pregnant with multiple fetuses (twins, triplets, and more) need to be especially conscientious about their nutritional status throughout their pregnancy. They have a higher risk of low birth weight babies, preterm birth, gestational diabetes mellitus, and anemia. It is important to maintain good nutritional status and adequate amounts of weight gain, especially at the beginning of pregnancy (due to the risk of preterm delivery).

Multiples diets

Diet suggestions for multiples are based on observational data or data extrapolated from singleton pregnancies. There are no set DRIs for multiple births.

Micronutrient needs

Because the risk of anemia is higher with multiple births, a separate iron supplement may be suggested. Iron needs for multiples increase to 30 mg from supplemental sources. Otherwise, mothers of multiples do not need to consume additional supplemental micronutrients. Taking more than one prenatal supplement each day is not recommended unless advised by your health-care practitioner.

Guide to...
Extra energy needs for multiples

The Institute of Medicine recommends that women with more than one fetus consume higher amounts of calories to support fetal growth and development:

- Calorie needs for multiples: an additional 150 calories per fetus (450 additional calories per day above pre-pregnancy intake).

- Weight gain recommendations for twins: 35 to 45 lbs (16 to 21 kg) total weight gain, with 1.5 lbs (0.7 kg) per week in the second and third trimesters.

- Weight gain recommendations for triplets: 50 lbs (23 kg) total weight gain.

- Women who are overweight and obese should gain at the lower end of the range, and women who are underweight prior to pregnancy should gain weight at the upper end of the recommended range.

- Women may find it difficult to consume all the calories required to gain the suggested amount of weight and, if so, should focus on eating only nutrient-dense foods and add three snacks a day to ensure that all of the required nutrients are consumed.

- There is no evidence that taking more than one prenatal supplement can benefit multiple births and, in fact, there may be a risk in doing so as some vitamins (such as vitamin A) are teratogenic in high doses.

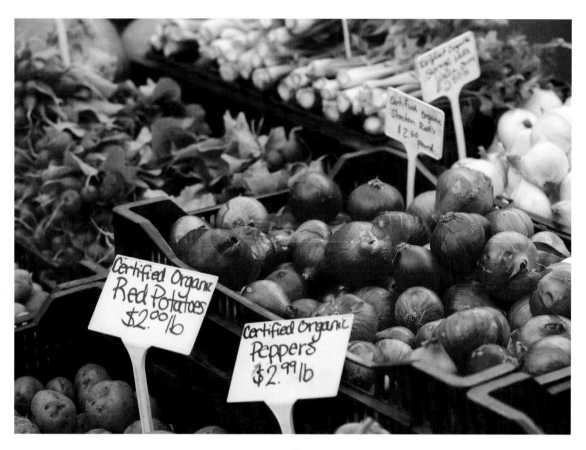

Organic foods

Organic foods are becoming more popular as health concerns about additives, pesticides, antibiotics, and growth hormones used in food production are increasing. Organic foods are grown without conventional fertilizers, pesticides, antibiotics, and hormones and are processed without food additives. It makes sense to eat organic foods for the safety of the mother and fetus, but organic foods may be deficient in key nutrients.

Nutrient adequacy

In pregnancy, we rely heavily on the fortification of certain foods to obtain adequate amounts of key nutrients, so be careful to read the label of organic foods to ensure that they contain these key nutrients in adequate amounts. For example, not all organic milk will be fortified with vitamin D or vitamin A in the same amounts as conventional milk, and not all organic white flours will be fortified with folic acid and iron at the same levels as conventional foods. In addition, organic foods have not been tightly regulated, so you cannot be certain that a food labeled as organic truly follows organic farming processes.

Food allergies and avoidance

While you are pregnant, you may have food allergies to cow's milk products, gluten-containing grain products, corn and soy foods, eggs, shellfish, or peanuts. Although these allergies will not necessarily be passed on to your child before birth or make your child susceptible to the same allergies later in life, we do know that a child's risk of allergy is increased if a member of the immediate family has an allergy to any food or suffers from asthma. If you must avoid certain foods, work with a dietitian to ensure that you do not compromise healthy weight gain and deplete micronutrients.

Food additives

Processed foods often have ingredients added to enhance their color, flavor, or texture and to improve their shelf life. These additives and preservatives may not necessarily affect you or the fetus, but to be sure, avoid or limit them in your diet.

Nitrites

Nitrites are used as food preservatives and color enhancers in a variety of foods, including cured meats and fish, some baked goods, and some vegetables (preserved beets, corn, and spinach). There are concerns about

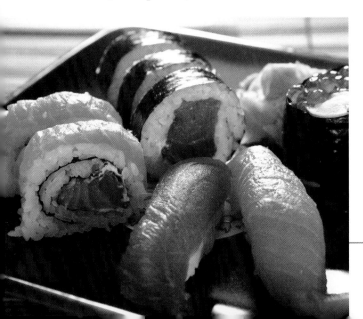

nitrites increasing the risk of certain cancers if consumed in large amounts. However, there are few data to make any recommendations about nitrite consumption during pregnancy, and at this time it is suggested to consume these foods in moderation.

Monosodium glutamate

Monosodium glutamate (MSG) is a sodium (salt) derivative used as a flavor enhancer. As with nitrites, there are health concerns with MSG, but MSG does not seem to cross the placenta, so there are no recommendations to avoid MSG specifically during pregnancy. If you have high blood pressure, you may want to consider limiting foods containing MSG because the sodium content is very high.

Foods to avoid or limit

- Unpasteurized cheeses (listeria)
- Deli meats (toxoplasmosa gondii)
- Raw fish (parasites)
- Big fish (mercury)

For more information on food-borne toxins, see Part 13, Managing Medical and Environmental Risks (page 453).

Food preparation safety

To prevent food poisoning and the possible transmission of toxic substances across the placenta, be sure to prepare your food safely and to the highest hygiene standards. If in doubt, throw out any possibly contaminated food.

HOW TO...

Prevent food-borne illnesses

1. Always wash your hands and all cooking utensils, including cutting boards, with hot soapy water before and after preparing foods.
2. Use separate utensils and cutting boards for raw and cooked meats. Use separate utensils and cutting boards for other foods, such as breads, fruits, and vegetables.
3. Do not eat food that has been out of the refrigerator for more than 2 hours.
4. Keep all hot foods hot (140°F/60°C) and cold foods cold (40°F/4°C).
5. Keep meats in the coldest part of the refrigerator.
6. When defrosting foods, do so in the refrigerator (not on the counter), and cook them as soon as they have defrosted.
7. Do not reheat or refreeze foods that have been cooked from frozen.
8. Consume pasteurized foods and beverages rather than unpasteurized options.
9. Do not eat raw meats or fish, including sushi, sashimi, oysters, or clams.
10. Cook fish until it easily flakes with a fork.
11. Avoid raw eggs, including those in baking batter, dressings, sauces, and beverages.
12. Cook all egg whites and yolks until firm.
13. Wash all fruit and vegetables before eating them.

Recommended safe minimum internal cooking temperatures

Follow these guidelines to make sure that meats are well cooked. A meat thermometer can help ensure that the internal temperature of the meat has reached a safe temperature.

Beef steaks and roasts	145°F (63°C)
Fish	145°F (63°C)
Pork	160°F (71°C)
Ground beef	160°F (71°C)
Egg dishes	160°F (71°C)
Chicken breasts	165°F (74°C)
Whole poultry	165°F (74°C)

F.A.Q.

We answer many questions from pregnant women and their partners. Here are some of the most frequently asked questions. Be sure to ask your health-care providers any other questions that may arise. If they don't have the answers, they will refer you to a colleague who does.

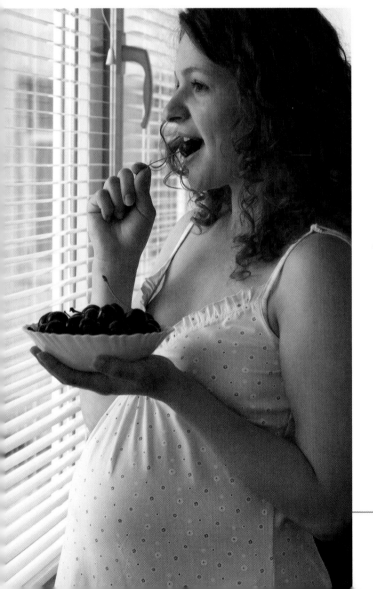

Q: Do I really need to take prenatal vitamin supplements if I'm eating a balanced diet?

A: As with most things, it depends. If you are already careful about nutrition and eat a balanced diet, you're probably getting all the nutrients you and your baby need. But most women — particularly those with dietary restrictions or food intolerances — can benefit from taking a prenatal vitamin and mineral supplement. Besides, prenatal supplements offer vitamins and minerals that you can't always absorb in adequate amounts from food, for example two of the crucial nutrients pregnant women require — folic acid and iron. Just as important as taking a supplement is finding one that includes no more than the recommended amounts of nutrients like vitamin A, which can be harmful to you and the fetus if you take too much.

Q: Why do I crave some foods that I never liked before and avoid others I used to like?

A: Many women say that they knew they were pregnant when they started to crave strange foods or could no longer eat their favorites. Foods craved typically include salty carbohydrates, such as potato chips, and pickles, while food aversions typically include foods with a strong odor and foods from the meat and alternatives food group.

There is no harm in giving in to your cravings or aversions, as long as you are not consuming so much or so little of these foods that it contributes to excessive weight gain or loss, or that because of consuming a large amount of the foods, you are not hungry for other food groups. Research suggests that the cravings may result from nutrient deficiencies.

Q: *What is pica? Is it dangerous for the fetus?*

A: Pica is the craving of non-food substances, and it tends to occur most often in pregnancy. The most commonly craved non-foods during pregnancy include dirt, clay, soap, chalk, and paint chips. It is thought that the cravings are a result of a nutrient deficiency (for example, iron, calcium, or magnesium), but this has not been determined by research.

In some cultures, this practice is accepted. However, consuming non-food substances may have an impact on fetal growth. Some substances may cause maternal gastrointestinal illnesses (constipation or bowel obstruction), breakdown of tooth enamel, or poisoning, as seen in consumption of lead found in paint. Speak with your health-care provider to ensure that your cravings are safe and that you are not nutrient deficient. Also be mindful that the consumption of certain non-food substances is not displacing nutritious foods.

Q: *Should I stop eating peanuts during my pregnancy?*

A: Avoiding peanuts and peanut products during pregnancy is not thought to reduce the risk of your child being allergic to this food. The decision is yours. On the one hand, peanuts and peanut butter are rich sources of protein and iron, making them a good snack choice during pregnancy and lactation. On the other hand, peanuts are not an essential food group and can be avoided without jeopardizing your health or the fetus in any way. However, other foods that may cause allergies, such as eggs, milk, or wheat products, belong to essential food groups. Don't compromise your own nutritional status by avoiding these foods when there is no proven benefit to you or your child.

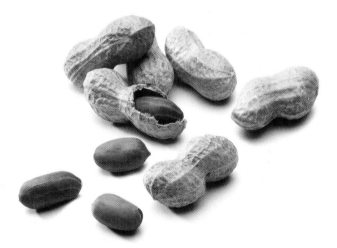

What's next

Get ready to be punched and kicked as the arms and legs of the fetus develop — one of many physical thrills in the course of your pregnancy!

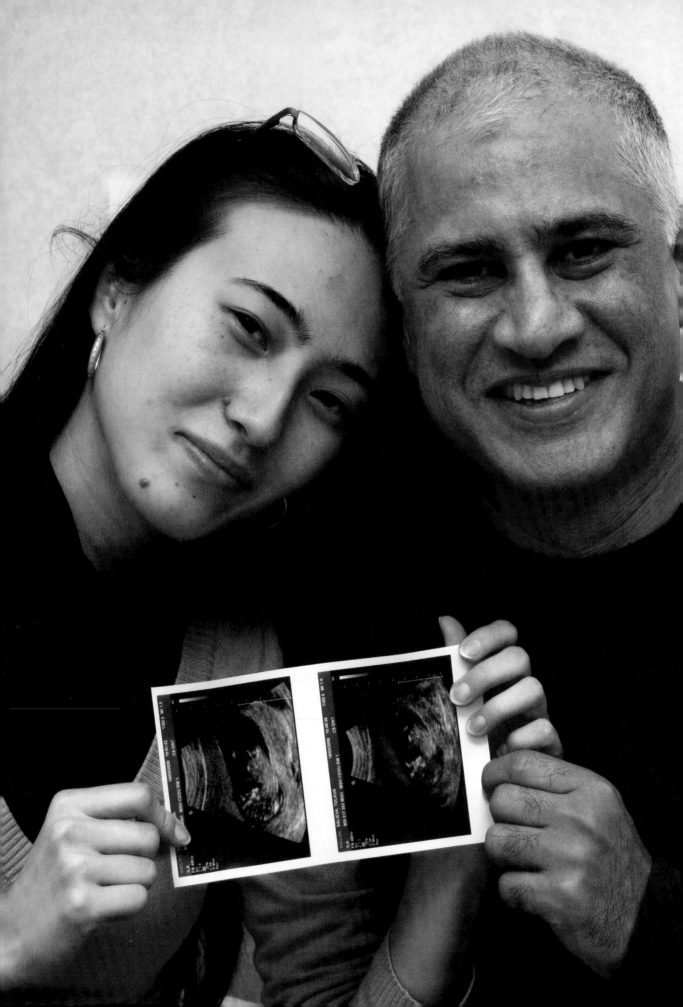

Part 4

First Trimester Progress

Month 2 to 3 (Week 4 to 12)

Dividing your time... and your cells

For the 9 months of your pregnancy, your attention is going to be focused on 3-month periods known as trimesters. By convention, your pregnancy is dated from the first day of your last period, but conception takes place after this, generally at week 2, and you probably won't even know you are pregnant until the end of week 4, when you miss your next period. The first trimester occurs between month 0 and 3 (weeks 0 and 12), but, for you, the first trimester really only lasts for 8 weeks, between weeks 4 and 12!

Early activity

But a lot is going on in those early weeks. The cells of the embryo are dividing, growing, and changing into a fetus, developing all the body parts that will be present in your baby. By the end of the first trimester, all the essential organs are formed — they just need to grow and develop further during the next 32 weeks!

In the first 10 weeks of gestation, a fetus develops from a single fertilized egg into a ball of cells, then into a tadpole-like embryo, and finally into a fully formed fetus that is more than 3 inches (8 cm) long, with arms that wave and legs that kick.

Ten tips for a healthy first trimester

1. Keep on taking your prenatal vitamins.
2. Still no alcohol.
3. Stick to your diet for healthy weight gain.
4. Explore ways to manage morning sickness and other physical aggravations.
5. Take care of yourself... okay, go ahead and spoil yourself with some new clothes, a facial, and a manicure.
6. Don't let your sex life lag. Try some new positions that don't cause discomfort.
7. Don't douche — ever!
8. Evaluate your need for genetic screening and testing.
9. Take a trip. It may be your last solo adventure for a long time.
10. Enjoy the excitement of a new pregnancy!

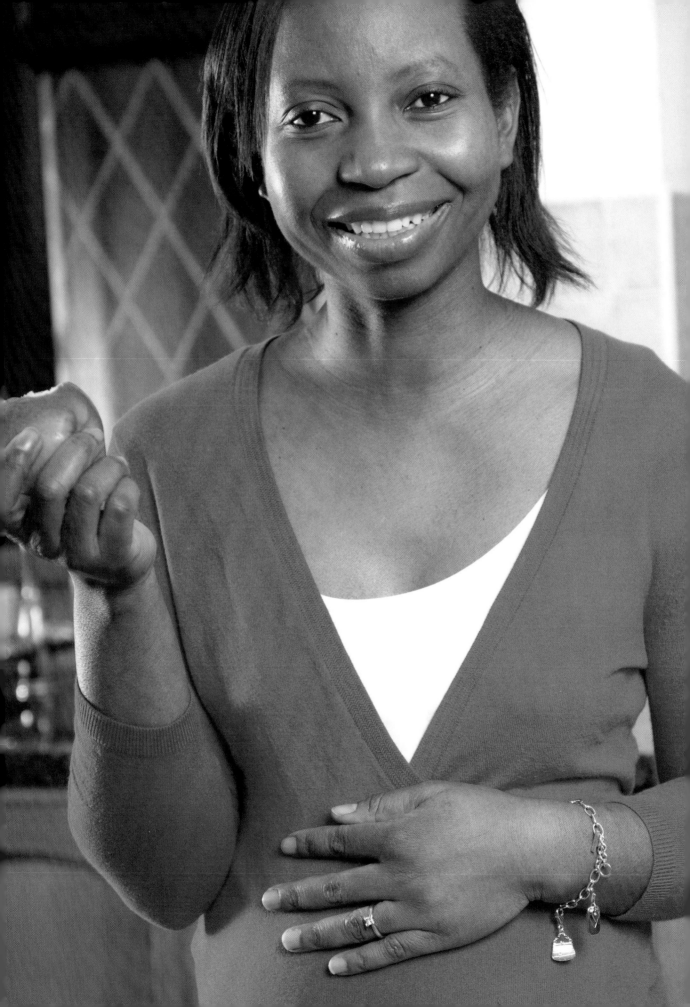

Fetal growth and development

Due to the peculiarities of pregnancy dating, by the time you miss your period and realize you are pregnant, you are already 4 weeks along in your pregnancy, but the embryo is only 2 weeks old. An enormous amount of growth is already underway, with significant development milestones passed every week.

Pregnancy milestones

At week 4

Cells that will grow to become the embryo have begun to separate from the developing placental tissue, which is implanting itself in the wall of the uterus.

At week 5

Organ systems are beginning to differentiate and organize themselves into primitive nerve tissue, gut tissue, and heart tissue.

At week 6

- The embryo elongates to $\frac{1}{8}$ inch (3 mm) and curves into a C-shape.
- The heart starts to form and even to beat.
- Arm buds become visible, and a tail begins to form.
- Internal organs (liver, pancreas, gallbladder, and spleen) begin to develop.
- The bowels become distinct from the urinary tract.

Embryo at 6 Weeks

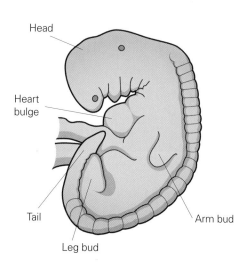

Head

Heart bulge

Tail

Leg bud

Arm bud

Embryo at 8 Weeks

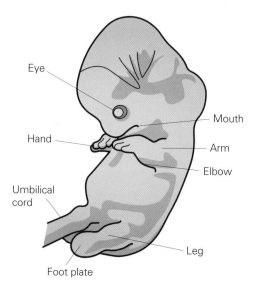

Eye

Hand

Umbilical cord

Foot plate

Mouth

Arm

Elbow

Leg

At week 7

- The embryo is now ¼ inch (0.5 cm) in length.
- The brain is developing.
- The eyes and nose begin to develop.
- Leg buds appear.
- The hands begin to differentiate from the arms.
- A primitive form of blood begins to circulate.

At week 8

- The embryo is ½ inch (1 cm) long.
- Lungs begin to form.
- Hands and feet have digits but are still webbed.
- The gonads begin to develop.

At week 9

- The embryo is ¾ inch (2 cm) long.
- Nipples and hair follicles are developing.
- All essential organs have begun to form.
- On ultrasound scans, the embryo can be seen to move.

At week 10

- The embryo is now called a fetus. The fetus is 1.2 inches (3 cm) in length.
- The face continues to develop, including eyelids and ears.

At week 11

- The fetus is 2 inches (5 cm) long.
- Tooth buds develop.
- Limbs are long and thin.
- The eyelids close.

At week 12

- The fetus is 3.2 inches (8 cm) long.
- The head is half the size of the entire fetus.
- The face is well formed.
- Blood cells are produced in the fetal liver.
- The genitals are formed.

Embryo at 10 Weeks

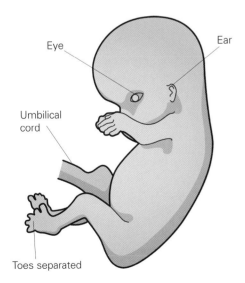

Eye

Ear

Umbilical cord

Toes separated

Embryo at 12 Weeks

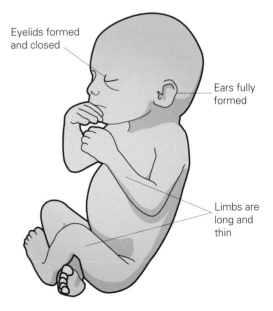

Eyelids formed and closed

Ears fully formed

Limbs are long and thin

Looking and feeling pregnant

During the first trimester, your body and emotions are going through their own changes to enable you to carry your baby safely to term. Some of these physical and emotional changes can be a bit disconcerting, but if you know what's going on, you can take them in stride.

Nausea and vomiting in pregnancy

Approximately 80% of pregnant women will experience at least some nausea and vomiting, commonly called morning sickness. For most women, it begins around 6 weeks after the last period and begins to subside by the end of the first trimester, but for an unlucky few it persists longer, sometimes right until delivery.

Causes and cures

Medical researchers don't know for sure what causes this nausea, but they suspect it may be related to high levels of the pregnancy hormone (ßHCG), estrogen, or progesterone. This may be why nausea can be worse with a twin pregnancy – the hormone levels are usually higher. Progesterone can slow down the way your stomach moves and processes food, making nausea worse. The bacterium *Helicobacter pylori*, which can cause stomach ulcers, may be involved in some cases. There are some other less common causes of vomiting in pregnancy, so make sure you talk to your doctor or midwife about your symptoms, especially if they do not seem typical or if there are any other symptoms (such as pain, diarrhea, jaundice, and headaches).

There is no shortage of home remedies for nausea and vomiting. Some are effective, some not. Attend to your eating habits, try ginger and acupressure, and if the condition persists or worsens, see your health-care providers, who can prescribe effective and safe medications.

Ginger

Ginger is an old remedy that has been shown to be effective in some clinical studies. You can take ginger in the form of teas,

Did You Know?

Beginning to show

During the first trimester, you may begin to "show" as your uterus grows to accommodate the growing fetus. Your uterus will grow from the size of your fist at conception to the size of a large grapefruit by 12 weeks. It will change from an organ contained wholly within your pelvis to one you can feel just above your pubic bone. By 12 weeks, most women notice a thickening of their waist, especially if this is a second or third pregnancy.

Guide to...

Eating habits for relieving nausea and vomiting

Although there are no specific foods to recommend for managing nausea and vomiting, you might be able to ease symptoms by changing the way you eat.

- Don't worry too much about eating a balanced diet at this time. Eat what appeals to you and what you can keep down. The fetus is going to grow regardless of what you eat, because it will feed on nutrients already stored in your body. You can make up for any dietary deficiencies when you are feeling better.

- Try to eat frequent, small meals, even just a mouthful or two every hour. Keeping a little food in your stomach at all times may help.

- If your nausea is worse in the morning, try to eat a few crackers before you even get out of bed. Sometimes dry crackers or toast can help calm your stomach.

- Try eating salty foods, such as pretzels or potato chips, to help settle your stomach.

- Try eating food cold instead of hot — it doesn't smell as strong. Sometimes smells can trigger nausea and vomiting. You may have to avoid cooking odors.

- Try to drink small amounts of fluids throughout the day. You may want to avoid drinking immediately around meal time. Sour drinks, like lemonade, may settle your stomach more than water.

- If you are having difficulty with food, try a nutritional supplement like Boost or Ensure — mix it with ice in a blender and eat it a few spoonfuls at a time.

---

preserves, powder, capsules, and ginger ale. If you use capsules, try 250 mg up to 4 times a day. Ginger is believed to be safe at this dosage, although no formal safety studies have ever been done.

Acupressure

Acupressure above your wrist, on the inner surface, has been shown in some studies to be helpful. You can buy special wristbands to wear (for example, Sea-Bands) that apply pressure at this point or use something as simple as the eraser on the end of a pencil.

Safe medications

If these measures are not helping, the nausea is getting worse, or you are vomiting frequently, you should talk to your doctor, who might recommend the first-line anti-nausea medication Diclectin. Diclectin is a combination of doxylamine, an antihistamine, and pyridoxine (also called vitamin B_6). This drug is safe in pregnancy; it will not harm the fetus.

If Diclectin does not control your nausea and vomiting, do not despair! There are other medication options:

- Gravol (dimenhydrinate) over-the-counter pills or rectal suppositories
- Phenergan (promethazine)
- Largactil (chlorpromazine)
- Stemetil (prochlorperazine)
- Reglan (metoclopramide)
- Zofran (ondansetron)

Severe vomiting

Severe vomiting (hyperemesis gravidarum) affects up to 1% of pregnant women. If you have severe vomiting for more than a few hours, you may need intravenous fluids for rehydration and to replace lost salts and vitamins. Some women are admitted to

Symptoms of dehydration

If you have these symptoms, seek emergency care:

- Your mouth is dry, not moist
- Your urine is dark and comes infrequently or in small amounts only
- You feel faint and dizzy, especially when you stand up
- You may have the sensation that your heart is racing, or if you measure your heart rate, it is more than 100 beats per minute

hospital for treatment, while others might be sent home to have a visiting nurse come to administer IV fluids and medications. Rarely, a woman will need to receive nutrition through a tube placed into her stomach or through an intravenous line.

Did You Know?

Morning misnomer

"Morning sickness" is the common name for nausea and vomiting in pregnancy, but the "morning" designation is really misleading. Some women find that their nausea is indeed worse in the morning, but for others, nausea can be worse in the afternoon or evening. Some women do feel sick all day, and sometimes there is no pattern to the symptoms.

Constipation

As if you didn't have enough to worry about ... the hormonal changes in pregnancy can make you more constipated, as can the growing uterus and the pressure it exerts on your bowels. The iron in your prenatal vitamins doesn't help either. Most women experience constipation at some stage of pregnancy, but it is most common in the first and third trimesters.

Fiber remedies

The best way to treat constipation is to improve your intake of dietary fiber, increase your fluid consumption to 12 cups (3 L) each day, increase your physical activity, and try to have a bowel movement once a day.

If fiber is increased without increasing fluid consumption, constipation worsens as bulk is added to stool without extra water to help soften bowel movements. Increase fiber slowly. If you don't, your digestive system may produce a lot of gas as it adjusts to the new diet.

If you need to, you can use a bulking agent, such as Metamucil. You could also use a stool softener, such as docusate sodium, if your stools get very hard. Ideally, you wouldn't use a stool softener for more than a few days, but some women need one for longer periods of time. Avoid using laxatives.

If the iron in your prenatal vitamins makes the problem worse, take a few days off, but try to keep taking folic acid (at least until 12 weeks).

Heartburn

Heartburn (esophageal reflux) affects between 30% and 50% of pregnant women. It is likely due to hormonal changes that trigger the relaxation of the esophageal sphincter, which usually keeps stomach acid in its place, or the expansion of the uterus in the third trimester. Heartburn can be uncomfortable, and, in more severe cases, it can negatively affect dietary intake and weight gain.

HOW TO...

Manage Heartburn

Changes in your posture, your eating habits, and even your clothing can alleviate heartburn symptoms. Specific drugs are also effective and safe.

Lifestyle changes

1. Sit up straight when you eat and don't lie down or slouch for 1 hour after eating.
2. Don't chew gum, drink from straws, or talk while eating, to reduce potential air intake.
3. Limit high-fat foods because they take longer to digest. Choose lower-fat alternatives.
4. Limit foods with high levels of citric acid, such as tomatoes, oranges, and juice.
5. Eat small, frequent meals and avoid large meals in the evening, because heartburn often occurs at bedtime.
6. Sleep with the head of the bed elevated. Unless you have a hospital bed, this can be tricky. Putting more pillows under your neck won't help. Instead, place the legs of the headboard of your bed on one or two bricks so you lie at a slight slant.
7. Wear loose-fitting clothing, especially at the chest and waist.

Drugs for managing heartburn

Start with antacids such as calcium carbonate (for example, Tums) or aluminum hydroxide (for example, Maalox).

Move on to medications that reduce the amount of acid your stomach produces, such as ranitidine (Zantac), if needed. These medications are safe and available without a prescription in most places.

Gingivitis and dental health

Gingivitis is an inflammation of the gums that is common during pregnancy. It may occur at any time. The hormone progesterone increases blood flow to the gums. The higher blood blow leads to increased sensitivity to the bacteria in normal plaque build-up and inflammation of the gums, causing tender and bleeding gums. Poor dental health can increase the risk of preterm labor.

Maintain good oral health by brushing your teeth after all meals (especially if eating more often), use a fluoride toothpaste, floss every day, and limit foods that promote tooth decay — carbohydrate and sugar.

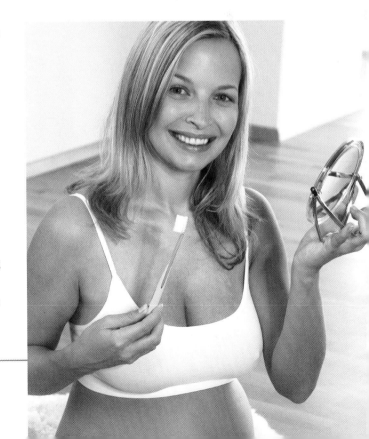

Did You Know?

Dental work cautions

1. **Complications:** Although the data are not conclusive, some studies have suggested that periodontal disease may be linked to pregnancy complications, such as preterm birth, low birth weight, and pre-eclampsia. It is still unclear whether or not treating pre-existing periodontal disease in pregnancy will reduce these negative outcomes.

2. **X-rays:** Try to avoid routine X-rays, but if you have a dental problem and an X-ray would be useful, it is safe if your abdomen is well shielded.

3. **Fillings:** Amalgam fillings should not be inserted or removed during pregnancy because they contain mercury, which could harm the fetus. If you need a new filling, ask your dentist to use a non-amalgam one.

4. **Cosmetic dentistry:** Many women today regularly whiten their teeth. There is no evidence that teeth-whitening systems are harmful to the fetus, but very few studies have been done. Most doctors would advise you to defer these treatments until after pregnancy.

5. **Checkups:** You should continue to visit the dentist for cleaning and check-ups as usual. If you need urgent dental work done, you should proceed. Local anesthetics are safe during pregnancy, although many dentists advise that you wait until you have completed the first trimester to have dental work done, if possible, to minimize a theoretical risk of pain medications causing birth defects. In reality, these risks are very small, and probably greatest in the first 4 weeks of pregnancy.

Fatigue

Many women feel an overwhelming sense of fatigue in the first trimester. This is normal. Even though you don't look very pregnant yet, your body is doing a lot of work. Not only are you growing a fetus, your body is adapting to pregnancy by increasing your blood volume and your lungs' breathing capacity. Your hormone levels are high. You may not be sleeping well if you are getting up at night to empty your bladder or if you are feeling nauseous. All of these things contribute to your profound sense of tiredness.

Listen to your body. Slow down. Sleep. Cut back on any unnecessary activities. Try to eat well and exercise a little bit. Make sure you are taking your prenatal vitamins, and, if you have anemia, take extra iron supplements. Have faith that the worst of the fatigue usually ends after the first trimester — at least until the end of the third trimester!

Sore breasts

Many women notice a significant amount of breast tenderness. You may be in agony if someone even gently bumps into your chest. You may also find your breasts increasing significantly in size, and it may seem as if you need to buy a new bra every week. These symptoms tend to be the worst in a first pregnancy. The tenderness should diminish as the pregnancy progresses, although the size doesn't.

Resign yourself to it — buy a good supportive bra and enjoy being buxom. Your breasts are doing this for a good cause — they're getting ready to feed your newborn.

Frequent urination

You may feel as if you need to urinate every 5 minutes. As your uterus grows, it is putting pressure on your bladder, reducing its effective capacity. Your kidneys are also working more efficiently, making more urine in response to your increased blood volume.

What can you do about it? Not much. Don't stop drinking fluids in an effort to reduce how often you need to urinate. That will only make you dehydrated.

Headaches

The increased estrogen levels in pregnancy are probably the cause of the headaches that some women experience. Some of those who get migraines develop more frequent and worse migraines in pregnancy. The migraines tend to abate about halfway through the pregnancy.

Make sure that you don't have numbness in any of your limbs, or any weakness associated with the headaches. If you are, see a doctor right away. If not, try taking acetaminophen (Tylenol), which is safe in pregnancy. You may need a narcotic medication, such as codeine, but you should talk to your doctor about that before you take anything. For more information on pain relief, see Part 7, Birth and Newborn Planning (page 259).

Emotions

Your hormones are going crazy! Your emotions may be, too, both because of all the changes in your life that having a baby entails and because of the hormones. As your moods change, you'll need to ask for lots of understanding from your loved ones.

Twin rollercoaster

Your physical well-being as well as your emotional condition are challenged when you carry twins. Often, one state feeds into the other. Your body is changing so rapidly that it limits your ability to do the things you could do before pregnancy, and this is difficult to cope with. Wrapped up in all of this is the fear of how to give birth to more than one child and care for them down the road. To say that dealing with all of this is difficult is a gross understatement.

Talking with your caregivers will help. There are support groups for parents of multiples in most communities. The assistance of a social worker may offer some support to get you over the rough spots. Sometimes a referral to psychiatry is necessary where there is a backdrop of pre-existing problems worsened by the gestation of multiples.

Did You Know?

Mixed emotions

The first weeks of pregnancy can be an emotional time. Some women are thrilled to be pregnant, and while others may be pleased, they may have some reservations because of personal, professional, or medical issues. Others may not be happy about it at all. It can also be an anxious time. We know that miscarriage rates are highest in the first trimester, and you may be worried about this possibility. This may affect your decision to share your news with friends, family, and co-workers. Or it may not....

Many women begin to feel unwell, with nausea, vomiting, and fatigue in the first trimester, which can temper the pleasures of being pregnant.

Personal care and comfort

Pregnancy can be exhausting, leaving little time to care for yourself. Between changes in your appearance and fluctuations in your mood, you don't always feel good about yourself. Take time to flatter yourself by wearing attractive and comfortable maternity clothing, and pamper your skin, hair, and body. Taking special care of your personal hygiene can make a big difference in the way you look and feel about yourself. You'll feel clean, healthy, and radiant inside and out.

Maternity clothing

Maternity clothes have been known for their utility, not their elegance, but this is changing as more manufacturers recognize the desire of pregnant women to not only feel comfortable but look good in their maternity clothing.

Fit

Maternity clothes fit differently than your regular clothes — it's not just a matter of buying clothes in bigger sizes. Maternity skirts and dresses are usually made longer in the front than the back, so that they drape with an even hemline. Nevertheless, some of your regular clothes — loose dresses and tops — may work for you well into your pregnancy. Give them a try before shopping for new ones.

Cost

Maternity clothes can be expensive, especially considering the relatively short time you will be wearing them. Buy only what you really need and consider borrowing from family or friends or shopping at secondhand maternity clothing stores, where you can often find high-quality merchandise at bargain prices. When you don't need them anymore, pass them on to the next expectant mother.

Skin care

All of a sudden your skin may be breaking out in pimples. This is a common reaction to the hormonal changes in pregnancy. Understandably, you may be unhappy at this change in your complexion.

What can you do about it? Do everything you did as a teenager … wash your face often and drink lots of water. But do not use the acne drug Accutane, because it is known

---

Did You Know?

Start time

When you choose to start wearing maternity clothes depends a lot on how soon your regular clothes begin feeling tight and uncomfortable. For some women, that happens as early as the end of the first trimester. Other women are able to get by wearing their regular clothes until about 6 months.

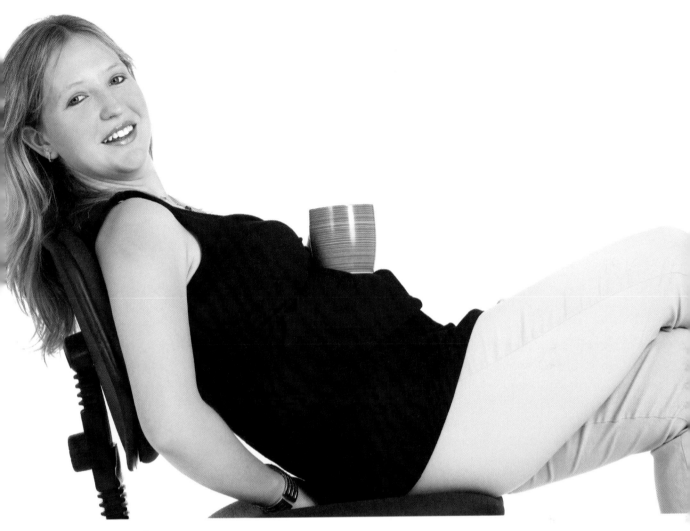

HOW TO...

Take care of your skin in pregnancy

1. Make sure you dress in light, breathable fabrics, such as cotton, especially in the warm months. The glands of your skin may become more active during pregnancy, so you might tend to perspire more. You might also feel warmer due to increased blood flow.

2. Take frequent baths or showers. Baths in warm (not too hot) water are refreshing and relaxing — and can help prevent insomnia. If your skin feels dry, use moisturizing cream or lotion.

3. Take care to apply sunscreen with a protection factor (SPF) of at least 15 and regularly use moisturizing lip balm. Hormonal changes might cause your skin to react differently to the sun.

4. If your face breaks out during pregnancy, blame it on your hormones! You can fight acne as you did when you were a teenager — cleanse and hydrate your face a few times a day, and drink plenty of water. But speak to your health-care provider before using any acne treatments, because some of them (for instance, Accutane) have been shown to be harmful to the growing fetus.

to cause serious birth defects, and avoid face creams with tretinoin (or Retin-A) in them because of a relationship between tretinoin and Accutane. Instead, your doctor can prescribe clindamycin, an antibiotic ointment or cream that is perfectly safe in pregnancy. The acne typically resolves itself during or after pregnancy.

Hair care

Hair tends to become oilier during pregnancy due to the overactive oil glands of the scalp and may require more frequent shampooing. Many pregnant women also notice that the texture of their hair changes — straight hair often begins to curl, curly hair begins to straighten, and dry hair may become increasingly brittle. Frequent conditioning and experimenting with a new style or cut may help you cope with these changes.

Safety concerns

Having your hair colored will not harm the fetus. Chemicals used in hair dyes are absorbed by the body only when applied to your hair. Highlighting is also safe.

However, hair dye might react differently with your skin and hair than it did before you became pregnant. To avoid unexpected color results, have your hair colored professionally at a salon.

As with coloring your hair, there is little evidence to suggest that having your hair permed or straightened while you are pregnant is harmful. However, the results may surprise you — and not necessarily in a good way. Because the texture of your hair changes during pregnancy, your perm, for instance, may leave your hair looking frizzy instead of wavy. For this reason, you

Did You Know?
Douching is unsafe
A vaginal douche involves rinsing or cleaning the vagina by forcing water or another solution into the vaginal cavity. Douching is never advised, and particularly not in pregnancy. If air gets into the fetal bloodstream or your own, it can be fatal.

Regular vaginal douching changes the chemical balance of the vagina and can increase your susceptibility to infections that can spread up from the vagina through the cervix, uterus, and fallopian tubes. In addition, regular users of vaginal douches face increased risk of developing pelvic inflammatory disease (PID) — a chronic condition that can lead to infertility. Don't douche. Ever.

might want to wait until after you have had your baby to have your hair permed or straightened.

Vaginal care

Hormonal changes mean that normal vaginal secretions are usually intensified during pregnancy, due to increased blood circulation to the pelvis. Some women may feel damp (or unclean) as a result. There is no need for concern unless the discharge is itchy, has a foul odor, or is any color except white or clear. When bathing or showering, use warm water and gentle unscented soap to cleanse your perineum. So-called feminine hygiene products, such as soaps, powders, and sprays, should be avoided because they may lead to irritation of sensitive tissues.

Sex during pregnancy

For some women, sex in pregnancy is fabulous; their libido is on the rise, vaginal lubrication usually increases, and they may be more orgasmic than ever before. Other women report decreases in their libido and anxiety about sex in pregnancy. Both responses are normal, but if anxiety is your main issue, perhaps allaying some of your concerns about sex in pregnancy can help you join the first group!

Safety concerns

Is it safe to have sex during pregnancy? The answer, in most cases, is yes. If your pregnancy is low-risk, sex is considered safe throughout all stages, but if you are at risk for certain complications, you may be advised against sexual intercourse. Otherwise, your challenge is to accept fluctuations in your desire and, as your belly grows, to find a comfortable position. Maybe the best part is … you don't have to worry about contraception, although, if necessary, protect yourself against sexually transmitted infections with a condom.

Some people are concerned that the activity of the penis in the vagina will somehow bother the baby. Don't worry. The cervix is a few centimeters long and protects the baby well, as does the sac of amniotic fluid surrounding the baby. Other people worry that the mild uterine contractions associated with orgasm may precipitate labor. Again, don't worry. There is no evidence that orgasm leads to labor. Some people have even argued that the hormones released by your brain after sex, which contribute to a sense of well-being, may benefit the baby as they cross the placenta.

Desire

While sex is safe during most pregnancies, many pregnant women find that their libido fluctuates quite a bit over 9 months and that, as their bodies get bigger, sex

Risk factors in sexual intercourse

If you have any of the following issues, you should not have sex. In some cases, orgasm may be okay but not vaginal intercourse. Check with your doctor.

- Threat of miscarriage, with spotting, cramping, or both
- History of preterm labor
- Unexplained vaginal bleeding, discharge, or cramping
- Leakage of amniotic fluid

- Placenta previa (a condition in which the placenta is located near or over the cervix)
- Incompetent cervix (a condition in which the cervix is weakened and dilates, or opens prematurely, raising the risk for miscarriage or premature delivery)
- Presence of active sexually transmitted diseases (STDs), such as herpes, genital warts, chlamydia, or HIV, in you or your partner that could be transmitted to your baby

Did You Know?

Waning and waxing libido

In the first trimester, many pregnant women are not interested in having sex because of fatigue, nausea, breast tenderness, and other pregnancy-related issues. Often, as fatigue and nausea subside during the second trimester, sexual desire returns, sometimes stronger than ever. In many cases, it fades again during the third trimester as the uterus grows larger. Your partner's desire for sex is likely to ebb and flow as well. Some feel even closer to a pregnant partner and enjoy the body changes that pregnancy brings. Others may experience decreased desire for a variety of reasons. Communication with your partner will help you to deal with these issues.

becomes more challenging and possibly uncomfortable. You and your partner need to keep the lines of communication open regarding your sexual relationship. If intercourse is uncomfortable or otherwise unappealing, talk about other ways to achieve intimacy — for example, through kissing, caressing, or holding each other.

Masturbation (mutual or solo) and oral sex might work out for you if intercourse is not easy. While oral sex is safe, avoid air being blown into the vagina. This could cause a bubble of air to enter the uterus and, theoretically anyway, a blood vessel, causing an air embolus — a rare but potentially fatal event.

Multiples cautions

Although there are no specific contraindications for having intercourse during pregnancy with multiples, there may be circumstances where this is inadvisable.

If there is a history of pregnancy loss or premature labor, sexual intercourse is not advised. The biggest risk to twins or higher multiples is premature labor. The survival of twins born at 28 weeks gestation is so much greater than twins delivered at 25 weeks.

If you get a lot of uterine activity as a result of intercourse, it is not advised.

Comfortable positions

When you do have sex, you will probably need to experiment with different positions until you find what's most comfortable and satisfying. Many couples find that these work best:

- Woman on top
- All fours (man behind woman, rear entry)
- Sitting, woman on top
- Lying on the side ("spooning")

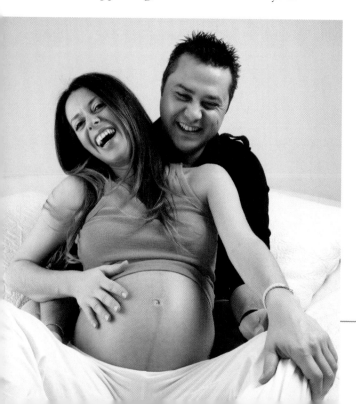

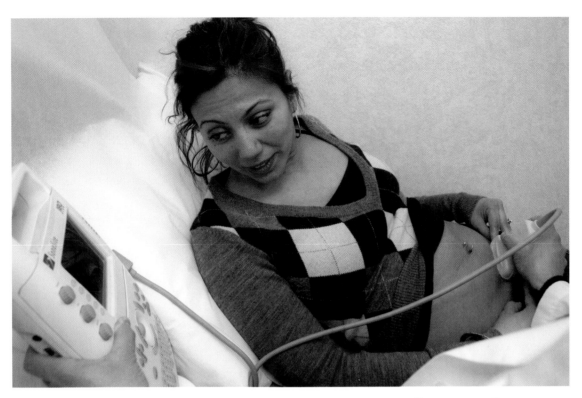

First trimester medical check-up

Typically scheduled at 12 weeks or earlier, your first trimester appointment will probably be quite long. At this visit, the doctor or midwife will take your medical history, perform a physical exam, discuss your care plan, organize some tests, and try to answer all of your questions.

Topics for discussion

When you sit down with your doctor or midwife to discuss your pregnancy-care plans, you may want to review your schedule of appointments and take care of some related practical questions before turning to your medical concerns.

- How long will my prenatal appointments be?

- Who will I see at each appointment?
- Will there be any trainees (medical students, student midwives, or resident doctors) involved in my care?
- Where do your deliveries take place?
- What sort of nursing care is available during delivery? Is there one-to-one nursing care?
- What kind of pain medication is available for delivery?

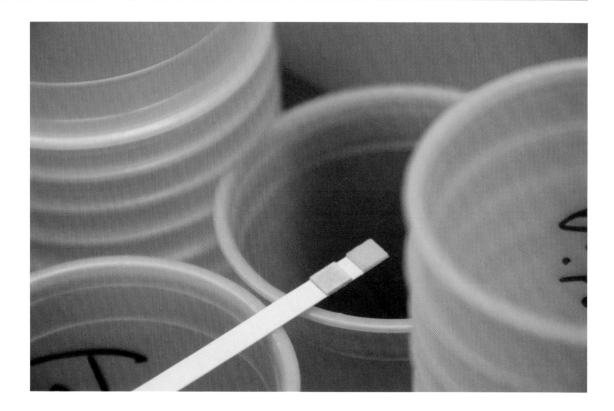

Medical history checklist

At your first trimester appointment, your doctor or midwife will take your medical history. A well-informed patient is a doctor's or midwife's delight. Be prepared to provide the following information:

- **Date of your last menstrual period:** Include the dates your period began and ended. This allows your health-care provider to make her own estimate of your due date and schedule monthly and then weekly appointments.
- **Your pregnancy progress:** Note any problems you have had in this pregnancy so far (especially nausea or bleeding).
- **Your obstetric history:** If applicable, describe previous pregnancies, deliveries, miscarriages, and abortions. Details of each of these events will help your

doctor or midwife assess some of the risk factors in your current pregnancy.

- **Your medical history:** List any medical problems you have that may affect your pregnancy. You might want to review the discussion of pre-existing or chronic medical conditions in Part 1, Planning Your Pregnancy (page 46), and Part 13, Managing Medical and Environmental Risks (page 431).

Did You Know?

Doptone

Your pregnancy care team will likely listen to the fetal heart beat with a doptone, a portable machine used for this purpose. Ask to listen in. You've heard nothing like this before in your life!

- **Your surgical history:** Describe any past surgeries, including your response to the anesthetics involved. They might have an affect on your pregnancy-care plan.

- **Your psychiatric history:** Give your health-care providers a history of any anxiety conditions or episodes of depression so they can assess your risk of similar problems in pregnancy and the postpartum period. They will be prepared to monitor your mood if necessary.

- **Your family history:** Take stock of the genetic make-up of both you and your partner and the ethnic background of ancestors. This is particularly relevant if there is any history of inherited disorders. You might want to review the discussion of genetic diseases in Part 1, Planning Your Pregnancy (page 41), and Part 13, Managing Medical and Environmental Risks (page 429).

- **Your medications:** List any over-the-counter and prescription medications you are taking. You might bring the prescription, pill bottle, or medication packaging with you. Note any allergies you may have to medications.

- **Your immunization history:** Make a report on your history of infections and vaccinations, including rubella (German measles), varicella (chicken pox), parvovirus (fifth disease), toxoplasmosis, herpes, hepatitis C and B, HIV, and syphilis. You might want to review the discussion of infectious diseases in Part 1, Planning Your Pregnancy (page 52), and Part 13, Managing Medical and Environmental Risks (page 439).

Physical and internal examinations

After taking a thorough medical history, your health-care provider will perform a physical exam, paying special attention to your weight and blood pressure. Your doctor may also do an internal exam in order to do a Pap smear and take cervical cultures to screen for infection. A urine sample will be collected to look for protein levels (a marker of how well your kidneys are working) and bladder infections.

Routine blood tests

Your health-care providers will take a blood sample to test for:

- Blood count, specifically hemoglobin levels, which may indicate anemia

- Blood type, especially to determine if you are Rh negative, which may indicate risk of disease

- Rubella (German measles), hepatitis B, syphilis, and HIV exposure and immunity

- Parvovirus, toxoplasmosis, and varicella (chicken pox) exposure and immunity, depending upon your history and risk factors

- Sickle cell disease or thalassemia, if advisable because of your ethnicity

For more information on Rh disease and genetic diseases, including sickle cell disease and thalassemia, see Part 13, Managing Medical and Environmental Risks (page 429).

Genetic screening and diagnostic tests

At your first medical check-up, you will typically be offered the option of various non-invasive screening tests and invasive diagnostic tests for some inherited genetic diseases, such as sickle cell disease and thalassemia, and non-inherited chromosomal disorders, such as Down syndrome and trisomy 13 and 18. These tests are designed to identify problems the mother and the fetus may encounter during pregnancy and after birth.

Screening vs. diagnostic tests

Non-invasive screening tests are used to determine the possibility of an uncommon disease or disorder in an individual who has no symptoms or reason for concern. These tests are not able to determine for certain if the disease or disorder is present. They present no risk to the fetus.

Invasive diagnostic tests are used to confirm the presence or absence of a disease or disorder in an individual at risk, either because of a positive screening test or because of a strong clinical suspicion of a problem. Because tissue or fluid must be obtained to do the diagnostic tests, these tests present a small risk to the fetus.

Some sort of prenatal screening and diagnosis is offered to every pregnant woman, but screening for these diseases is optional, and not all conditions can be diagnosed. You will need to consider your values and preferences when deciding what sort of prenatal screening to undergo, if any.

Inherited genetic disease screening

If there is no specific family history of genetic disease and testing wasn't done prior to pregnancy, doctors usually consider non-invasive screening tests on mothers to look for the possibility that she is a carrier of certain genetic diseases, such as thalassemia, sickle cell disease, and Tay-Sachs, which are more common in some ethnic populations. For more information on these genetic diseases, see Part 1, Planning Your Pregnancy (page 41), and Part 13, Managing Medical and Environmental Risks (page 429).

Ideally, you would have been tested earlier, but it can be done now. In general, the tests for sickle cell anemia and

Did You Know?

Risk analysis

With genetic screening, you and your doctors are exploring two risk questions:

- What is the risk of this baby having an *inherited* disease, based upon your personal and family history of disease and your ethnic heritage?

- What is the risk of this baby having a specific *non-inherited* disease, specifically Down syndrome and trisomy 18?

thalassemia are easily done in any lab. Tests for some of the other diseases are more complicated and may not be available everywhere. Check with your pregnancy-care team.

Non-inherited chromosomal disorder screening

Beginning in the first trimester, your care team can also screen for non-inherited chromosomal disorders in the fetus, specifically trisomy 13, trisomy 18, and trisomy 21 (Down syndrome).

Sometimes, as the egg and sperm are combining, the wrong number of chromosomes can end up in a developing embryo. Most of the time, this embryo does not survive and there is an early miscarriage. But sometimes an embryo can survive with an extra chromosome.

Down syndrome is an example of this — a child with Down syndrome has an extra copy of chromosome 21, three copies instead of two. This is called trisomy 21. It is occasionally possible for a fetus to survive with three copies of chromosome 18 (trisomy 18) or 13 (trisomy 13).

Down syndrome

Down syndrome is characterized by some typical physical features, particularly involving the head, neck, and limbs. Not every person with Down syndrome has all the features. These features can include a flat face, small mouth, protuberant tongue, slanted eyes, short neck, small hands, a side-to-side, or transverse, crease across the palm, and 50% of the Down population has heart problems as well. The most significant result of Down syndrome is intellectual impairment. It is present in all people with

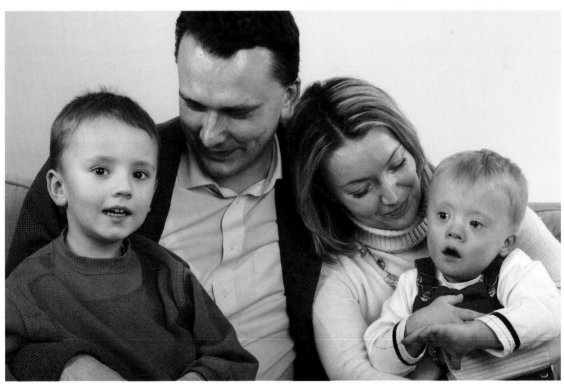

Down syndrome, but the severity can vary widely from mild to severe. In general, life expectancy is shortened, but many people with Down syndrome now live into their 50s.

Trisomy 13 and Trisomy 18

These conditions are associated with numerous physical abnormalities and severe mental retardation. Fetuses with one of these trisomies usually die in utero, and if they survive to birth, they usually die within a few months.

Risk of chromosomal abnormalities in live-born infants at term

Maternal age in years	Risk of Down syndrome	Risk of any chromosomal abnormality
20	1 in 1650	1 in 530
25	1 in 1250	1 in 480
30	1 in 950	1 in 390
35	1 in 385	1 in 180
40	1 in 100	1 in 65
45	1 in 30	1 in 19
Adapted by permission from the Genetics Education Program.		

Non-inherited chromosomal disorder diagnostic tests

The only way to know for certain if the fetus has any of these chromosomal disorders is to test the fetus directly. To do this, cells must be obtained that have the same genetic make-up as the fetus. These cells can be found in the amniotic fluid and in the developing placenta.

There are two invasive diagnostic tests available — amniocentesis and chorionic villus sampling (CVS). Fetal cells obtained by these tests can also indicate inherited genetic disorders. Unfortunately, both of these tests are associated with a small risk of miscarriage. To avoid the risk of miscarriage associated with amniocentesis and CVS, non-invasive screening tests have been developed. If you do decide to undergo fetal chromosomal testing, your health-care provider or genetic counselor will recommend the type that's best for you.

Amniocentesis

Perhaps the better known of the available genetic diagnostic tests, amniocentesis (more casually known as an amnio) is an invasive procedure. A very fine needle is inserted through the abdomen and into the uterus so that the amniotic fluid can be extracted and tested. The procedure is performed by an obstetrician using ultrasound as a guide. Most women feel no pain with the procedure.

Amniocentesis can be done anytime in a pregnancy after about 16 weeks gestation, although for genetic diagnostic testing, it is usually done around 16 to 18 weeks. After an amniocentesis, it will normally take about 3 weeks to get a final result, although in some places a rapid test called FISH (fluorescent in situ hybridization) will provide preliminary results the next day.

Amniocentesis and Chorionic Villus Sampling Procedures

Amniocentesis

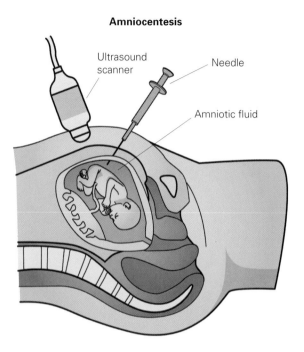

Ultrasound scanner

Needle

Amniotic fluid

Chorionic Villus Sampling

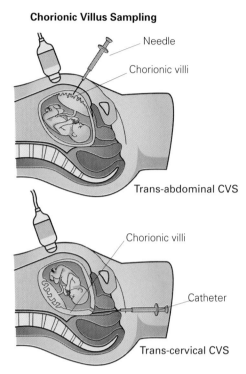

Needle

Chorionic villi

Trans-abdominal CVS

Chorionic villi

Catheter

Trans-cervical CVS

Chorionic villus sampling

With chorionic villus sampling, samples of cells are extracted from the chorion (chorionic villi), a membrane that surrounds the embryo before the placenta is fully formed. Chorionic villi cells are part of the developing placenta.

There are two methods that can be used to extract the sample, depending on the location of the placenta. If the placenta is at the front of the uterus, a needle is passed through the abdomen; otherwise, a trans-cervical CVS is performed. A catheter is passed through the cervix into the uterus and the sample is taken from there.

Like amnio, there is an increased risk of miscarriage. The risk is a little bit higher with trans-cervical CVS. The risk of miscarriage as a consequence of CVS is quoted by different sources as anywhere from 1 in 100 to 1 in 200.

CVS is normally done between the beginning of the 12th week and end of the 13th week of pregnancy. The accuracy of CVS for the purposes of chromosomal analysis is comparable to amniocentesis — approximately 99%.

Did You Know?
Accuracy and safety of amniocentesis

Amniocentesis is more than 99% accurate in detecting nearly all non-inherited chromosomal disorders and can also detect inherited genetic disorders and neural tube defects. Most studies looking at the increased risk of miscarriage associated with amniocentesis seem to conclude that 1 out of every 200 to 400 pregnancies will miscarry due to the amniocentesis procedure.

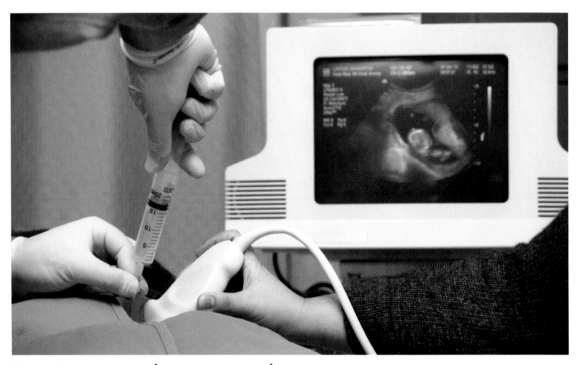

Non-invasive chromosomal screening tests

To avoid doing unnecessary invasive diagnostic tests, non-invasive screening tests have been developed that use a combination of ultrasound scans and blood tests. They are only screening tests, not the highly accurate diagnostic tests. They will indicate if there is a risk of having a baby with Down syndrome, but cannot confirm that the baby will have it. If the screening test is positive, you may choose to undergo an invasive diagnostic test, such as amniocentesis or CVS.

Chromosomal screening tests include first trimester screening (FTS), integrated prenatal screening (IPS), serum integrated prenatal screening (SIPS), and quadruple screening. The test you choose will depend on the gestational age and the urgency in receiving results. If your first medical appointment is after 14 weeks, the only option is the quadruple screen. And not all tests may be available everywhere.

■ Amniocentesis — amniotic fluid being withdrawn

Weighing screening options

For example, FTS will provide you with a result sooner than IPS, but you sacrifice some accuracy in order to get a result sooner — FTS will detect only 80% to 85% of fetuses with Down syndrome — meaning that 15% to 20% of babies with Down syndrome will have a normal FTS result. There is also a higher chance of having an abnormal result, even in a normal baby without Down syndrome, which might lead you to choose an amniocentesis and face the risk of miscarriage that goes along with an amnio. IPS will also report upon your risk of an open neural tube defect. If you choose FTS, you will be offered a separate blood test at 15 to 20 weeks to determine your risk of having a baby with an open neural tube defect.

Non-invasive chromosomal screening tests

	First trimester screening (FTS)	Integrated prenatal screening (IPS)	Serum integrated prenatal screening (SIPS)	Quadruple screening
Timing of 1st blood sample	11–14 weeks	11–14 weeks	11–14 weeks	None
Nuchal translucency ultrasound*	11–14 weeks	11–14 weeks	None	None
Timing of 2nd blood sample	None	15–20 weeks	15–20 weeks	15–20 weeks
Results available	12–15 weeks	16–21 weeks	16–21 weeks	16–21 weeks
Detection rate (Of every 100 pregnancies with Down syndrome, about _____ will be detected)	80–85%	85–90%	80–90%	75–85%
False positive rate (Of every 100 pregnancies tested, about _____ will have a positive result on this test, but further testing will reveal NO Down syndrome)	3–9%	2–4%	2–7%	5–10%

* The nuchal translucency ultrasound measures the thickness of the skin fold at the back of a fetus's neck. It must be measured between 11 and 14 weeks of pregnancy. Ultrasound technicians need special training to do this test, so it may not be available everywhere. If ultrasound is not available, then SIPS or quadruple screening can be done.

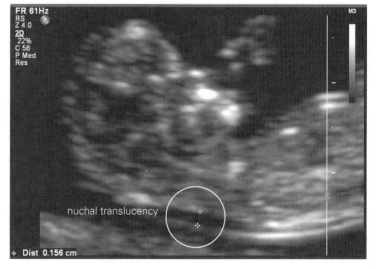

Adapted by permission from the Genetics Education Program.

Did You Know?

Twins testing

Because the protein levels in twins are different than in singletons, we cannot do the FTS, IPS, and quadruple screening tests in multiple pregnancies. In order to determine the risk of Down syndrome, the nuchal translucency of each twin is measured. However, CVS and amniocentesis can be used in twin pregnancies (making sure the two samples are from two different twins is the tricky part!)

Ultrasound tests

Many fetuses with trisomy 21, 18, or 13 will have abnormalities that are detectable by routine ultrasound at 18 to 20 weeks. Non-invasive ultrasound can also detect congenital heart defects, kidney problems, bowel problems, and brain and other abnormalities. Some of these conditions have a genetic basis and some do not.

To test or not to test

Always remember that these prenatal diagnostic and screening tests are optional.

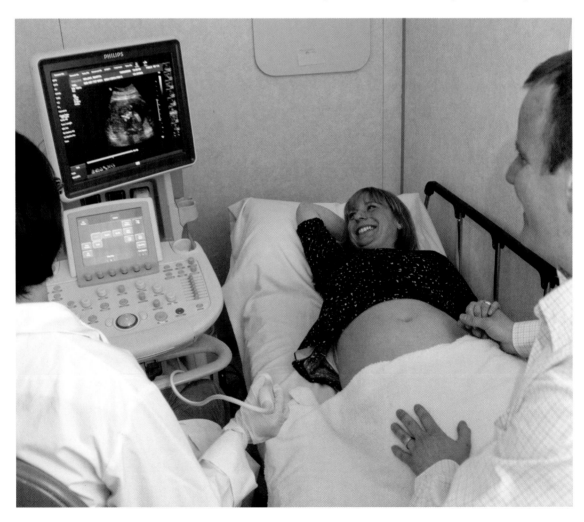

Discuss their pros and cons with your doctor or midwife. Genetic screening may be something that you and your partner feel strongly about. Perhaps you don't want to risk losing the pregnancy during an invasive procedure, or maybe you feel that no matter what is discovered, you wouldn't terminate your pregnancy. Obviously, the decision to undergo genetic screening is a serious one, particularly if there is a family history of a genetic

Guide to...

Making a decision about screening

You and your partner might want to consider these questions when weighing your genetic screening options:

- Would information about the current health of the fetus make a difference to you?

- If the fetus was found to have a severe problem, would you continue the pregnancy?

- Would you consider an abortion?

- If you did not choose termination, would foreknowledge about the condition help you prepare for the birth of your child?

- Would your religious beliefs play a role in guiding your decision?

- How would you rate the quality of life of a child with significant physical or intellectual disabilities? Would this factor into your decision-making process?

- If you had a child with significant physical or intellectual disabilities, how would this affect your life? How would it affect the lives of other people in your family?

disease or chromosomal disorder. You and your partner should discuss this between yourselves and with your health-care provider. Make sure you have all the information you need and take the time to consider your options — as well as your feelings — carefully.

Non-chromosomal conditions

Prenatal screening programs can also determine the fetal risk of open neural tube defects. The neural tube is a component of the fetal brain and spinal cord. Open neural tube defects, such as anencephaly and spina bifida, are non-chromosomal conditions that occur when the fetal nerve and brain tissue is not properly covered by the spine, skull, and overlying skin during fetal development.

In the second trimester, these defects are indicated by elevated levels of a protein called alpha-fetoprotein in your blood and in the amniotic fluid. Most open neural tube defects can also be diagnosed by an ultrasound at 19 weeks gestation or earlier. For more information on neural tube defects, see Part 1, Planning Your Pregnancy (page 48).

Miscarriage

Unfortunately, miscarriage in the first trimester is a common event. Almost 20% of recognized pregnancies miscarry, and the percentage is higher if you include unrecognized pregnancies that are over before the woman realizes she was pregnant.

A miscarriage means that the embryo or fetus does not implant or develop properly and dies. Although this can happen at any time in the pregnancy, it most commonly occurs in the first trimester. After 15 weeks, the chance of a normal pregnancy miscarrying is less than 1%.

Symptoms of a miscarriage

One of the first symptoms of a miscarriage is bleeding and, sometimes, cramping. Sometimes the bleeding can become quite heavy, and you pass some big clots or pieces of tissue. The tissue usually represents the developing gestational sac and placenta. Usually, once the sac has been passed, the bleeding slows down significantly, more like what you would expect with a heavy period. It will then taper off over a period of about a week. You can expect a normal period again 4 to 6 weeks later.

Missed abortion

Sometimes, a woman can have a miscarriage and not have any bleeding or cramping. The medical term for this is a "missed abortion." This diagnosis is usually made following an ultrasound that shows an embryo without a beating heart. If this happens, there are three management options:

- Do nothing. Eventually, most women will miscarry without assistance. Some women do not wish to deal with the uncertainty of not knowing how long this will take. It could take several weeks.
- Undergo a D&C (dilation and curettage). During the procedure, the non-viable pregnancy tissue is removed from the uterus through your cervix. Many, but not all, doctors arrange for you to be asleep under an anesthetic during this procedure.
- Use medication to induce your uterus to contract and expel the non-viable pregnancy tissue. Misoprostol works quite well if the pregnancy is not very advanced, that is, less than about 9 weeks, and if you feel you will be able to cope well at home with any bleeding and cramping.

Did You Know?

Miscarriage causes

About 50% of miscarriages are associated with abnormalities in the genetic make-up of the embryo. The chromosomes containing the genetic material from the egg and sperm did not come together properly, and the embryo was never destined to grow into a normal baby. In the other 50% of cases, factors involved may include other fetal abnormalities or problems related to the mother's health, such as uterine fibroids, hormone imbalances, and infections. In most cases, the cause of a miscarriage is never determined precisely.

Guide to...

Managing a miscarriage

At home

Some women are comfortable staying at home and dealing with the bleeding and cramping themselves. That is fine as long as the bleeding is not too heavy, but seek emergency care if you soak more than two sanitary pads an hour for more than 2 hours. You do not need to collect the tissue you see to show your doctor; there are no tests that need to be done on the tissue. If you need to take some medication for the pain, you could take some acetaminophen (Tylenol). It is advisable to avoid ibuprofen. Although ibuprofen will slow down the cramping pain, it will also slow down the uterine contractions that are necessary to get rid of the pregnancy tissue.

With your doctor or midwife

If you are having any bleeding, you need to contact your doctor. How urgently you need to do this depends a little bit on how much you are bleeding. If you are just spotting a little bit and have no cramping, your doctor may arrange for you to have an ultrasound to check the state of your pregnancy. Unfortunately, there is no specific treatment available to prevent a miscarriage from occurring.

In an emergency

If your bleeding is heavy (more than two pads per hour for more than 2 hours), you will need to seek emergency care right away. To stop the bleeding, a D&C is sometimes necessary to remove the pregnancy tissue from your uterus. Once the tissue is removed, your bleeding will settle down.

After a miscarriage

If you have a miscarriage, it is normal to feel quite sad about it. Pregnancy loss can have a much more far-reaching impact on the emotions of a woman and her partner than many expect.

People may encourage you to shrug it off and move on, but it is advisable to take the time you need to grieve the loss of the potential baby. In some places, support groups and counseling are available if you find that you need help coping with your loss. Eventually, you will feel ready to move on and try to conceive again.

Did You Know?

Conceiving again

The good news is that having one miscarriage does not automatically reduce your chances of having a successful pregnancy in the future. If you wish to try to conceive again, there is no reason to wait. Traditionally, women have been advised to wait for two to three normal menstrual cycles before trying to conceive again, but there does not seem to be any harm in conceiving sooner. If you have multiple miscarriages (three or more) there may be a more significant problem, and tests are warranted to determine the cause. You should speak with your health-care providers if this is the case.

Abnormal pregnancies

While most pregnancies progress to term without complications, some pregnancies are not normal and will never culminate in the development of a baby. These abnormal pregnancies are usually diagnosed in the first trimester.

Ectopic pregnancy

One of the most dangerous first trimester pregnancy complications is ectopic pregnancy. This occurs when the embryo implants outside of the uterus, most often in the fallopian tube. It can also implant on the ovary and other parts of the abdomen, but this is extremely rare.

The fallopian tube is not a muscular structure (as the uterus is) and cannot expand as the pregnancy progresses. The growing fetus will eventually rupture the tube, often causing a significant amount of bleeding into the abdominal cavity. If a ruptured ectopic pregnancy is not attended to quickly and properly, a woman could bleed to death.

Did You Know?

Stopping the pregnancy

If you have an ectopic pregnancy, the fetus will never go on to become a live baby. Doctors are sometimes asked if the pregnancy can be transferred into the uterus so that it can grow normally. Unfortunately, this is not possible. The pregnancy tissue must be removed or stopped from growing using surgical methods or by injecting a medication to stop the developing pregnancy.

Symptoms of an ectopic pregnancy

Symptoms of an ectopic pregnancy start about 6 weeks after conception. These include abnormal bleeding and spotting and lower-abdominal pain, but if the tube ruptures, this pain will be extreme and you may lose consciousness. If you have mild pain or spotting, you should see your doctor to arrange for tests. If you have severe pain, feel dizzy, or lose consciousness, you should get to an emergency department. However, some women have no symptoms and the diagnosis is picked up when an ultrasound is done for other reasons.

Tests

If an ectopic pregnancy is suspected, your health-care providers will test for the pregnancy hormone (ßHCG). Typically, in an ectopic pregnancy, the ßHCG level will not be increasing properly, so the level is abnormally low for the gestational age. In an ectopic pregnancy, the pregnancy sac will be seen in the tube, not in the uterus, and, sometimes, it will also show blood in the abdomen. If an ectopic pregnancy is suspected, it is important to have an early ultrasound to determine if the pregnancy is in the uterus or in the tube.

Medical management

If the ectopic pregnancy is discovered early in the first trimester and you are not in pain, it can be managed medically instead of surgically. You can be given an injection of methotrexate, a medication designed to stop the pregnancy tissue from continuing to develop. After this injection, your pregnancy hormone level will be followed closely until it goes down to zero. If you receive methotrexate, it is important to do all the recommended blood tests and stay in contact with your doctor.

Surgical management

Approximately 85% of ectopic pregnancies can be resolved with medications, but there is still a small risk that you will need surgery. If the fallopian tube is ruptured, it must be removed in order to stop the bleeding and remove the pregnancy tissue. This procedure is called a salpingectomy. In most cases, it can be done laparoscopically (using small incisions). After the operation, the pregnancy hormone must be monitored until it goes down to zero, as some of the tissue may have been left behind.

Molar pregnancy

A molar pregnancy is also known as a tumor of the placental tissues. Most of the time,

these tissues are benign, but they can spread to other parts of your body. There are two types of molar pregnancies: complete moles and incomplete moles.

In a complete mole, there are no fetal parts, only an abnormal placenta; the ultrasound shows a pattern that looks like a bunch of grapes. In a partial mole, there is both an abnormal placenta and a fetus, although the fetus is usually chromosomally very abnormal and fetal death usually occurs early in the pregnancy. Rarely, a baby will be born alive, but this child will have multiple congenital problems and will not survive.

The diagnosis is usually confirmed by ultrasound reviews and hormone levels. The treatment involves a surgical D&C to remove the abnormal placental tissue. In the majority of cases, this will be all that is necessary.

Molar pregnancy monitoring

It is important to track the pregnancy hormone levels for at least 6 months to ensure that the levels go down to zero and stay down for at least 6 months. If the levels do not go down, or if they rise, it suggests that the placental tumor is not all gone and chemotherapy may be necessary. This delay is often very frustrating for women who wish to have a child, but it is important for their long-term health.

Guide to ...

Signs of a molar pregnancy

- Abnormal first trimester bleeding
- Very high level of pregnancy hormone
- Uterine size larger than it should be for the gestational date
- Because of the high pregnancy hormone levels, considerable nausea and vomiting

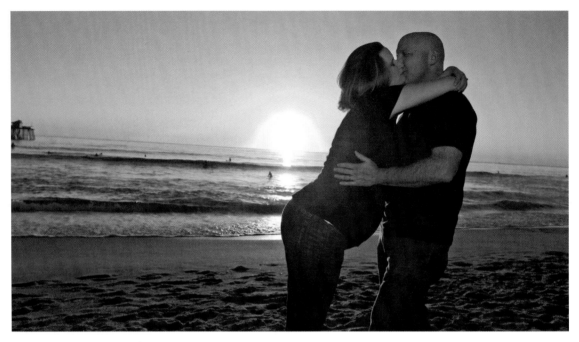

Traveling safety

The fear of complications often deters pregnant women from many activities, including traveling.

Some pregnancy complications might make traveling risky for you and your baby, but for the most part, travel during pregnancy is a great idea. It is a lot easier than traveling with a baby!

Still, if you're considering taking a trip, it is probably wise to discuss it with your doctor or midwife. Make sure that wherever you go, you will have access to emergency care if needed, and insurance to pay for it. Also remember that airlines may not let you board if you look so pregnant that they are worried you might go into labor and deliver on board! Check with your airlines and travel health insurers about gestational age limits and whether you need certificates from your doctor.

Guide to...

Travel cautions

Pregnant women experiencing complications are advised not to travel. Some of these complications include:

- Cervical problems, such as incompetent cervix
- Vaginal bleeding
- Multiple fetuses — depending upon the number of fetuses and the gestational age
- High blood pressure
- Pre-eclampsia
- Possible premature labor
- History of preterm delivery in a previous pregnancy

Working safety

If you're having a low-risk, normal pregnancy, you may certainly continue working. Of course, the kind of work you do will factor into your decision on whether to keep working and for how long. Audit your workplace to make sure that you minimize any health and safety hazards. The important thing is that your job and work environment do not endanger either you or your baby.

Duration

How long you remain working is another decision you'll have to make. You've probably heard stories about indomitable women who have worked right up to labor. You may or may not want to go that route. Remember that toward the end of your pregnancy, you might find yourself tiring more. If you can afford to start your maternity leave a week or two before your due date, consider using it to rest, prepare, and indulge yourself. You won't have much time for that with a new baby in the house.

While most women are able to work throughout their pregnancies, in some circumstances — including a previous preterm delivery, , high blood pressure, a history of miscarriage, or multiple fetuses — it might be best to stop. Your health-care provider will be able to advise you on whether you need to consider taking a work break.

Health and safety

If you think your job might involve potential hazards relating to your pregnancy, talk to your health-care provider about it. While workplace health and safety policies vary from company to company, certain basic accommodations are required by law, both in the United States and Canada. For further information on legislated rights in both countries, see the Pregnancy Care Resources list (page 466). Health and safety issues related to pregnancy are not just about physical problems, but also mental fatigue, stress, and traveling on the job.

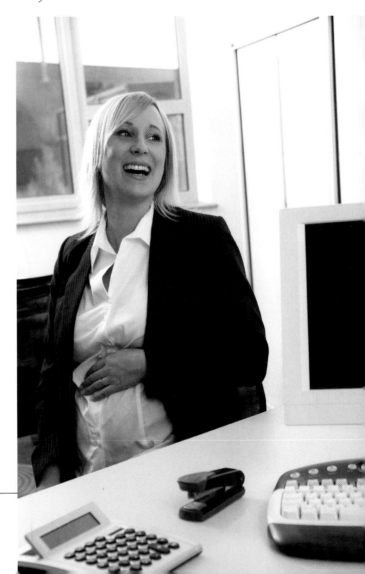

F.A.Q.

We answer many questions from pregnant women and their partners. Here are some of the most frequently asked questions. Be sure to ask your health-care providers any other questions that may arise. If they don't have the answers, they will refer you to a colleague who does.

Q: *When should I tell people (my boss, my parents, my friends) that I am pregnant?*

A: This is a very personal decision. Some women tell everyone the minute they know they are pregnant. They want to share their good news! Some women prefer not to announce their pregnancy widely until the second trimester. Perhaps these women have had an early miscarriage or know about the increased risk of miscarriage in the first trimester. They may want to keep a miscarriage private if it occurs. Other women want their friends and family to know if they have had a miscarriage so that they feel free to share and express their grief. There is no right answer. Think about how you will feel if you lose the pregnancy. Who would you want to share that information with? If the answer is very few people, then hold off on your big announcement until after your 12-week ultrasound, or even until after you know the results of any genetic tests you may choose to do.

Q: *Does my nausea and vomiting harm the fetus?*

A: You would think that nausea and vomiting can't be good for the fetus. In fact, unless the nausea and vomiting is very severe, pregnancies associated with nausea and vomiting have better outcomes than those without. There are fewer miscarriages, premature deliveries, very small babies, and stillbirths. The fetus steals the nutrients it needs from your body, regardless of your dietary intake, so even if you aren't eating much, the baby should be fine. Do keep taking folic acid, though, either in a maternal vitamin (if you can tolerate it) or on its own.

Q: *Can I sleep on my back or my stomach?*

A: Yes. As your uterus grows bigger, there is a possibility it may compress a blood vessel returning blood into your heart when you lie down on your back. This has been a long-held belief, but in reality, as long as you do not feel dizzy lying on your back, then plenty of blood is going to your brain, and a similar amount will be traveling to the baby. So, if you feel dizzy lying on your back, roll to the side or on to your stomach, as long as you are comfortable. You will not harm the baby by doing this. And you may not be able to do it for much longer.

Q: *Why do some couples choose to undergo prenatal screening and diagnosis and some don't?*

A: Many couples want to reassure themselves that the pregnancy is normal. They also want to know about significant problems early in the pregnancy so they can inform themselves about their nature. Sometimes they will use this information to prepare themselves and their families for a baby with significant health challenges. Sometimes they will use this information to make a decision about ending a pregnancy in which the fetus has significant problems.

Other couples know that they are not going to end a pregnancy no matter what the problem is. Or they do not want to face the anxiety that an abnormal screening test may bring. Some couples are worried about genetic screening because they have heard it is associated with miscarriage and do not want to take that risk. Only invasive diagnostic tests are associated with miscarriage, however.

Q: *Will a Pap smear harm my baby?*

A: No. A Pap smear scrapes a single layer of cells off the top of your cervix to screen for pre-cancerous cells. A normal cervix is $1\frac{1}{2}$ to 2 inches (4 to 5 cm) long at this point, so the Pap smear is well away from where the fetus is growing. You may have some bleeding or spotting after the Pap smear, but this is normal and will stop in a few minutes. Post-Pap smear spotting does not have anything to do with a miscarriage.

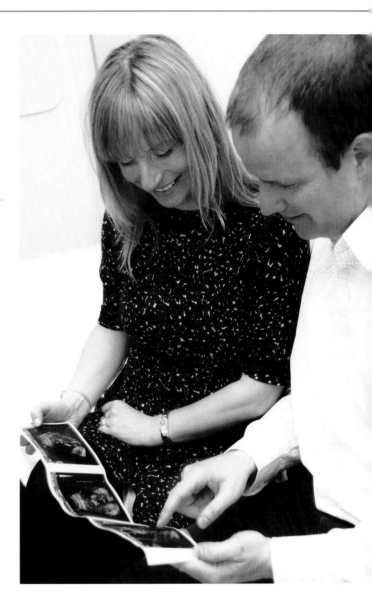

What's next

Now that the fetus is working out regularly inside your uterus, it's time to begin your own exercise program to get fit for the weeks to come. Flexibility, strength, and endurance — you will need them all.

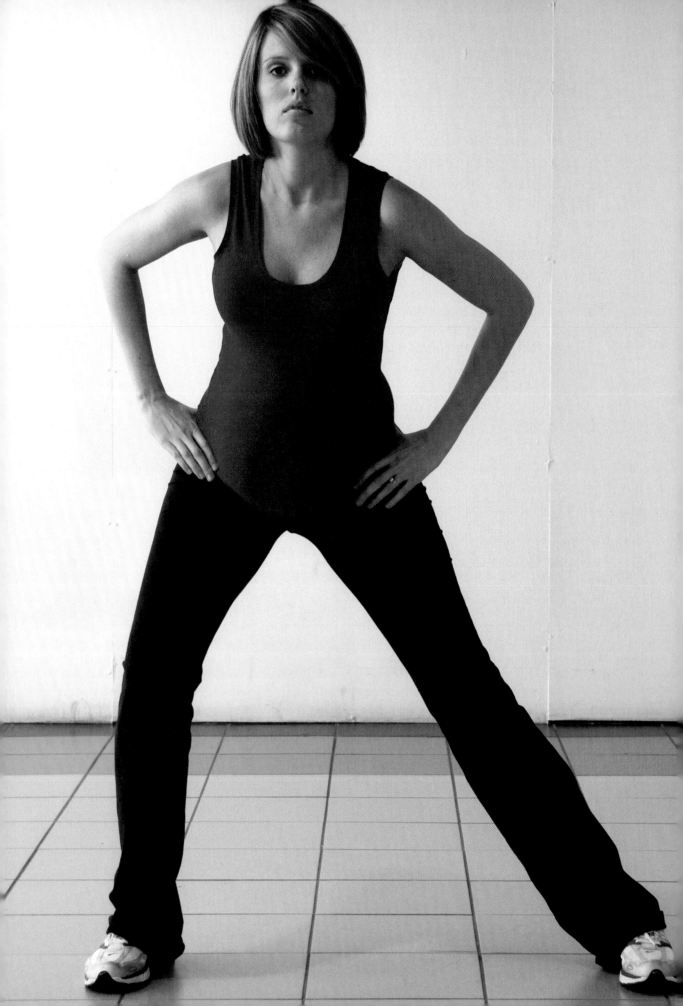

Part 5

Exercising Safely During Pregnancy

Not so fragile

"Can I exercise safely?" This is one of the most frequently asked questions when women are pregnant. Many women are already exercising and want to continue — but they want to do it safely and not put their pregnancy at risk. Other women feel that if they are going to gain weight in a pregnancy, they should start exercising early to combat the effects. The age-old belief that a pregnant woman is in a "fragile state" when expecting and should avoid exercising is incorrect, unless there are complications that place the mother or child at risk. Today, women have adopted a new outlook on exercising while pregnant.

Fitness and strength

The general goals of exercise in pregnancy are to improve your cardio-respiratory fitness and to strengthen the muscles and joints most affected by your pregnancy. The changes your body undergoes during this time challenge your ability to breathe effectively and to carry your baby to term. Specific exercises can help you meet these cardiovascular, respiratory, and musculoskeletal challenges.

Exercise throughout your pregnancy will not only help your physical well-being but also strengthen your emotional health. The physical energy and mental focus you gain through an exercise program help you continue your daily tasks with strength and confidence during pregnancy, prepare you to push effectively during labor and delivery, and get you ready for the life-changing experiences of motherhood.

Ten tips for exercising safely and successfully during pregnancy

1. Before starting any exercise program during pregnancy, consult with your health-care provider.
2. Remember that your body is changing and that any exercise routine will need to accommodate these changes.
3. Avoid any exercises that involve jumping, falling, or jarring movements or quick changes in direction.
4. Warm up with exercises that invigorate your circulation before starting flexibility and stretching routines.
5. Cool down with diaphragmatic breathing and light aerobic exercises after strength and resistance routines.
6. Exercise within 65% to 85% of your target heart rate range.
7. Know the warning signs of over-exercising. Don't push these limits.
8. Exercise conscientiously but not compulsively. If you miss a day now and then, don't sweat it.
9. If you are carrying more than one baby, that's a workout in itself, so it is not unusual to have to cut back on activity as the pregnancy progresses. By the time you reach week 24, you will be at the size of a mother carrying a singleton close to term!
10. Have fun!

Guide to...
Pregnancy fitness
These guidelines for exercise in pregnancy are supported by the American College of Obstetricians and Gynecologists (ACOG) and the Society of Obstetricians and Gynaecologists of Canada (SOGC). The American College of Sports Medicine recommends at least 30 minutes of physical exercise daily to derive health benefits from exercise.

Exercise benefits
Thirty minutes of exercise every day can help to
- Decrease backache, constipation, bloating, and swelling
- Prevent and treat gestational diabetes mellitus
- Improve energy, posture, and overall mood
- Promote muscle tone, strength, and endurance
- Improve sleep
- Return to pre-pregnancy weight more easily

Safe exercises
Exercises considered safe during pregnancy:
- Walking (outside or on a treadmill)
- Swimming
- Cycling (on a stationary bike)
- Aerobics (low-impact and water aerobics)
- Jogging

Exercises to avoid during pregnancy
- Jumping, jarring movements or quick changes in direction
- Sports involving balance and a risk of falling (downhill skiing, horseback riding, gymnastics)
- Scuba diving (may have an effect on the fetus)
- Contact sports (such as soccer, hockey, and basketball)

Safe practices
- Do not exercise hard in hot, humid weather.
- Wear a bra that fits well and provides support.
- Drink lots of water to help prevent overheating and dehydration.
- Consume enough calories for healthy weight gain for each trimester of your pregnancy.
- Stop if you feel pain, have uterine cramps, or see any bleeding.

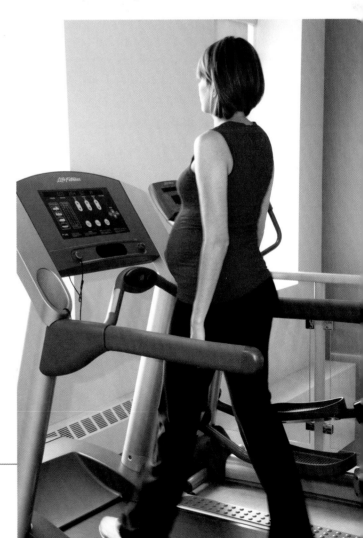

Body changes and challenges

Exercising during pregnancy offers a few additional challenges because of changes affecting your cardiovascular, respiratory, and musculoskeletal systems.

Heart rate and blood volume

In pregnancy, there is an increase in your heart rate and a big increase in the amount of blood flowing in your veins. Your blood vessels will be dilated more than usual to cope with the volume of blood. Because your growing uterus pushes on the inferior vena cava (the big blood vessel that brings blood back to your heart), activities that require you to lie on your back for long periods of time are not recommended. This pressure can make you feel faint. As long as you roll

over when you feel faint, blood supply to the fetus will not be affected.

Breathing

There is less oxygen available for exercise because your growing uterus also presses on your diaphragm, which is your largest breathing muscle. The increasing restriction of your diaphragm will force you to take more shallow breaths than you took prior to pregnancy. Focusing on deep "belly" breaths that expand your diaphragm will help keep this muscle strong and prepare you for the breathing required during labor. In fact, this diaphragmatic breathing technique is recommended whether you're pregnant or not.

Bones and muscles

The most noticeable physical change during pregnancy is seen in the musculoskeletal system. Each trimester, the fetus grows and the uterus expands, and this puts new stress on your bones, muscles, and joints. With this stress comes a change in your posture. Pregnancy requires strong muscles, large and small.

Joints

All women gain weight during pregnancy. This added weight increases the pressure on

Did You Know?

Shifting center of gravity

As your belly gets bigger, your center of gravity shifts forward to maintain an ideal distribution of internal and external loads placed on your body. The change in body shape and size makes for an increased risk of losing your balance and falling. (It is much more common for a pregnant woman to complain of tripping or falling.) To compensate for this shift, most pregnant women increase the curve in their lower back by letting their pelvises tip forward. Engaging in a prenatal resistance exercise program can counterbalance the postural changes and muscular imbalances that occur during pregnancy.

your joints during exercise. This may cause discomfort in healthy joints and possibly even damage those that may already be diseased, with arthritis, for example.

Pregnancy hormones loosen your joints to allow the baby to fit through your pelvis successfully, but the hormones loosen all the ligaments and joints of your body, not just the ones in your pelvic area. Therefore, it's important that you protect all of your joints during exercise in pregnancy. This also means that during pregnancy, you will experience a newly expanded range of motion. This is due to the laxity of the joints, not your muscles. Activities that involve quick changes in direction should be done with caution because your loosened joints increase the risk of injury. Strengthening the muscles surrounding the joints can help reduce this risk.

Multiples advice

If you are pregnant with twins or other multiple gestations, exercise is only recommended early in your pregnancy. Low-impact activities are best; these include walking, swimming, yoga, and water aerobics. Keep well hydrated by drinking plenty of water before your session.

Carrying more than one baby is such a workout that you may need to adjust your activity, not only with respect to exercise but also for other daily routines. Additional rest periods will be required to get you off your feet. Consider taking a nap during the day.

Breathing will become more difficult as a multiple pregnancy advances, because the babies are taking up more room and your diaphragm is being pushed up. This

Did You Know?
Changes in posture during pregnancy

Pelvis
To accommodate new stress on your bones, muscles, and joints, your pelvis will tilt forward, creating increased lumbar curve to your lower spine. The pelvis not only tilts forward, it also spreads in preparation for the baby's passage through the birth canal.

Feet
Fallen arches are a result of the hormones released during pregnancy. They place more stress on the instep of your foot and affect the knee-to-foot angle.

Upper body
Due to hormonal changes, your breasts become larger, in preparation for nursing your baby. The surrounding soft tissue attachments to the enlarged breasts cause your shoulders and upper back to round forward. This creates a forward head position, spreading of the shoulder blades, and rounding of your mid-back.

Back
Backaches are a very frequent complaint during pregnancy. Maintaining a healthy posture through exercise will reduce the chances of suffering back discomfort.

sense of "shortness of breath" is also a result of your heart working harder to pump more blood. Modify your activity during the day to compensate for these demands on your body.

If you are dizzy or feel any pain or heart palpitations, stop exercising immediately.

Preparing for an exercise program

Before starting an exercise program, ask your health-care provider to assess your overall health, obstetrical history, and medical risks. Consider your age, general physical condition, exercise history, obstetrical history, risk factors for heart disease, muscle and joint problems, previous injuries, use of medication, and the presence of chronic conditions, lung disease, or physical disabilities. With the help of your health-care providers, you can develop an exercise routine for all three trimesters that best suits you.

Types of exercise

There are three types of exercise you should integrate into any pregnancy exercise program — flexibility, strength, and aerobic exercises.

Flexibility and stretching exercises

Flexibility exercises include mobility, stability, and range of motion routines. Due to the increased laxness of your joints, be careful when doing flexibility exercises. There have been no documented long-term detrimental effects observed on the baby during this type of exercise.

Guide to...

Starting a program

- If you haven't exercised before, set a goal of 30 minutes of exercise a day.
- Start with 5 minutes each day.
- Add 5 minutes of exercise each week until the 30-minutes-a-day goal is reached.
- Start and end each session with 5 to 10 minutes of warm-up and cool-down exercises, such as slow walking and diaphragmatic breathing.
- As a rule of thumb, if you still feel good, continue increasing the intensity of your exercise; if you do not, decrease your exercise until it is tolerable.

Strength and resistance exercises

Strength exercises include resistance and weight training routines. Smaller weights with multiple repetitions through a full range of motion are considered ideal in pregnancy. Start with 5-pound (2.25 kg) dumbbells or even a can of soup.

Aerobic exercises

Aerobic exercise, also known as cardiovascular training, consists of any activity that uses large muscle groups in a continuous, rhythmic manner. This includes walking, swimming, cycling, and rowing. Activities such as skiing and cycling are great aerobic exercises, but they carry risk related to the possibility of falling. Swimming is an excellent aerobic exercise because it decreases the pressure on your joints, does not involve

Contraindications to exercise

Absolute contraindications

If any of the following conditions are present, do not start (or immediately stop) exercising:

- Ruptured membranes (your waters have broken)
- Preterm labor
- Hypertension or pre-eclampsia
- Incompetent cervix
- High-order multiple gestation (triplets or more)
- Placenta previa
- Persistent second or third trimester bleeding
- Uncontrolled Type I diabetes or other serious cardiovascular or respiratory disorders

Relative contraindications

If any of the following conditions are present, consult your health-care providers before starting or continuing exercise:

- Mild to moderate cardiovascular or respiratory disease
- Twin pregnancy after the 28th week
- Excessive shortness of breath
- Chest pain
- Lightheadedness, dizziness
- Painful uterine contractions
- Leakage of amniotic fluid
- Vaginal bleeding

lying on your back for prolonged periods, and reduces the risk of overheating. And balance and falling are not a worry.

Intensity

If you have not been exercising regularly, increase the length of time you exercise and how hard you work gradually. Pregnancy is not a time to markedly improve physical fitness, but rather it is a time to maintain it. Most pregnant women find that their fitness levels decline as the pregnancy progresses.

You can gauge the intensity of your workout by determining your target heart rate range, which involves taking your pulse and recording it. If you're a beginner, start your routine at the bottom end of your range and increase it to the top. Don't overdo it.

Go slowly

If you were sedentary prior to getting pregnant, be cautious about starting a cardiovascular routine without supervision. Go slowly. If you took part in exercise programs before pregnancy, continue exercising through the first trimester, but slow down to avoid overheating and dehydration.

Did You Know?

Basal metabolic rate

Your basal metabolic rate (the energy you "burn" to stay alive) is higher in pregnancy. You must, therefore, be very careful not to get overheated during exercise. This is more likely to happen if you are exercising in a warm climate. You should drink enough water to maintain a good level of hydration.

HOW TO...

Calculate your target heart rate range

To calculate your target heart rate range:

- Subtract your age from 220 to arrive at your age-predicted maximum heart rate (MHR)
- Multiply this number by 0.65 (65%) and 0.85 (85%) to arrive at your target heart rate range

For example, if you are 30 years old:

- 220 – 30 = 190 MHR
- 190 × 0.65 = 123
- 190 × 0.85 = 161

Therefore, the lower end of your heart rate range is 123 beats per minute and the higher end is 161. Aim to start your exercise routine at the lower end of the range and end the routine at the higher end.

Talk test

If calculating your heart rate to gauge the intensity of your workout is inconvenient, try the "talk test." Increase your exercise intensity to the point where conversation is difficult but not impossible.

Glossary of exercise terms

Body core (torso)	Middle section of the body, from the shoulders to the groin. Core muscles provide stability, balance, and flexibility.
Dumbbell	Handweights of a fixed weight used as part of resistance exercise, unlike barbells with adjustable weights used in weight training
Intensity	A measure of how hard you are exercising, indicated by your heart rate compared to your maximum heart rate
Functional exercises	Exercises that mimic everyday activities at work and at home, focusing on body core flexibility and strength
Machine exercises	Exercises done on machines with adjustable weights that create resistance and guide range of motion
Range of motion (ROM)	Distance between the flexed (bent) position and the extended position of a joint
Repetition (rep)	One complete range of motion for a movement or resistance exercise
Resistance	An opposing force
Rest	Time period between sets of repetitions
Set	A fixed number of repetitions
Stability ball (Swiss or exercise ball)	Inflatable ball used for support during exercises, usually 2 to 3 feet (60 to 90 cm) in diameter
Tempo	Speed of a repetition of a resistance movement, with a slow tempo preferred because it requires concentrated strength throughout the range of motion

General exercise routine

Let us emphasize that if you are pregnant and did not exercise consistently prior to getting pregnant, consult with your health-care provider before starting any new routine.

Warm-up

Start your exercise routine with a 5- to 10-minute circulatory system warm-up. The warm-up increases your heart rate, which dilates your blood vessels, allowing more oxygen and blood to be delivered to your body's working tissues and your fetus. Examples of effective circulatory warm-up exercises are walking, cycling, elliptical machine training, and rowing at a slow to moderate pace.

Flexibility and stretching exercises

Once the circulatory warm-up is completed, a few range of motion and balance exercises will increase your flexibility, mobility, and stability. These exercises improve your posture, lubricate your joints, and increase your coordination.

Range of motion exercises for your pelvis (lower body) and shoulder girdle (upper body) prepare you for childbirth and child care in the early postpartum days. As the alignment of your body changes in pregnancy, your ankles and feet become less stable and your walking pattern and weight distribution change. The goal of balance and stability exercises is to increase your awareness of your ankles and feet and their respective joints and ligaments. These exercises reduce the chances of injury to these joints — and reduce your chance of falling.

Stretches should only be taken to the point of mild tension, never pain. Hold each stretch for a maximum of 30 seconds.

Strength and resistance exercises

Because the load on your musculoskeletal system increases throughout the 40 weeks of your pregnancy, functional training (rather

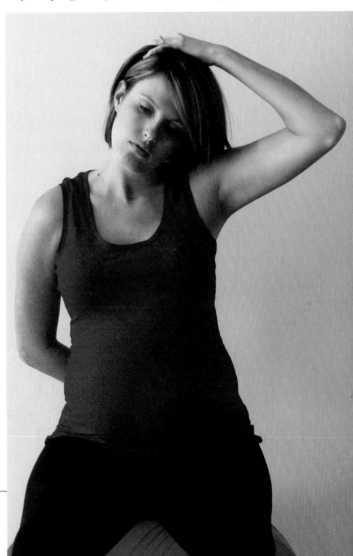

than machine training) is recommended. Functional exercises use multiple muscle groups by linking muscle chains, whereas machine training isolates a targeted muscle.

A functional prenatal program prepares you for each trimester and its associated physical and physiological changes. It will also help you deal with your changed posture. Functional exercises also prepare you for motherhood and all its related tasks, such as putting the baby in a crib. The baby is now an external load that your body must learn to adapt to holding. These strength exercises will teach your body to be more functional, preparing you to execute your daily tasks, prenatal and postnatal, with more ease.

Aerobic exercises

The cardiovascular, or aerobic, portion of your exercise routine should be done after the strength and resistance training so you do not exhaust your working muscles. Cardiovascular conditioning can be done 3 to 5 times per week at an intensity that allows you to carry on a conversation without becoming breathless.

Cool-down exercises

Once you have finished your routine, gradually allow your heart rate and breathing to return to normal, where talking can be performed with ease. Cool down using diaphragmatic breathing and slower versions of warm-up exercises, such as slow walking, stationary bicycling, and light stretching. This will help prevent muscle injury.

Kegel exercises

Kegel exercises help maintain bladder control during and after pregnancy and strengthen the muscles of the pelvic floor (which will help you during labor and delivery). To do a Kegel exercise, pretend you are stopping the flow of your urine "mid-stream" by pulling up on your pelvic floor and contracting your bladder. You can do Kegels slowly or quickly — slowly by holding the contraction for a count of three or quickly by tightening and quickly relaxing the muscle continuously. Try doing Kegels in sets of 10 repetitions (10 times in a row) at least 3 or more times a day. Kegel exercises should be done several times a day, and not just during pregnancy, but for the rest of your life.

Diaphragmatic breathing exercises

Like Kegel exercises, diaphragmatic breathing (or "belly breathing") should be done several times and become a lifelong habit. Diaphragmatic breathing exercises involve placing one hand on your chest and the other on your belly. As you breathe in (inhale), your belly should rise, rather than your chest. As you breathe out (exhale), your belly should fall. Do this several times a day until your body does it automatically. Most people were taught to do the reverse when they breathe — "Chest out! Stomach in!" — which prevents both maximal oxygen uptake and complete movement of the lungs.

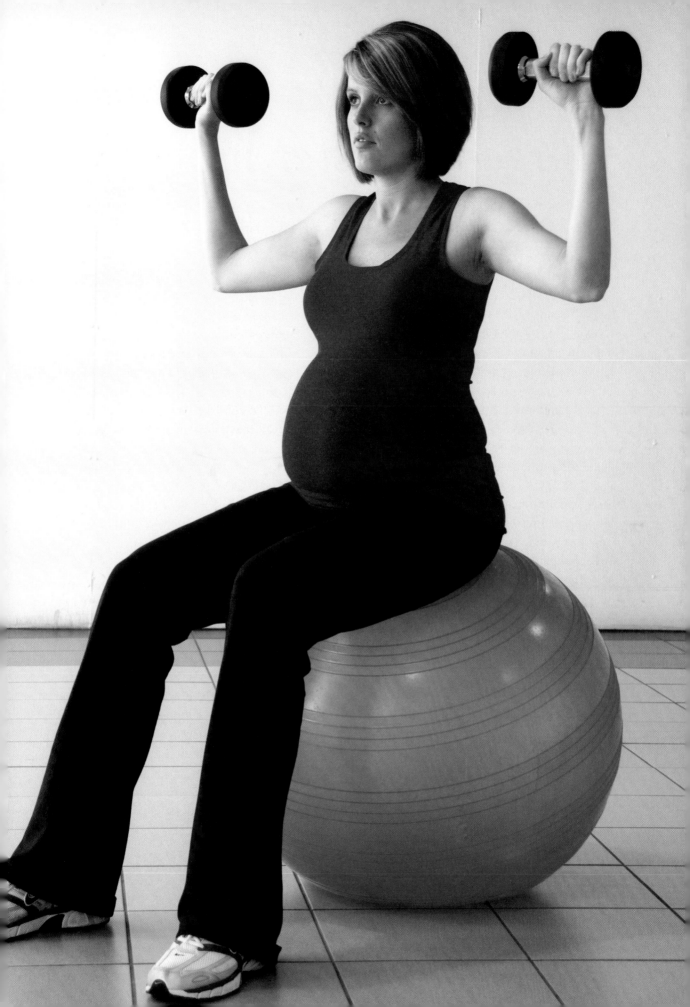

Three-trimester program

Following are three routines — one for each trimester — that you can follow regularly. These routines are designed for a moderately active woman.

Objectives

- **First trimester routine:** The objective of this routine is to prepare your body for the postural and muscular changes that occur during pregnancy.
- **Second trimester routine:** The objective of this routine is to further prepare your body for the postural and muscular changes that occur during pregnancy, with greater emphasis on body core stability.
- **Third trimester routine:** The objective of this routine is to prepare your body for your increasing body weight and changing shape during this trimester. You will find that certain exercises are becoming more difficult. Modify your program based on how you feel. In a word, if it doesn't feel good anymore, stop doing it. Most women find they cut back their exercise routine during this trimester. Let your body tell you when it is time to stop exercising due to fatigue, but still continue to maintain a regular workout schedule, even if it is less intense. Non-weight-bearing activities, such as cycling or swimming, may be the most comfortable options.

Staging

For all three routines, begin with a 5- to 10-minute circulatory warm-up in order to prepare your body and prevent injury. Follow this with flexibility and stretching exercises, strength and resistance exercises, and aerobic conditioning. Finish up with some cool-down exercises. Don't forget your Kegels and breathing routines.

Guidance

Discuss these routines with your health-care providers before starting them and consider consulting a physiotherapist or certified fitness coach to guide you at the beginning. In most exercises demonstrated here, a coach helps with positioning and spotting to prevent injury. Also consider exercising at a fitness center, where you will be matched with the best equipment. Once you feel safe in these exercises, you can practice at home, substituting professional equipment with home-made weights (cans of soup) and benches (stools and chairs), for example. Your partner makes a great spotter, once properly trained!

If you do not feel confident in doing these exercises at home, don't. Go to the gym and ask for a coach.

First trimester flexibility and stretching exercises

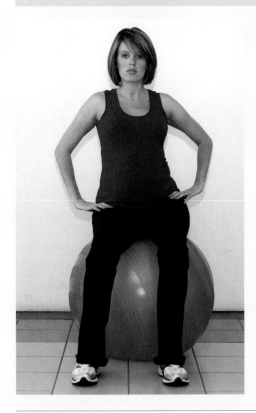

Pelvic rocking (front to back) seated on a stability ball

Reps: 10 / Duration: 6 sec

Instructions for One Repetition

1. Sit up straight on a stability ball. Have both feet flat on the floor with your hands on your hips in front of you.
2. To a slow count of 3, tilt your pelvis forward, bringing your tailbone up and arching your lower back.
3. To a slow count of 3, tilt your pelvis back, flattening your lower back.
4. Repeat this rocking motion in a continuous manner.

Benefits

- Makes the pelvis and lower back act in conjunction
- Warms up the lower back, stimulating blood flow to the area
- Relieves lower-back stress caused by prolonged standing or sitting

Shoulder press seated on a stability ball

Reps: 10 / Duration: 6 sec

Instructions for One Repetition

1. Sit upright on a stability ball, with your shoulders back. Keep both feet flat on the floor.
2. Keep your pelvis tilted back to flatten your lower back. Tighten your lower abdominals by pulling your navel back to your spine.
3. Hold a small weight in each hand at shoulder level, elbows out and bent 90 degrees.
4. To a slow count of 3, press the weights toward the ceiling by straightening your arms.
5. To a slow count of 3, return the weights to shoulder level to complete one repetition.

Benefits

- Reduces the stresses on your upper spine due to the increased breast size
- Maintains the mobility of the spine and shoulder girdle
- Allows the joints to move through their full range of motion
- Strengthens the arms and shoulders

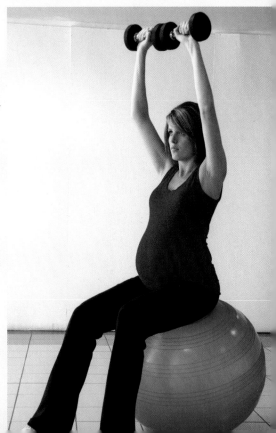

Ankle and foot awareness

Reps: 1–2 RL (right/left) / Duration: 15–30 sec

Instructions for One Repetition

1. Stand on one foot. (Use one hand to support yourself against a wall or chair if necessary.)
2. Keep your pelvis tucked in, with your hip bones facing forward.
3. Maintain alignment of the following three points: protruding bone at the front of your pelvis (anterior superior iliac spine); knee cap; second toe.
4. Hold the position for 15–30 seconds.
5. Repeat on the other side.

Benefits

- Reduces stress on the arches of the feet
- Helps the foot adapt to the unequal contours of the ground by distributing body weight and altering the curvature of the arches
- Strengthens muscles around the joints in order to reduce injury caused by hormones that relax the soft tissue stabilizers

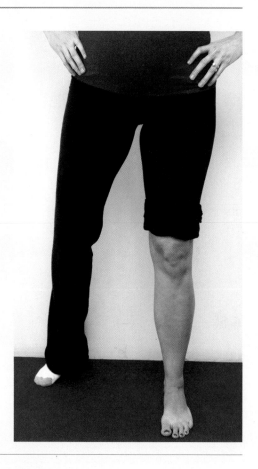

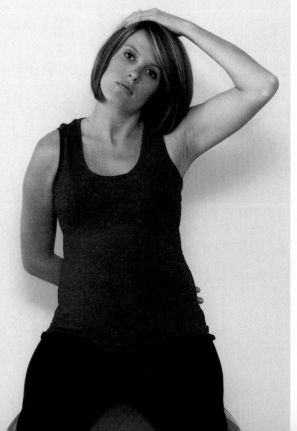

Lateral neck stretch

Reps: RL / Duration: 30 sec

Instructions for One Repetition

1. Sit or stand straight with your shoulders relaxed.
2. Tilt your head to your left side without bending it forward, bringing your left ear to your left shoulder.
3. Use your left hand to apply a gentle pressure to increase the neck stretch.
4. Place your right hand behind your back to increase the stretch.
5. Repeat on your right side to complete one repetition.

Benefits

- Reduces the stiffness and aches commonly felt in the neck as the center of gravity shifts forward
- Maintains a normal range of motion and proper alignment in the tissues of the neck that are being pulled forward due to the common postural deviations associated with pregnancy, such as a forward head posture, rounded shoulders, and increased arch in the lower back

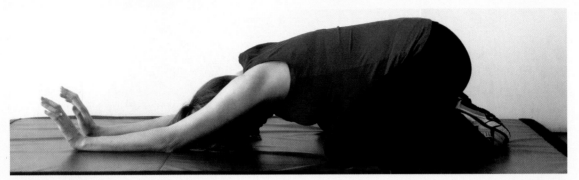

Back stretch

Reps: RL / Duration: 30 sec

Instructions for One Repetition

1. Kneel on a mat in an upright position, with your feet together and your toes pointing behind you. Lower yourself down to sit on your heels.

2. Settle back on your heels with your arms extended above your head, palms down.

3. Bend forward to rest your forehead on the mat, keeping your chin tucked.

4. Sit on a block or a blanket to reduce the strain on your knees or to make this stretch more comfortable.

Benefits

● Releases the tension placed upon the lower back musculature caused by the growing belly

● Prevents lower back discomforts associated with an increased lordosis (swayback) of the lumbar spine

Quadriceps and hip flexor stretch

Reps: RL / Duration: 30 sec

Instructions for One Repetition

1. Stand with both feet on the floor, hips facing forward and pelvis tilted back. Shift your weight and find your balance so you can stand on one foot, with your knee slightly bent.

2. Slowly bend your other knee and bring your foot up to your buttocks. Reach your hand back and grasp that foot by the toe.

3. Keep your hips forward and your body upright and straight (if necessary, extend your free hand to help you keep your balance).

4. Hold the position to a count of 30, slowly return to the standing position, and repeat on the other side.

Benefits

● Maintains the proper mechanics of the pelvis during the walking pattern

● Prevents injury to the muscles, allowing them to absorb the forces of impact during gait without placing undue strain on the spine, particularly the lower back

● Reduces tension in the lower back

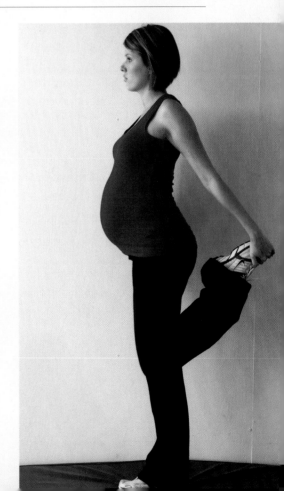

First trimester strength and resistance exercises

Choose weights that allow you to do 1 or 2 sets of 12 repetitions with some effort. These weights may be 5 pounds (2.25 kg) or they may be as low a weight as a can of soup that you can comfortably hold in your hand. The key is to be able to do the movements in a slow and controlled manner that takes your muscles to the point of fatigue. Progress to 2 sets of 15 repetitions. Once 2 sets of 15 repetitions can be completed with less effort, increase the amount of weight and go back to 2 sets of 12 repetitions.

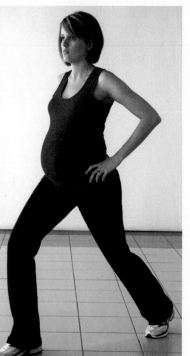

Stationary lunge

Rest: 45 sec / Reps: 12–15 RL (right/left)

Tempo: Moderate / Sets: 1–2

Instructions for One Repetition

1. Stand with both feet together, your pelvis tilted slightly back, and your lower abdominals tightened.
2. Take a long step forward and check your balance. Keep your toes forward, your hips facing forward, your chest up, and your spine straight.
3. Bend your knees and lower your body, lifting your back heel to allow you to drop lower.
4. Keep your lower abdominals tightened.
5. In a slow and controlled manner, lower your back knee toward the floor (keep your knee directly below your hip). Hold the position without touching the floor.
6. Maintain weight distribution over your heel and mid-foot.

Benefits

- Improves alignment of the leg relative to the pelvis, lower back, and foot
- Increases leg strength needed for the extra weight

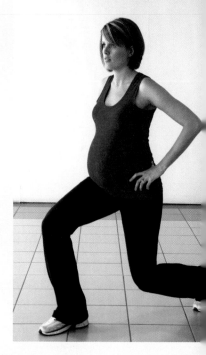

Lower abdominal draw-ins

Rest: 45 sec / Reps:10–12

Tempo: Hold 3 sec / Sets: 1–2

Instructions for One Repetition

1. Lying on your back on a mat, place one hand on your chest and the other on your stomach.
2. Inhale and expand your stomach only.
3. Exhale by pulling your stomach in.
4. Then draw your navel to your spine and hold for 3 seconds.

Benefits

- Strengthens the lower abdominals, which help decrease the strain placed on the lower back
- Helps during labor by strengthening the lower abdominals
- Supports the uterus

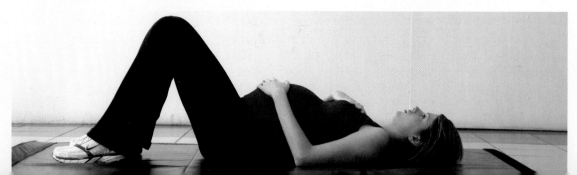

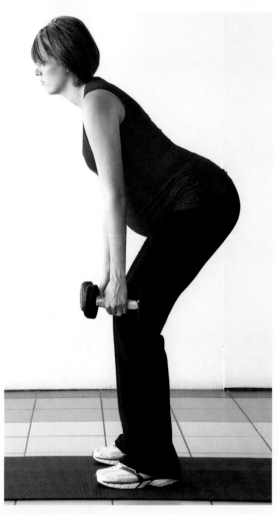
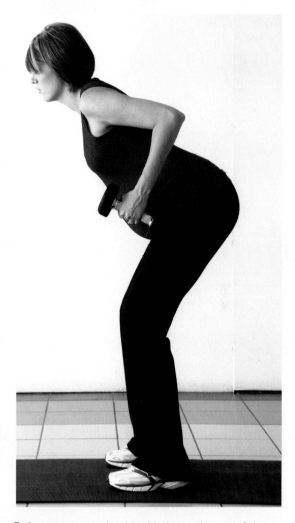

Bent-over row

Rest: 45 sec / Reps: 12–15

Tempo: Moderate / Sets: 1–2

Instructions for One Repetition

1. Holding a small weight in each hand, stand with your back straight.

2. Tilt your pelvis back and pull in your lower abdominals to set your core. Draw your navel in toward your spine to support your lower back.

3. Bend your knees slightly and then bend your torso forward at your hip joint, making an angle between 60 and 90 degrees.

3. Hold each weight with the palms of your hands facing each other, arms hanging down.

4. To a slow count of 3, raise your hands and bring the weight to your bottom ribs, until your elbow bends past 90 degrees.

5. Squeeze your shoulder blades at the top of the movement.

6. Slowly lower the weight back to starting position.

7. Keep control of your shoulder joints throughout execution.

Benefits

- Prevents the shoulder blades from winging and shoulders from rounding

- Prepares the back for all the bent-over activities you will engage in once the baby is born, such as sitting and nursing the baby or bending over and playing with your child

- Enables the muscles surrounding the thoracic spine to maintain natural spinal curvature

- Develops postural endurance in back muscles

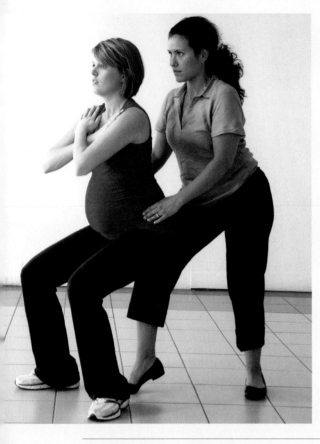

Squat

Rest: 45 / Reps: 12–15

Tempo: Moderate / Sets: 1–2

Instructions for One Repetition

1. Stand with your feet shoulder-width apart and arms crossed in front of you. Put your hands on the opposite shoulders. Keep your chest up and your spine natural.
2. Tighten your abdominals by pulling your navel to your spine.
3. Look forward (you may use a chair as a guide).
4. Breathe in, then lower yourself into a squat (imagine you are sitting on a chair) as you breathe out. Have a coach or spotter support you with her knee.
5. Lower yourself to a comfortable angle so you do not place undue stress on your knees.
6. Breathe in as you return to the starting position.
7. Ensure your knees remain behind your toes and your torso remains upright.
8. Maintain proper leg alignment: hip, knee cap, and second toe should all remain in alignment.

Benefits

- Strengthens the muscles in your buttocks
- Develops an essential movement pattern
- Trains the lumbar spine and upper back

Oblique crunch (side lying on a ball)

Rest: 45 sec / Reps:12–25 RL (right/left)

Tempo: Moderate / Sets: 1–2

Instructions for One Repetition

1. Place the stability ball close to a wall. Sit upright on the ball and turn your feet sideways to brace them against the wall.
2. Position yourself on your left side with your left hip on the ball. Hold your hips square (belly button facing forward) and use your left arm to stabilize yourself on the ball.
3. Put your top leg back and your bottom leg forward to brace and stabilize yourself more effectively
4. Use the muscles in your side to lower your body. Pause. Then raise your body (bring lower ribs to pelvis).
5. Change position and repeat on your other side.

Benefits

- Strengthens the muscles that help maintain the pelvis in place
- Helps support the growing uterus by acting as a girdle for the uterus

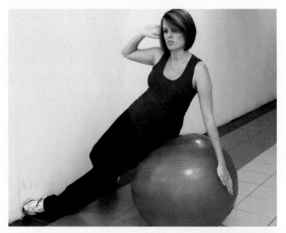

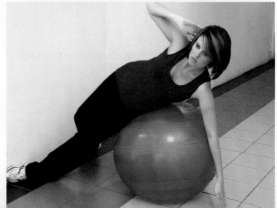

Dumbbell chest press with a bridge (lying on a ball)

Rest: 45 sec / Reps: 12–15

Tempo: Moderate / Sets: 1–2

Caution: Do this exercise with the help of a fitness coach or trained spotter.

Instructions for One Repetition

1. Position your upper back on the stability ball.

2. Lower your hips toward the floor, keeping your back on the ball, feet shoulder width apart.

3. With your elbows bent, hold small weights at shoulder level. Your palms should be facing.

4. Slowly lift the weights straight up toward the ceiling while simultaneously lifting your hips up to a "bridge" position.

5. Lower the weights with elbows out, maintaining wrist position over the elbows. Simultaneously lower your hips back to starting position.

6. Lower the weights until your wrists are level with your shoulders.

Benefits

- Strengthens the muscles in your buttocks
- Teaches the hip, pelvis, and core to stabilize while the hamstrings and thighs are moving dynamically
- Strengthens the posterior muscles
- Aids in the prevention of poor posture

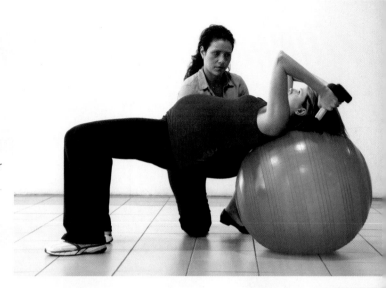

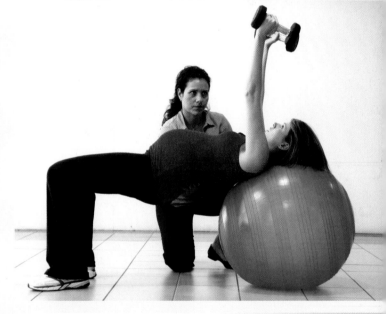

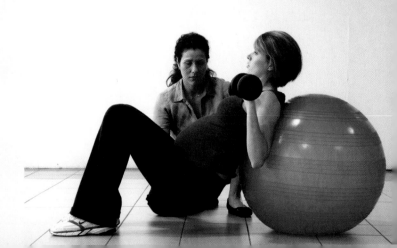

Second trimester flexibility and stretching exercises

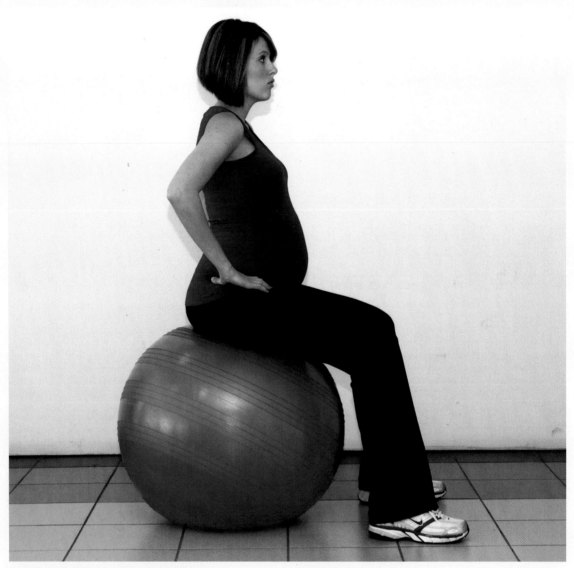

Pelvic rocking (side to side) on stability ball

Reps: 8–10 / Duration: 10 sec

Instructions for One Repetition

1. Sit up straight on a stability ball, with both feet on the floor and your hands on your hips.

2. Keep your torso as still and straight up as possible as you lift your right hip as high as is comfortable.

3. Drop your right hip and lift your left. Steps 2 and 3 are one repetition.

Benefits

- Makes the pelvis and lower back act in conjunction

- Warms up the lower back, stimulating movement and blood flow to the area

- Relieves the stress placed on the lower back from prolonged stationary activities, such as standing or sitting for long periods

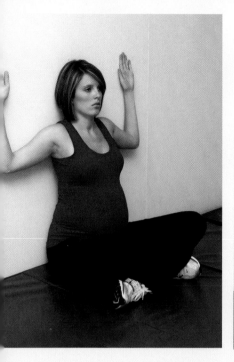
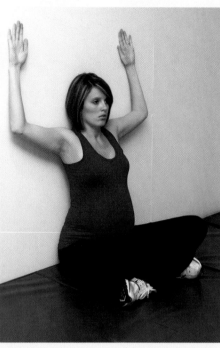
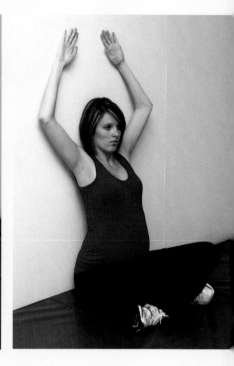

Shoulder girdle (seated on mat)

Reps: 4–6 / Duration: 10 sec

Instructions for One Repetition

1. Sit against a wall with your head, shoulder blades, lower back, and buttocks touching the wall.
2. Keep your lower back against the wall by slightly drawing your navel in toward your spine and tilting your pelvis back.
3. Raise your hands and put your shoulders back until your elbows are at 90 degrees and your shoulders, forearms, wrists, and hands are against the wall.
4. Breathe in and, as you breathe out, slide your arms up the wall toward the ceiling.
5. Breathe in as you lower your arms back to starting position. Breathe out.
6. Maintain all points of contact with the wall throughout the exercise; if you are arching your back, reposition your pelvis and abdominals.

Benefits

- Reduces the stresses placed on the thoracic spine due to the increased breast size
- Maintains the mobility of the thoracic spine and shoulder girdle
- Allows the joints to move through their full ROM using breathing

Chest stretch (against wall)

Reps: RL (right/left) / Duration: 30 sec

Instructions for One Repetition

1. Stand comfortably in a doorway or next to a wall with your arm on the door frame or wall, elbow at shoulder height and bent at 90 degrees.
2. Gently turn your body away from the door frame or wall and hold the stretch for 20 seconds.
3. Repeat on the opposite side

Benefits

- Relieves tension in the neck
- Improves posture
- Improves breathing
- Decreases kyphosis by increasing the range of motion

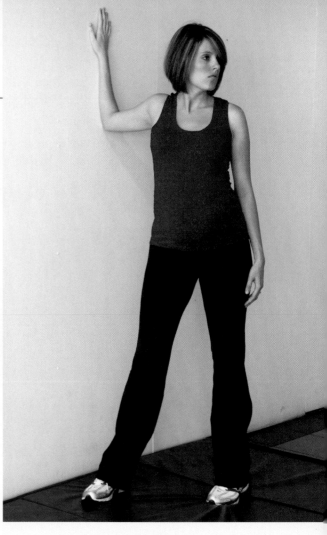

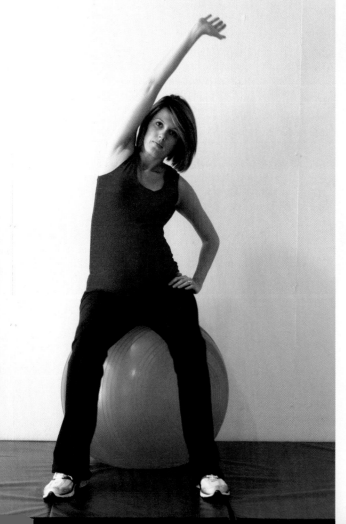

Side stretch (seated on a ball)

Reps: RL / Duration: 30 sec

Instructions for One Repetition

1. Sit up straight on the stability ball with your pelvis tilted slightly back and your feet flat on the floor.
2. Stretch your left arm overhead and then slowly stretch sideways, reaching to the right. Do not lean forward.
3. Flex your hand to enhance the stretch. Hold for 30 seconds.
4. Repeat on your right side.

Benefits

- Relieves tension in the deep muscles supporting the uterus
- Opens the ribcage for improved breathing
- Improves posture by stretching the side-bending muscles

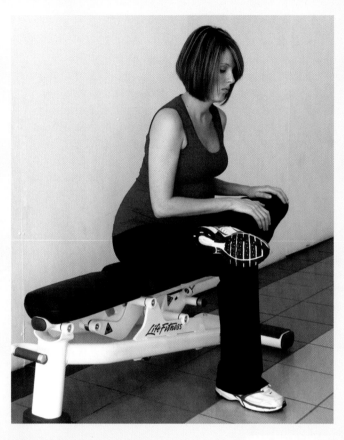

Piriformis stretch

Reps: RL / Duration: 10 sec

Instructions for One Repetition

1. Sit up straight in a chair or on a bench, then cross your legs and place your right ankle on top of your left knee.

2. Keeping your back straight, slowly lean your chest toward your right calf while gently pressing down on your right knee with your right hand.

3. Try to maintain a 90-degree angle between hips and knees of both legs.

Benefits

- Helps maintain a healthy back
- Decreases the discomforts associated with sciatica
- Improves the walking pattern by reducing the load on the pubic symphysis
- Increases stability when bending forward and when going up and down stairs

Hip abductor stretch

Reps: RL / Duration: 10 sec

Instructions for One Repetition

1. Sit comfortably in a chair or on a bench. Cross your left leg over your right.

2. Place your right hand on your left knee to brace yourself.

3. Extend your left arm behind you to hold onto the back of the chair or bench and gently twist your body to the left. Hold for 10 seconds.

4. Repeat on the opposite side.

Benefits

- Reduces tension in the spinal column muscles
- Improves walking
- Decreases tension placed on the groin

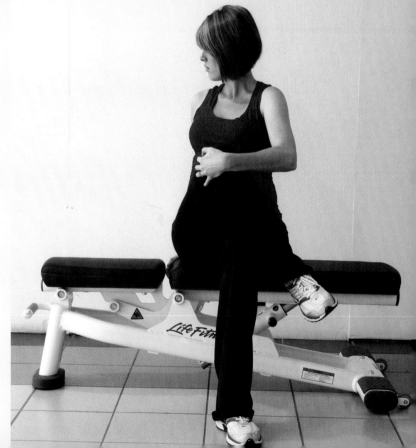

Second trimester strength and resistance exercises

Choose weights that allow you to do 1 or 2 sets of 12 repetitions with some effort. These weights may be 5 pounds (2.25 kg) or they may be as low a weight as a can of soup that you can comfortably hold in your hand. The key is to be able to do the movements in a slow and controlled manner that takes your muscles to the point of fatigue. Progress to 2 sets of 15 repetitions. Once 2 sets of 15 repetitions can be completed with less effort, increase the amount of weight and go back to 2 sets of 12 repetitions.

Bent-over reverse fly

Rest: 60 sec / Reps: 10–12

Tempo: Slow / Sets: 1–3

Instructions for One Repetition

1. Sit on a stability ball or a chair. Cross resistance bands under your feet. Bend over and lean your chest toward your thighs at a 30-degree angle. Pull your navel toward your spine.

2. Keep your spine and head in a natural position. Imagine a line running from your tailbone to your head.

3. The palms of your hands are facing each other, arms are slightly bent, and your feet are shoulder-width apart.

4. Open your arms and lift your wrists toward the ceiling. The only movement should come from your shoulder joints.

5. Squeeze your shoulder blades at the top of the movement.

6. Return to starting position in a slow and controlled manner and repeat.

Benefits

- Strengthens the posterior muscles of the shoulder to prevent rounded shoulders

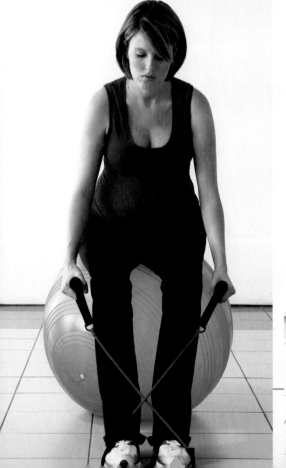
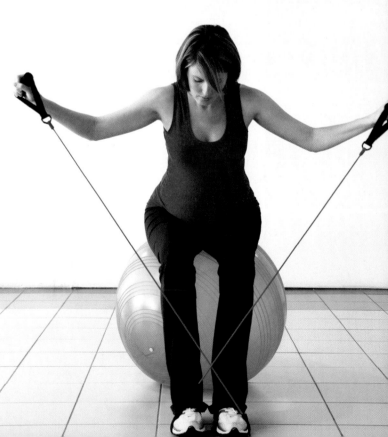

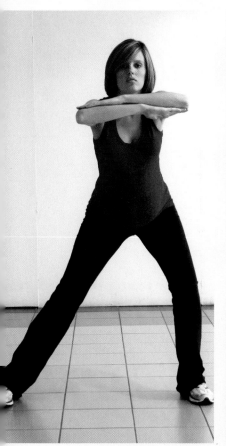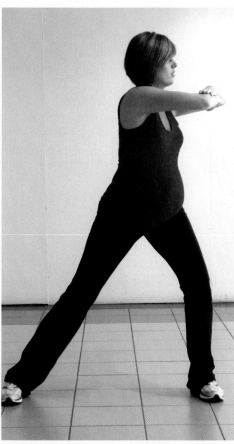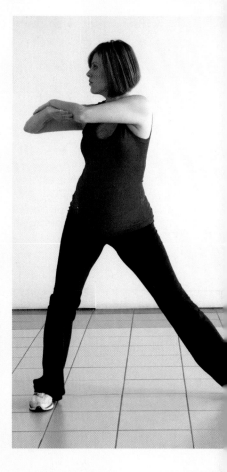

Lateral lunge with torso twist

Rest: 60 sec / Reps:10–12

Tempo: Slow / Sets: 1–3

Instructions for One Repetition

1. Stand straight with your feet shoulder-width apart, your hips facing forward, chest up with a natural spine.

2. Cross your arms in front of you at shoulder height or put your hands on your hips.

3. Stabilize your core by tilting your pelvis and pulling your navel to your spine.

4. Step out to the left, bending your left leg as you shift your weight onto it and stretch your right leg.

5. Rotate your upper torso to the left and sink further into the lunge, keeping your chest up and your hips forward at all times. Hold for 10 seconds.

6. Most of your weight should rest between the mid-foot and heel of the bent leg.

7. Repeat on the right side.

Benefits

- Strengthens the gluteal muscles, particularly the gluteus minimus and maximus

- Maintains the femur (thigh bone) in proper alignment with the hip bone (anterior superior iliac spine) and second toe

- Strengthening this area decreases the mechanical stress placed on the knee and ankle joints

Plié squat with dumbbell

Rest: 60 / Reps: 10–12

Tempo: Moderate / Sets: 1–3

Instructions for One Repetition

1. Stand with your feet wider than shoulder-width apart and toes pointing out approximately 30 degrees.
2. Holding a small weight with both hands, extend your arms. Keep your chest up with a natural spine and your navel pulled in to your spine as you set your core.
3. Breathe in; then lower yourself into a squat (imagine you are sitting on a chair) as you breathe out.
4. Lower yourself to a comfortable angle so you do not place undue stress on your knees.
5. Breathe in as you return to the starting position.
6. Ensure your knees remain behind your toes and your torso remains upright during the execution.
7. Maintain proper leg alignment: hip, knee cap and second toe should all remain in alignment.

Benefits

- Strengthens the gluteus muscles, particularly the gluteus minimus and maximus
- Maintains the femur (thigh bone) in proper alignment with the hip bone (anterior superior iliac spine) and second toe
- Strengthening this area decreases the mechanical stress placed on the knee and ankle joints

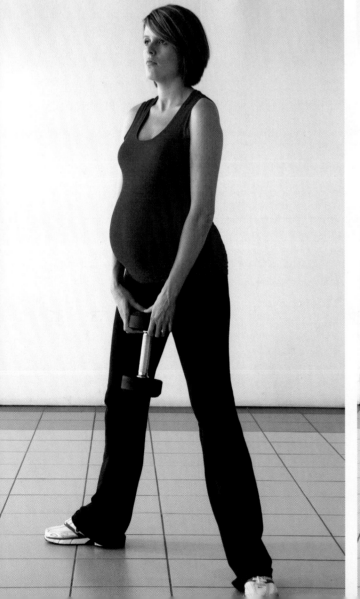
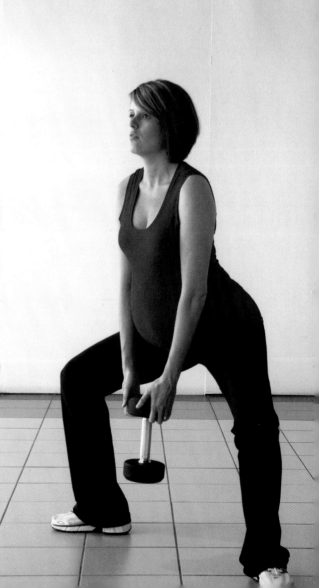

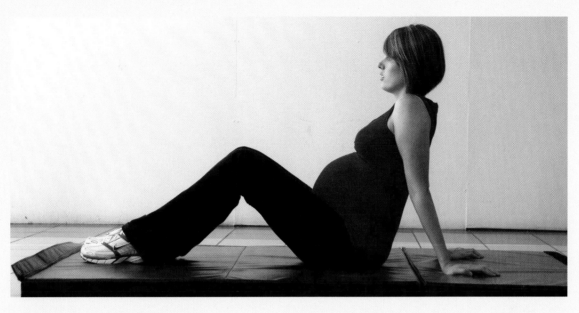

V-sit belly pull-ins (on a mat)

Rest: 45 sec / Reps:10–12

Tempo: Hold 5 sec / Sets: 1–2

Instructions for One Repetition

1. Sit on a mat on the floor with your knees bent and your feet flat on the floor.

2. Lean back so your body is angled approximately 45 degrees or to a comfortable position. Put your hands on the mat behind you and use your arms to support yourself from behind.

3. Breathe in.

4. As you breathe out, tuck your belly under (pull your belly toward your spine).

5. Breathe in.

Benefits

- Strengthens the lower abdominals, which help decrease the strain placed on the lower back
- Helps during labor by keeping the lower abdominal strong
- Supports the uterus

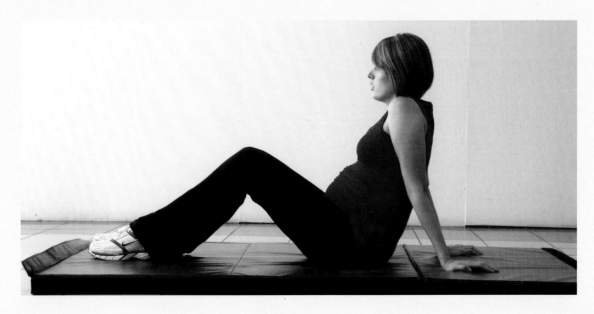

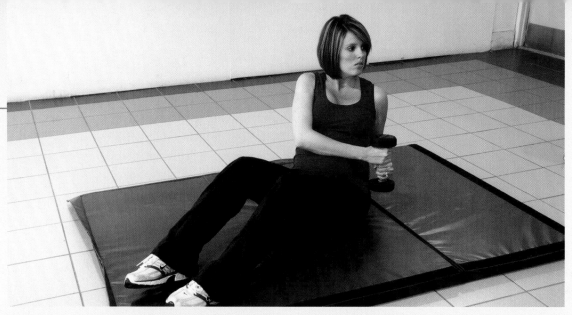

V-sit torso twist with dumbbell (on a mat)

Rest: 45 / Reps: 1–12 RL (right/left)

Tempo: Slow, controlled / Sets: 1–2

Instructions for One Repetition

1. Sit on a mat on the floor with your knees bent and your feet flat on the floor.
2. Set your body core by pulling your navel toward your spine.
3. Lean back so your body is angled at a comfortable position or at a maximum of 45 degrees.
4. Holding a weight with both hands in front of you, slowly twist your body to the left and then to the right while maintaining the "V" position.

Benefits

- Strengthens the quadratus lumborum muscle and external obliques, which help maintain the pelvis in place
- Helps support the growing uterus by acting as a girdle for it

---

Lying hip lift and hamstring curl (on a mat and ball)

Rest: 60 sec / Reps: 10–12

Tempo: Moderate / Sets: 1–3

Instructions for One Repetition

1. Lie on your back on the mat. Put your arms straight out on the mat, palms down. They will support you in this exercise.
2. Lift your feet and legs and pull the stability ball under your feet with the help of a coach or spotter.
3. Lift your hips, keeping your shoulders and head on the mat.
4. Bring your knees to your chest by rolling the ball toward you.
5. Continue to lift your hips toward the ceiling.
6. Lower your hips as you straighten your legs and roll the ball back.
7. Hold, then lower your body to the mat.

Benefits

- Teaches the hips, pelvis, and core to stabilize while the hamstrings and gluteals are moving dynamically
- Strengthens the extensor chain (posterior muscles)
- Aids in the prevention of poor posture

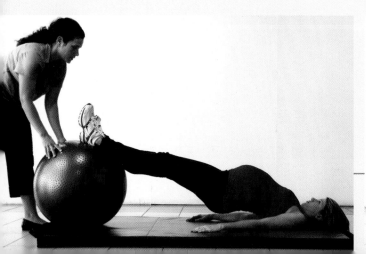

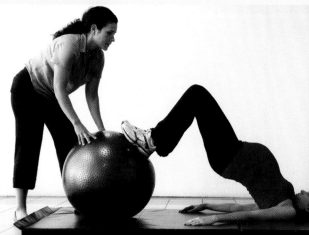

Third trimester flexibility and stretching exercises

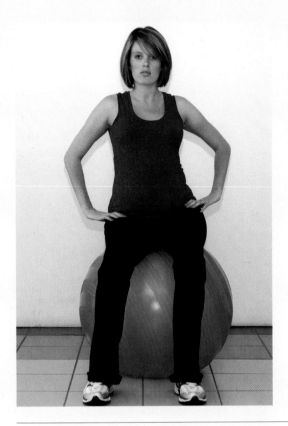

Pelvic rocking (figure-8) on a ball

Reps: 8–10 / Duration: 10 sec

Instructions for One Repetition

1. Sit up straight on a stability ball. Have both feet flat on the floor and your hands on your hips.
2. Slowly draw a figure-8 with your hips.

Benefits

- Makes the pelvis and lower back act in conjunction
- Warms up the lower back, stimulating movement and blood flow to the area
- Relieves the stress placed on the lower back from prolonged stationary activities, such as standing or sitting for long periods

Standing thoracic and shoulder girdle

Reps: 8–10 / Duration: 10 sec

Instructions for One Repetition

1. Stand with your arms stretched out to the sides at shoulder level, feet shoulder-width apart, knees slightly bent.
2. Turn your right arm palm up and your left arm palm down.
3. Reverse hand positions simultaneously; each time turn your head to look at your upturned palm.
4. Take a breath in while turning to the left; breathe out as you turn to the right.

Benefits

- Reduces the stresses placed on the thoracic spine due to the increased breast size
- Maintains the mobility of the thoracic spine and shoulder girdle
- Allows the joints to move through their full ROM

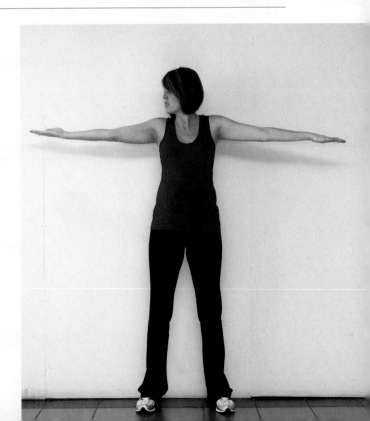

Medial arch awareness

Reps: 8–10 / Duration: 10 sec

Instructions for One Repetition

1. Stand on one foot. (Use one hand to support yourself against a wall or chair if necessary.)
2. Keep your pelvis tucked in, with your hip bones facing forward.
3. Maintain alignment with the following three points: protruding bone at the front of your pelvis (anterior superior iliac spine; knee cap; second toe.
4. Lift your big toe while keeping the rest of your toes on the floor.
5. Hold position for 15 to 30 seconds on each foot.

Benefits

- Reduces mechanical stress placed on the arches of the feet, particularly the medial arch (plantar fascitis)
- Allows the foot to adapt to the unequal contours of the ground by distributing body weight and altering the shape of curvature of the arches
- Strengthens the joints in order to reduce injury caused by hormones that relax the soft tissue stabilizers

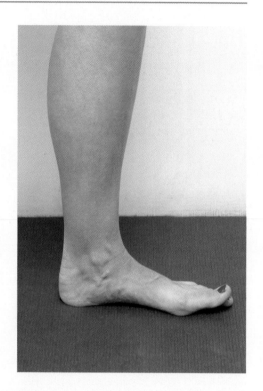

Levator scapulae stretch

Reps: RL / Duration: 30 sec

Instructions for One Repetition

1. Sit or stand in a comfortable position with your feet flat on the floor.
2. Put your left hand on the back of your head and gently pull your head forward. Point your chin to your underarm.
3. Place your right hand behind your back.
4. Repeat on the other side.

Benefits

- Reduces the stiffness and aches commonly felt in the neck and upper back muscles as the center of gravity shifts forward

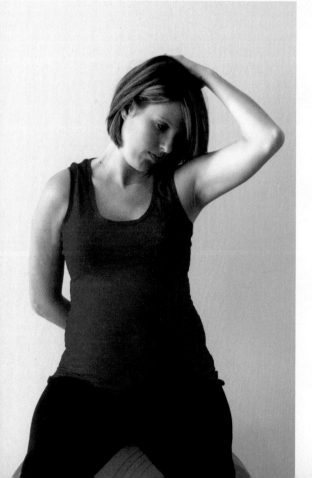

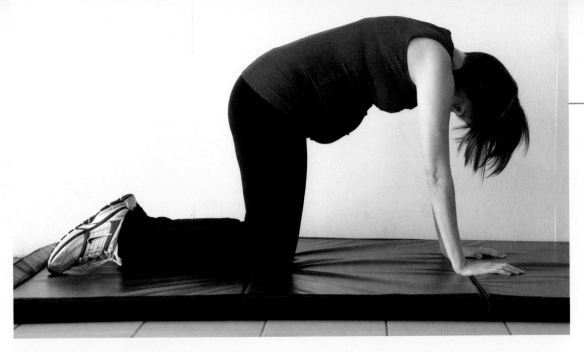

Back stretch (kneeling cat) on a mat

Reps: 10 / Duration: 10

Instructions for One Repetition

1. Get down on a mat on your hands and knees with your wrists directly under your shoulders and your knees directly under your hips.

2. Round your back, tucking your head down and your chin in, trying to create a "C" curve from head to tailbone.

3. Return to your starting position.

Benefits

- Increases mobility of the spine by stretching the spinal column, lower back, and upper back muscles

Biceps stretch

Reps: RL / Duration: 20 sec

Instructions for One Repetition

1. Stand beside a wall or in a doorway, facing left.

2. Stretch your right arm along the wall at shoulder height or hold on to the door frame.

3. Turn your body away from the wall or door frame.

4. Hold stretch for 20 seconds.

5. Repeat on the other side.

Benefits

- Decreases the tension of the tendons surrounding the anterior portion of the shoulder joint caused by rounded shoulders

- Improves posture

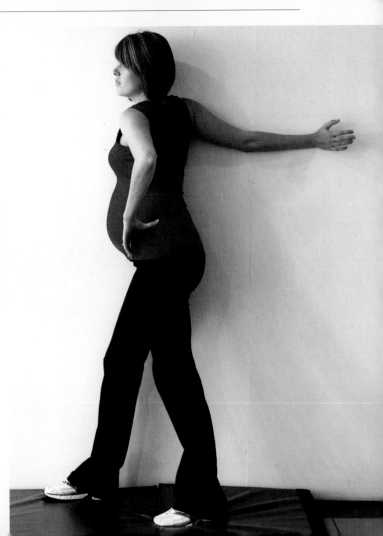

Third trimester strength and resistance exercises

Squats with ball against wall

Rest: 60 sec / Reps: 10–12

Tempo: Moderate / Sets: 1–3

Instructions for One Repetition

1. Place the stability ball between your lower back and a wall, with your feet shoulder-width apart and your hands on your hips.
2. Breathe in and roll the ball down the wall, lowering yourself into a squat (imagine you are sitting on a chair) as you breathe out.
3. Lower yourself to a comfortable angle so you do not place undue stress on your knees.
4. Breathe in as you roll the ball up the wall and return to starting position.
5. Ensure your knees remain behind your toes and your torso remains upright during the execution.
6. Maintain proper leg alignment: hip, knee cap, and second toe should all remain in alignment.

Benefits

- Strengthens the gluteus muscles
- Aids in the prevention of the pregnancy waddle
- Develops an essential movement pattern
- Trains the lumbar spine and upper back

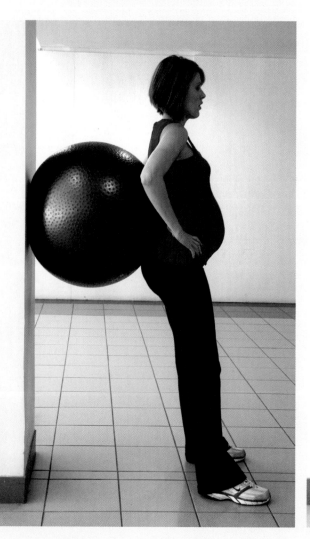

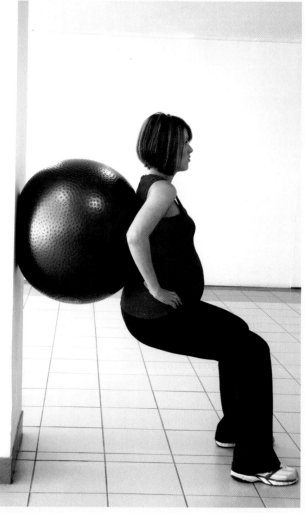

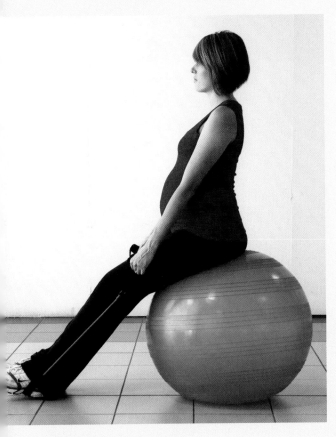 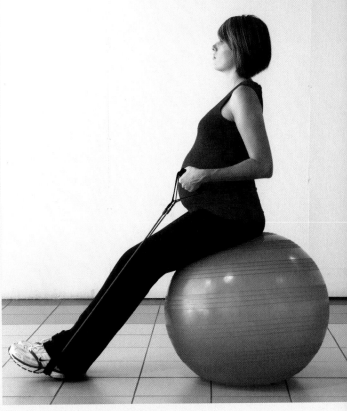

Seated row (on a ball)

Rest: 60 sec / Reps: 10–12

Tempo: Moderate / Sets: 1–3

Instructions for One Repetition

1. Sit on a stability ball in an upright position, chest up and shoulders back.
2. Anchor an elasticized band or tube under your feet by wrapping it around the soles of your shoes.
3. Draw your navel in toward your spine to set your core.
4. Pull the handles of the tubing back toward you without moving your torso.
5. Squeeze your shoulder blades at the end of the movement, then return to starting position (extended arm position).
6. Avoid locking your elbow joint when returning to starting position.

Benefits

- Prevents the shoulder blades from winging and shoulders from rounding
- Prepares the back for all the bent-over activities a woman will engage in once your baby is born, such as sitting and nursing the baby or bending over and playing with your child
- Encourages the muscles surrounding the thoracic spine to maintain its natural curvature

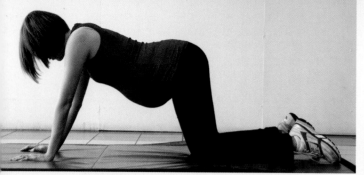
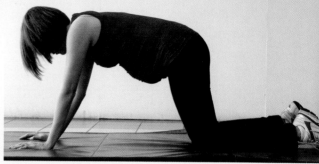

Kneeling belly pull-ins (on a mat)

Rest: 45 sec / Reps: 4–6

Tempo: Hold 3 sec / Sets:1–3

Instructions for One Repetition

1. Position yourself on the mat on your hands and knees with your wrists directly under your shoulders and your knees directly under your hips.
2. Breathe in (belly out). Hold for 3 seconds.

3. Breathe out (belly in). Hold for 3 seconds.
4. Pull your navel toward your spine and hold for 10 seconds.

Benefits

- Strengthens the lower abdominals, which help decrease the strain placed on the lower back
- Helps during labor by keeping the lower abdominals strong
- Supports the uterus

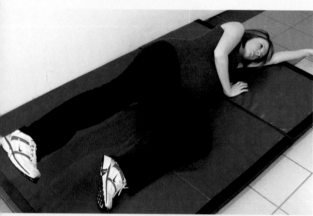

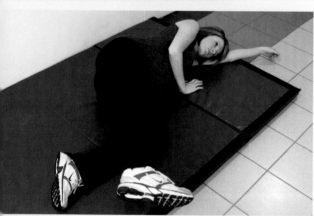

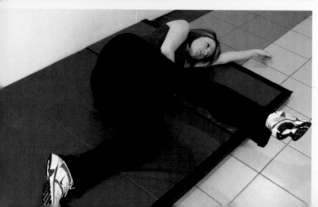

Leg lifts (side lying all three angles)

Rest: 45 sec / Reps: 12–15 on each side

Tempo: Moderate / Sets: 1–2

Instructions for One Repetition

1. Lie on a mat on your side with your shoulder, hip, knee, and ankle in a straight line.
2. Bend your bottom leg at 90 degrees or at an angle that stabilizes you on the mat.
3. Keeping your top leg straight, lift it toward the ceiling; tighten your buttocks at the same time.
4. Lower the leg slowly.
5. Ensure your hips remain parallel and in line with your shoulders throughout execution.
6. Avoid slumping your shoulders.

Benefits

- Strengthens the gluteus muscles, particularly the gluteus minimus and maximus
- Maintains the femur (thigh bone) in proper alignment with the hip bone (anterior superior iliac spine) and second toe
- Strengthening this area decreases the mechanical stress placed on the knee and ankle joints

Wall lean

Rest: 30 sec / Reps: 1

Tempo: Hold 30-60 sec / Sets: 1–2

Instructions for One Repetition

1. Standing with your back against a wall, lean your head against the wall. Use a towel to cushion your head.
2. Step away from the wall (approximately 12 inches/30 cm away), keeping only your head against the towel.
3. Tilt your head slightly back so you align your body in a straight line.
4. Hold the position for 1 minute.
5. When finished, bring one foot back, then the other, to slowly return to a standing position.
6. Avoid changing your position too quickly because it may cause dizziness.

Benefits

- Aids in the prevention of the forward head posture
- Decreases the strain on the neck muscles caused by poor posture

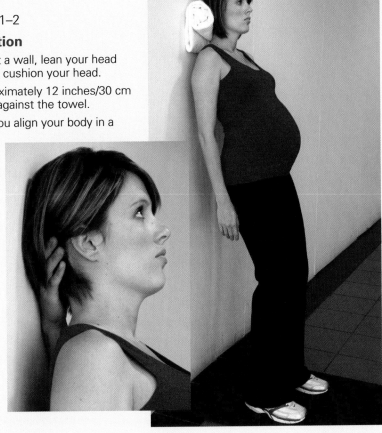

Kneeling alternate arm and leg lift

Rest: 45 sec / Intensity: Body weight

Reps: 4–6 RL / Tempo: Hold 3 sec / Sets: 1–2

Instructions for One Repetition

1. Position yourself on a mat on your hands and knees. Place your hands directly under your shoulders and keep your knees directly under your hips.
2. Lift your right arm and left leg simultaneously; hold the position briefly.
3. Repeat with opposite limbs (left arm and right leg).
4. Try to lift both to the same height.
5. Keep your thumbs up, fingers spread, and chin tucked (nose pointing down).
6. Avoid excessive curvature in your lower back.
7. Activate your buttocks.

Benefits

- Strengthens the posterior muscular chain
- Targets the muscles between the vertebrae
- Helps maintain a good working relationship between the upper and lower body

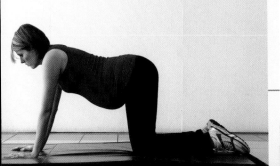
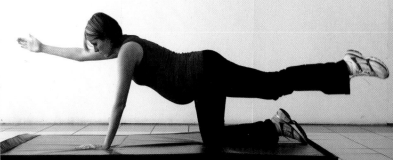

F.A.Q.

We answer many questions from pregnant women and their partners. Here are some of the most frequently asked questions. Be sure to ask your health-care providers any other questions that may arise. If they don't have the answers, they will refer you to a colleague who does.

Q: *Is it safe to lift weights during pregnancy?*

A: Yes, as long as you follow the guidelines discussed in this routine. Lift what feels comfortable without straining.

Q: *Can I lie on my back to do sit-ups?*

A: It's fine to lie on your back for sit-ups or other exercises. If you begin to feel dizzy, roll on to your side for a few minutes before resuming your routine.

Q: *Can I participate in a six-mile (10 km) run for fun?*

A: If you are already a runner before becoming pregnant, go ahead. Be sure to maintain good hydration and remember to stretch before and cool down after. If running is something new, now is not the time to begin training.

Q: *When can I begin to exercise after my baby is born?*

A: Whether your delivery was vaginal or Cesarean, you should always consult your health-care providers before beginning a postpartum exercise routine. When the go-ahead has been given, start by walking for 5 minutes and work your way up to 20 minutes of walking, 3 to 5 times per week. This routine can begin as early as 2 weeks after a healthy vaginal delivery.

If the delivery was Caesarean, you should wait at least 4 weeks before beginning an exercise program. Again, consult with your health-care provider first.

What's next

Now that you're feeling fit, you can keep up with the remarkable development of your fetus in the second trimester. There's no going back now…

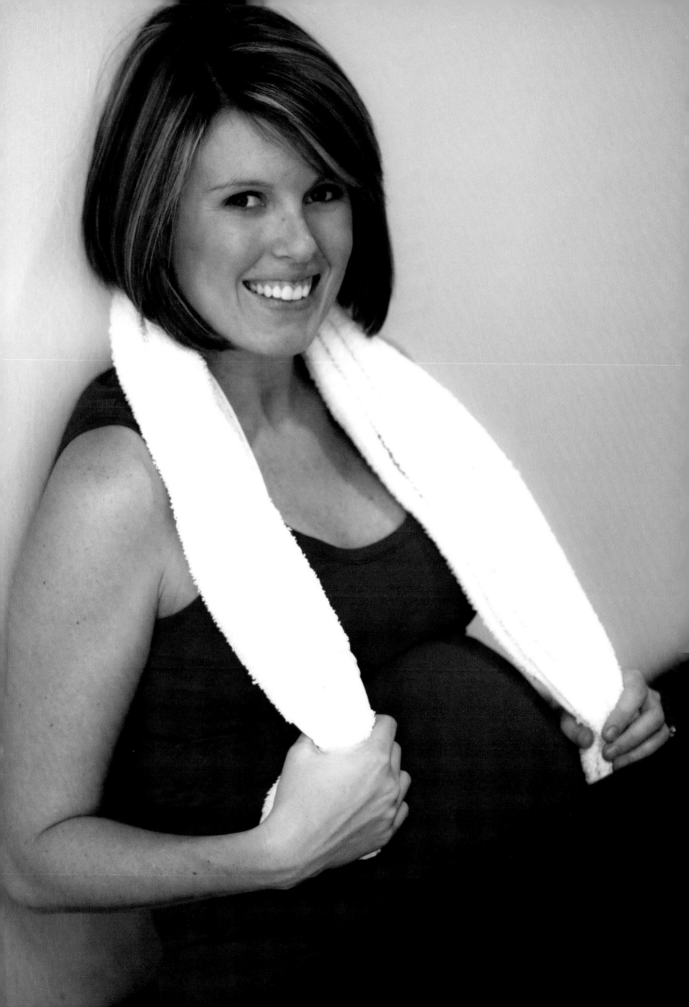

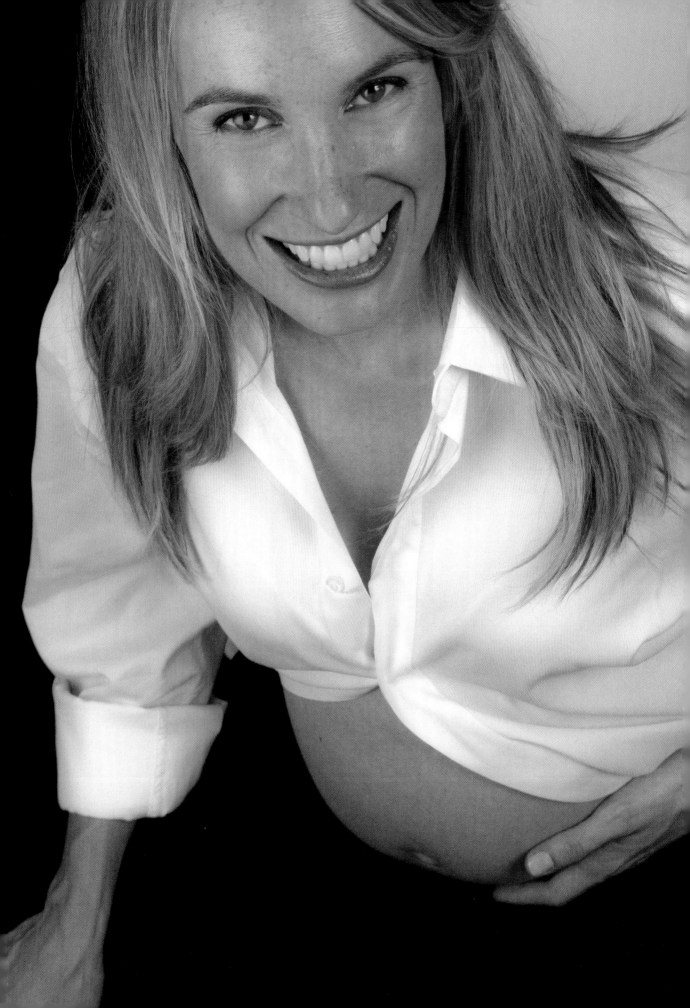

Part 6

Second Trimester Progress

Month 4 to 6 (Week 13 to 27)

It's for real!

During the second trimester, your pregnancy will begin to seem more real to you. The fetus will be very active, kicking his legs and moving his arms, even doing flips, although you probably won't feel those until about 20 weeks because the fetus is too small. But you will be able to see these gymnastics on an ultrasound. It's common to have an ultrasound between 18 and 20 weeks, and you will see lots of movement at that time. You may even be able to learn the gender of the fetus (if you want to!).

Ten tips for a healthy second trimester

1. Share the good news with family and friends if you haven't already.
2. Consider enrolling in an exercise class designed for pregnant women or modify your exercise routine to accommodate your pregnancy.
3. Eat well, ensuring you are getting plenty of iron and calcium.
4. Continue taking your prenatal vitamins.
5. If flu season is coming up, get a flu shot.
6. Continue to avoid alcohol, cigarettes, and any recreational drugs.
7. Try to get plenty of sleep.
8. Don't neglect important relationships in your life. You will need all the support you can get once the baby is born!
9. Enlist the help of your family and friends as you start to prepare a healthy home environment for your baby.
10. Relax and enjoy the second trimester — often women feel their best in this trimester!

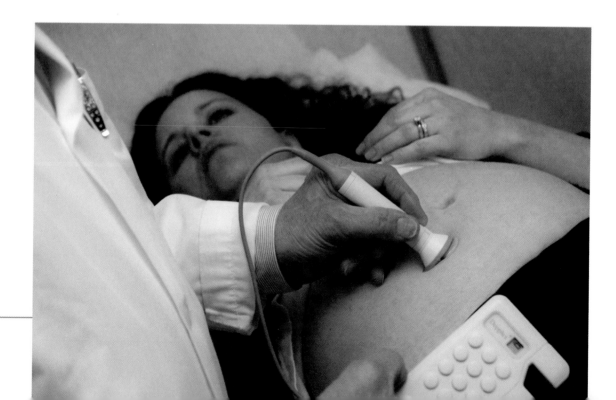

Month 4 fetal growth and development

There are very few new structures that develop from this point on — the most important aspect of fetal development is now growth! The fetus is recognizably human and has all his organs in place.

Pregnancy milestones
At week 13

- At week 13, the fetus is 3.4 inches (8.5 cm) long from crown to rump and weighs 1.6 ounces (45 g).
- The face is developing, with a tiny chin, ears, and nose.
- The eyes are moving to the front of the face.
- The hands are developing and soon will be able to grip — perhaps the nearby umbilical cord.
- The head is growing to accommodate the developing brain.

At week 16

- At week 16, the fetus is 5.5 inches (14 cm) long from crown to rump and weighs 5.3 ounces (150 g).
- The toenails start to develop.
- The ears stand out from the head.
- The limbs are well developed.
- The head is in better proportion to the rest of the body.
- The fetus starts to swallow amniotic fluid, then filter it through the kidneys and turn it into urine.
- The bones are starting to harden.

Embryo at 16 Weeks

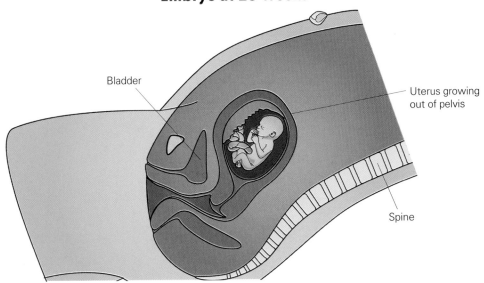

Bladder

Uterus growing out of pelvis

Spine

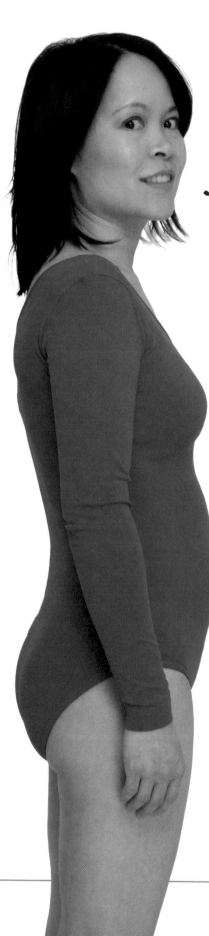

Looking and feeling pregnant

There's little chance of disguising it now — you look pregnant. Your waist is thickening, and you may not fit into your old jeans anymore. People will notice a "bump" soon, if they haven't already. Your uterus has grown, and you can now feel it above your pubic bone. By 16 weeks, the top of your uterus will lie about halfway between your pubic bone and your belly button. It's time to get out those maternity clothes you've bought and borrowed so you feel comfortable and give your body room to grow.

There are few surprises in how you feel early in the second trimester. Most women consider the second trimester the best part of pregnancy — the nausea and fatigue are reduced and the physical discomforts of the third trimester have not yet set in. Enjoy it!

- Your nausea (if you had any) might be starting to get better by now.
- Your breasts might be less sore, although they may continue to grow in size.
- Your energy might be beginning to return by this stage.
- You might feel some cramps or pain in your sides, which is generally attributed to the uterus growing and stretching the supporting ligaments.
- You might have a stuffy nose and even be more prone to nosebleeds because the blood vessels in your nose are enlarged and a little bit fragile.
- You might have more headaches than you used to — usually an effect of the increased estrogen levels in your body.
- You may be constipated.

Skin and nail changes

In addition to the skin pigmentation changes you saw in your early pregnancy, other changes now begin to become pronounced. You may also notice your nails growing more quickly than pre-pregnancy, but they may develop grooves, be brittle, and break more frequently.

Moles

You may see changes in your moles, mostly darkening and sometimes growing larger. While it is not clear if pregnancy affects moles adversely, some moles can be abnormal, and any unusual mole should be checked by a doctor and possibly biopsied to make sure that it is not a skin cancer.

Back pain

Back pain in pregnancy is understandably very common. Some of the pain can be attributed to changes in your posture and weight secondary to the pregnancy. Other sources of back pain can result from nerve compression from the fetus and uterus pushing on a nerve from the inside. Some women develop a particular pain called sciatica, which often begins in the lower back and radiates down one buttock into the back of the upper thigh.

Treating back pain

Although there is nothing that can be done to cure the pain, some treatments may reduce your pain:

- Try to be active and keep your back muscles in shape.
- Consider wearing a pregnancy belt, which is strapped under your belly to support your uterus and which takes some stress off your back.

Signs of an abnormal mole

- Changes shape, particularly if the borders become irregular instead of smooth and round
- Changes color, especially if the mole looks patchy or has multiple colors within it
- Becomes itchy or painful
- Bleeds or gets crusty
- Looks inflamed

- Try massage therapy and physiotherapy for specific exercises.
- If you need to take a medication for the pain, try acetaminophen. Avoid muscle relaxants.
- Try to remain optimistic — most pregnancy-related back pain will resolve after the pregnancy is over.

Did You Know?

Mask of pregnancy

The technical term for what's known as the mask of pregnancy is melasma, which occurs to some degree in up to 75% of pregnant women. Women who are affected develop hyper-pigmented (darker) brown or gray-brown patches on their faces. You can protect your face from the sun with sunscreen and a hat to try to prevent melasma, but since there are probably genetic factors involved, this may not be enough. Melasma usually fades after pregnancy, but not always. If it doesn't disappear, it can be treated with bleaching cream or chemical peels.

Carpal tunnel syndrome

Pregnant women who have some generalized swelling in their pregnancy feel numbness and tingling in their hands and fingers, especially during the night. Some of the nerves leading to the hands pass under the carpal tunnel, a dense, fibrous band of tissue that encircles your wrist. Compression of the nerves running through this tunnel is called carpal tunnel syndrome.

As long as you have not lost strength in your hands, this is not a serious problem, just an uncomfortable one.

What can you do? In severe cases, splints can be worn on your wrists to maintain them in a neutral position (that is, not bent forwards or backwards) to minimize the amount of pressure on these nerves; most people just wear them at night. It will get better after you deliver the baby.

Did You Know?

Veins, veins go away

The increased levels of estrogen in your body in pregnancy create havoc with veins, especially the ones you can see in your skin. Spider veins develop in 66% of Caucasian pregnant women and 10% of black women. They look like little red spiders, with branches leading out from a central area, and can appear around your eyes, as well as on your neck, face, chest, arms, and hands.

Varicose veins are another kind of vein that develops during pregnancy. These develop because of increased blood volume in pregnancy and because of pressure on your veins from your growing uterus. They are most commonly seen in your legs but can also be seen in the vulva. You can try to avoid developing varicose veins in your legs by wearing support hose, keeping your feet up, exercising, and avoiding being on your feet for long periods of time. There is not much you can do about varicose veins in your vulva, although support panty hose may provide some comfort. Hemorrhoids (dilated veins in your rectum) can be treated with medications. The good news is that varicose veins get a lot better after pregnancy, sometimes going away entirely.

Month 4 medical check-up

At your month 4 visit, your health-care providers will check your weight, blood pressure, and the protein level in your urine. They will check that your uterus is growing well by using their hands (palpating) to see where your uterus is reaching. You can listen to the fetal heart again using the doptone. There may be some blood test results to review with your health-care provider as well. The visit will probably be shorter than your first trimester visit. Be sure to bring a list of any questions that have arisen since your previous appointment. Record these in "My Pregnancy Diary" in this book.

Month 4 tests

Depending upon the kind (if any) of genetic screening you requested, there may be a follow-up diagnostic test at about 16 weeks.

If you have requested amniocentesis to test for any problems with the growth and development of the fetus, the procedure is usually scheduled during month 4.

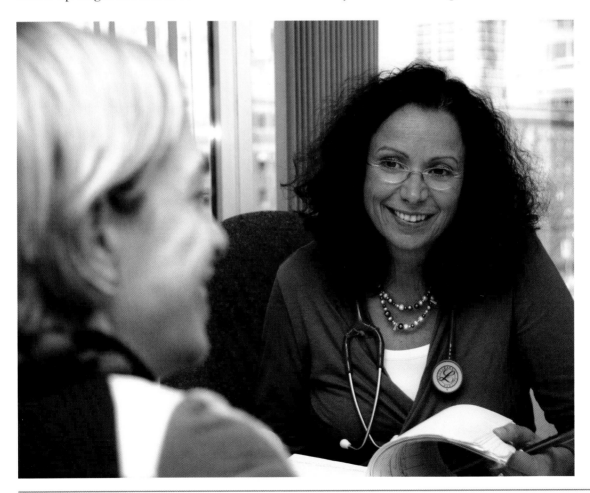

Rashes specific to pregnancy

The most common rashes in pregnancy share some features — they all have complicated names with lots of Ps in them, they start in pregnancy and disappear afterward, and they are often, but not always, itchy. Some people believe that these rashes are just variations on the same theme, but they are differentiated here.

Cholestasis of pregnancy

Choly what? In medicine, a word with "chole" in it refers to something related to your gallbladder. In this case, your gallbladder is not doing its job of pumping bile acids (otherwise known as the byproducts of liver metabolism) out of your liver and into your gut for excretion, or at least not doing it very well. These bile acids can accumulate in your liver, where they are absorbed into your bloodstream, travel to your skin, and make you very, very itchy. This condition usually appears in the second or third trimester.

Complications of cholestasis of pregnancy

Maternal: Some women have described this condition as an intolerable itch all over their bodies. Often it may be worse at night or on the palms of their hands and soles of their feet. In most cases, the itching usually resolves within a few days of delivering the baby and your blood returning to its pre-pregnancy levels. However, the chance of cholestasis of pregnancy recurring in a subsequent pregnancy is about 60% to 70%. In addition, there may be a slightly higher risk of developing gallstones in the future if you had cholestasis of pregnancy. About 10% of women with cholestasis of pregnancy will develop jaundice. If you suspect jaundice, your health-care provider will arrange for you to do some blood tests to check the levels of bile acids and other indicators.

Fetal: For the fetus, there are a few more potential complications. There is an increased risk of premature delivery, particularly in a multiple pregnancy, and

Did You Know?
Possible causes of cholestasis of pregnancy

It is not really known why some women develop cholestasis of pregnancy, although it does seem that genetic factors might play a role, since it can run in families and it is more common in some ethnic groups. For example, in the Araucanian Indians in Chile, cholestasis occurs in 15% of pregnancies! Elsewhere, the incidence can vary between 0.1% and 15% of pregnancies. Estrogen and progesterone hormones likely play a role, but exactly how and why is unclear.

an increased risk of fetal death prior to delivery. The risk of fetal death is extremely low, but it is still enough to warrant careful monitoring of the fetus, usually with an ultrasound at regular intervals, and to plan an early delivery at about 38 weeks. Unfortunately, we do not understand why this increased risk of fetal death exists.

Treating cholestasis

Treatment of cholestasis is usually with a medication called ursodeoxycholic acid (or Urso for short). It should help with the itching and keep the levels of your bile acids down. It is safe for use in pregnancy. Sometimes, an antihistamine medication is also prescribed specifically to help with the itching.

Prurigo of pregnancy

This rash usually begins in the second or third trimester, appearing as red bumps on the trunk and extensor surfaces of the limbs (that is, the kneecap side of the leg and the outside surface of the arm). The bumps can be grouped together and may look crusty or flaky. It affects between 1 in 300 and 1 in 450 expectant women. The rash generally resolves immediately after the baby is born, although in some women it can take up to 3 months to disappear. There are no risks to either mother or baby, although the rash may recur in subsequent pregnancies. Again, the usual treatment is antihistamine medication and corticosteroid creams to help with itching.

Pruritic folliculitis of pregnancy

This rash appears as red bumps and pustules on the torso and spreads to the arms and legs. It looks a bit like acne. It also appears in the second and third trimester, but seems to be more rare than prurigo of pregnancy. Otherwise it is treated the same way and, similarly, has no negative consequences for the mother or the fetus.

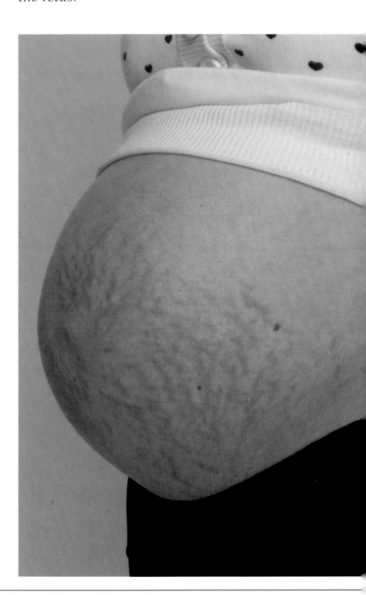

■ PUPPP red spots, worse in stretch marks

PUPPP

Going by the unwieldy name of pruritic urticarial papules and plaques of pregnancy, which, fortunately, is easily shortened to PUPPP, this condition is still relatively uncommon, affecting somewhere between 1 in 160 and 1 in 300 pregnant women. It is more common in first pregnancies and multiple pregnancies.

Most of the time, it starts close to full term, around 35 weeks, although on occasion it starts much earlier. Although PUPPP may get worse right after delivery, it generally resolves by 2 weeks postpartum. It has no effect on your baby, and no long-term effects on you, either. The chances of it recurring in another pregnancy are quite low.

PUPPP often starts as red spots within stretch marks, and from there it can spread to the whole abdomen, usually sparing the belly button area; sometimes it spreads to the arms and legs. It doesn't usually spread to the face, palms, or soles of the feet. Sometimes the red spots can all join together to form hives. It is extremely itchy.

This itchiness is usually improved with the use of antihistamines (like Benadryl or Atarax) and corticosteroid creams. Very rarely, oral corticosteroids are prescribed if the itching is severe.

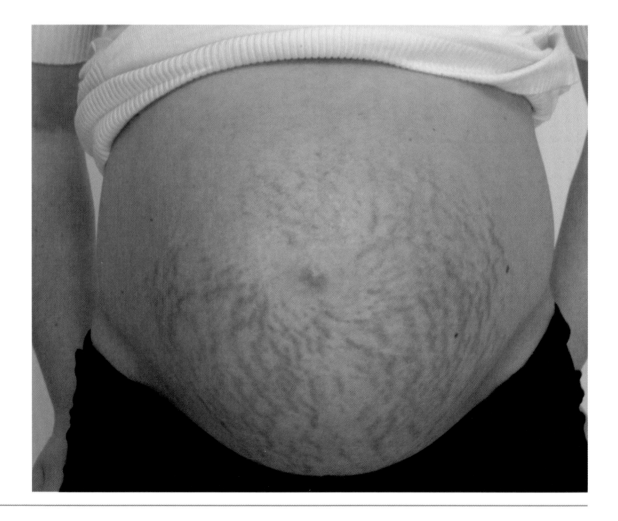

Month 5 fetal growth and development

There's no doubt now that the fetus is growing. To accommodate it, your belly is growing, too, quite noticeably. By 20 weeks, your uterus will reach your belly button! Significant milestones are reached in the development of the fetus, none more exciting than a nervous system that makes it possible for the fetus to communicate — by kicking you!

Pregnancy milestones

At week 20

- At week 20, the fetus is almost 7 inches (18 cm) long from crown to rump and weighs 10.6 ounces (300 g).
- The skin is covered in vernix, a white, creamy substance resembling cold cream that protects the skin from the amniotic fluid. (Imagine what your skin would be like if you sat in a waterbath for 10 months with no protection!)
- Hair is growing on the head and on the body. This soft, fine body hair is called lanugo and disappears by full term.
- The vagina is developing in girls, and, in boys, the scrotum is forming.
- The bones in the ears are hardening, and soon the fetus will be able to hear.

- The eyelids are still closed, but the eyes can move from side to side.

At week 24

- By week 24, the baby can survive if born prematurely.
- The brain and nervous system are developing rapidly. Once the nerves are coated in a protective sheath called myelin, the fetus will be able to pass messages around its body — messages of sensation transmitted to the brain and then messages to control movement from the brain to the limbs.
- Soon the fetus will be able to respond to a stimulus, such as touch through your belly, by kicking back.

Embryo at 20 Weeks

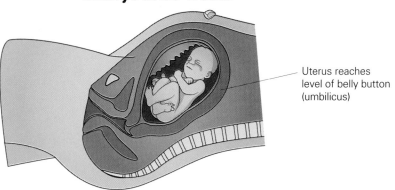

Uterus reaches level of belly button (umbilicus)

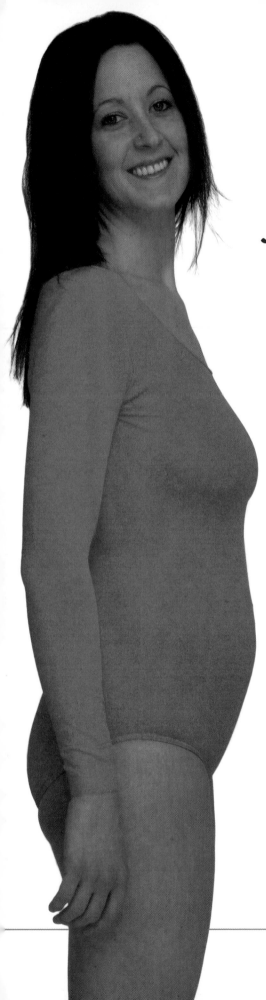

Looking and feeling pregnant

Beyond your growing uterus, there are few changes in your body at this stage that would cause new discomfort, but all the symptoms from earlier months may be present, slightly magnified — or slightly minimized (you hope!).

- You might be starting to feel a little bit slower and have trouble walking fast.
- You might find it harder to bend over and tie your shoes — your belly keeps getting in the way!
- You might have varicose veins in your legs.
- You might develop hemorrhoids.
- You might have leg cramps, especially at night.
- You might sometimes feel a bit dizzy.

Did You Know?

Edema

Retention of fluid (edema) in the lower extremities is commonplace in pregnancy and worsened by multiples. Prolonged standing will make this worse, as will a diet low in protein. Elevating your legs, when you can, above the level of the heart will help mobilize this excess fluid so that it may be excreted. Support hose may also assist.

Month 5 medical check-up

It's routine now. Just like your last visit, your health-care providers will check your blood pressure, urine, and weight. The growth of your uterus will be checked, and you will hear the baby's heart again. You can discuss any concerns and review any new test results.

Month 5 tests

The major test this month is an ultrasound image of the fetus. Ultrasound imaging has various names, including diagnostic ultrasound, ultrasound scan, and sonography. This test is also technically known as an anatomical scan (Level II ultrasound). You may also hear about 3-D ultrasound; it is literally three dimensional — you can see the facial features, for example, clearly. However, a skilled ultrasonographer can see all that is necessary for checking the development of the fetus on a regular 2-D ultrasound.

During this test, the ultrasound technologist and radiologist are looking at every part of your baby — from the brain right down to the toes! The scan can sometimes take quite a while because there is a lot to look at. During this ultrasound, you may be able to find out the gender of your baby as well. While it is very exciting to see your baby, remember that this is also a diagnostic test. The radiologist is looking to make sure that the baby is healthy. If there is any concern, this will be discussed with you and other tests may be needed.

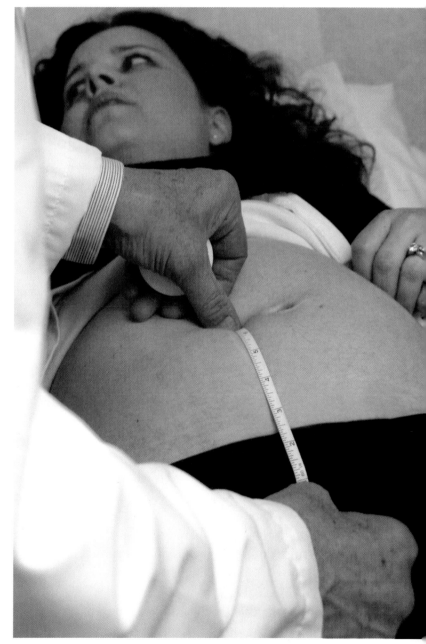

Ultrasound imaging

In ultrasound tests, a probe (transducer) is passed across the uterus, making a very high-frequency sound that echoes back information. The echoes are then displayed on a television screen showing a picture of the fetus, featuring the internal organs. This technology is similar to sonar, which uses sound waves to make pictures of objects underwater.

Many of the larger anatomical structures of the fetus can be seen, including the head, trunk, limbs, and placenta, as well as your uterus, cervix, and, on occasion, ovaries. The ultrasound shows movements of the arms, legs, and heart. This is an important diagnostic tool for both normal and complicated pregnancies.

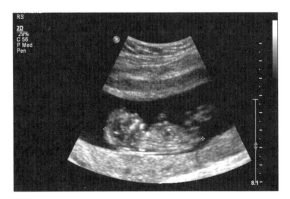

■ Fetus in late first trimester

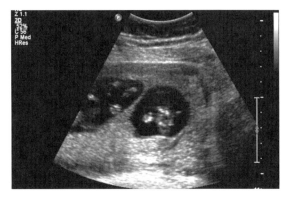

■ Fraternal twins in late first trimester

Kinds of scans

There are two basic kinds of scans. Routine scans are used to show that the pregnancy is proceeding as expected and detect any problems at an early stage. Routine scans are done during two periods in the pregnancy, between weeks 11 to 14 and weeks 18 to 20. Indicated scans (that is, suggested, or indicated, by other test results), also known as limited scans, are done at any time to evaluate problems that might arise during pregnancy and are quite specific in their procedures. Indicated ultrasound imaging is also used to guide various procedures, such as amniocentesis, CVS, and fetal blood transfusions.

Routine scan information

Routine scans are offered to every pregnant woman to confirm the healthy progress of the pregnancy and to detect any emerging problems:

11- to 14-week routine scan
- Pregnancy confirmed
- Fetal life established
- Gestational age and due dates estimated
- Twins detected and membranes examined
- Nuchal translucency (NT) (the fluid behind the baby's neck) measured to screen for potential problems

- Problems of the uterus (such as fibroids) and abnormal ovaries detected
- Baseline information about the fetus obtained to better manage problems that might arise later

18- to 20-week routine scan
- Anatomy of the fetus evaluated to look for visible birth defects
- Position of the placenta and cervix checked
- Fetal growth analyzed

Indicated scan tests
These scans are done in mothers who have the following risk factors or whenever a problem arises during the pregnancy:
- Bleeding
- Fetal heart not heard or movements not felt
- Uterus smaller or larger than expected for date in pregnancy
- High-risk for birth defects
- High-risk for fetal health or growth problems
- Fetal position concerns
- Gestational diabetes mellitus

Did You Know?
Ultrasound safety
Ultrasound has been in use for about 40 years, and no ill effects have been identified to date. Nevertheless, ultrasound is a form of energy. It is prudent to expose the developing fetus to ultrasound imagery only if there is a medical reason for the scan and benefit is to be expected.

Ultrasound procedure
Ultrasound scans are done by specially trained professional technologists (also called sonographers). Occasionally, a doctor will come in to check some findings. In all cases, the pictures are reviewed by a physician, who issues the report to your doctor or midwife. The procedure is simple and painless, in most cases requiring no special preparation. A complete examination takes about 30 to 60 minutes.

The ultrasound scan is a happy occasion in most cases. Some parents bring members of their family to watch. When the scan is finished, the technologist generally has a few minutes to show you images of the fetus and may print one out for you to take home.

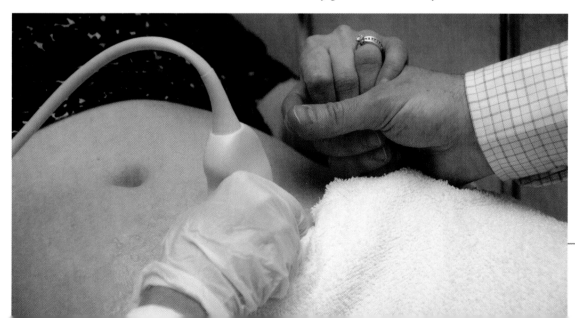

Ultrasound images of fetus

These ultrasound images were captured during a Level II anatomy ultrasound at about 19 weeks gestational age. They illustrate the normal features of a fetus at this age. They show not only a marvel of technology, but also the marvel of fetal development!

When you are looking at the pictures, keep in mind that on ultrasound, bone shows up as bright white, while fluid or water is darkest black. Muscle and other body tissues are seen as gray.

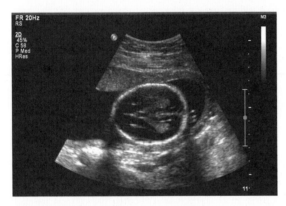

1. Cross section through the fetal skull and brain.

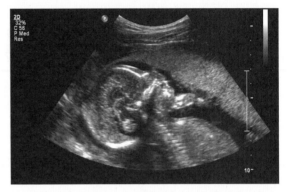

2. Fetus in profile, showing a lengthwise cross section of the brain, along with the bony (white) palate extending from the mouth into the center of the head.

3. Four chambers of the structurally normal heart. The heart is filled with blood, so we see the fluid inside the heart as black. The heart is the area that looks like four holes. You can also see one bright white bony rib on the bottom of the torso.

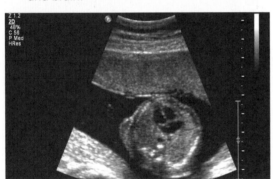

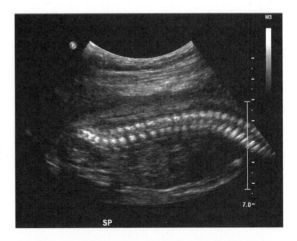

4. Normal nose and lips, face on. Because the nose and lips stick out from the face in the amniotic fluid surrounding them, they can be seen in isolation from the rest of the face.

5. Fetal spine showing each vertebrae.

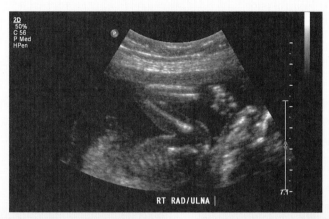

6. Fetal arm, bent at the elbow and raised to the head. It looks as if the fetus may be sucking its thumb.

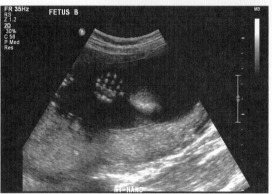

7. Open hand with the bones of the four fingers and a thumb clearly visible.

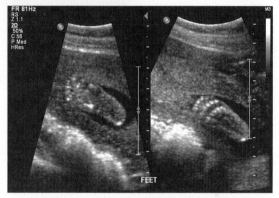

8. Fetal feet with each side of the image showing a different foot, ensuring that both left and right are normal.

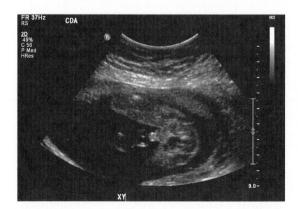

9. It's a boy!

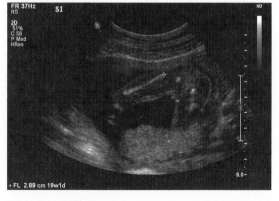

10. It's a girl!

Sometimes the most eagerly anticipated part of the Level II anatomy scan is finding out the gender! Above, left, the penis and testicles appear very clearly between the outstretched thighs. Above, right, the two folds of the female vulva are clearly seen.

Due date estimation

Ultrasounds allow your health-care providers to confirm your estimated due date. Measurements are taken of the fetus and charted beside the measurements of fetuses whose age is already known. This provides an approximate age and an estimated due date. Date assignment is most accurate in early pregnancy but declines in late pregnancy. That is one of the reasons your doctor may recommend an early scan at 11 to 14 weeks. Once the dates are set by the early scan, they must not be changed by later scans. The later scans just show how well the baby is growing. Still, remember that the fetus does not have a calendar and labor generally occurs only approximately on the estimated due date.

Guide to...

Ultrasound scans

- **Limited scan:** Done to evaluate specific, limited issues, such as the condition of the cervix or to follow up for structures not seen well at routine scan. Typically, patients will have had a complete scan that has evaluated the whole pregnancy and a limited repeat scan has been requested to answer a specific question.

- **Biophysical profile (BPP) scan:** Used in pregnancies where there is concern about the baby's growth and health. It is done after 26 weeks and evaluates indicators of baby's health such as movement, breathing, and the amount of amniotic fluid.

- **Measurement scan:** Can give a rough estimate of how much the fetus weighs and help determine if it is too small or too large for its age.

- **M-mode (movement-mode) ultrasound:** Used to make a trace of moving structures, such as the heart for an evaluation of heart rate.

- **Transvaginal scans:** Done with a special probe that is inserted into the vagina. This approach can allow evaluation of structures that are deep in the pelvis and cannot be seen using the abdominal approach. Target structures can include the cervix, ovaries, and fetal parts that are deep in the pelvis.

- **Doppler scans:** Make use of the fact that moving fluids, such as blood, change the echoes in a way that allows doctors to evaluate the speed and direction of blood flow (shown as colors on the pictures) and hear the pulsations. This is how a fetal heart monitor works. You can hear the repeating "whooshes" of pulsating blood.

- **3-D/4-D scans:** Project ultrasound information in three-dimensional or four-dimensional images. A special probe is used that makes a series of pictures side by side. Think of a loaf of bread. Standard 2-D ultrasound looks at it one slice a time and from one direction. With 3-D we can take a picture of the whole loaf and "slice" the loaf in any direction and look at these different slices. This ability to make pictures of the baby from any direction can be an important aid to doctors in limited situations. 4-D is a series of 3-D pictures taken during a time interval, which displays movements, much as a movie does, in a series of still pictures.

Did You Know?

Ultrasound procedures

- You should wear loose clothing so that you feel comfortable and can help the technologist move any clothing aside.
- Do not use skin creams that are sold to prevent stretch marks. These interfere with sound passing through the skin and create artifacts that make the pictures unclear.
- You will lie on your back or side.
- Some gel will be applied to your abdomen to allow sound waves to project more easily.

- The technologist will move the probe to look at different parts of the fetus and uterus, taking representative pictures.
- You will feel some pressure from the probe as the technologist tries to see some structures more clearly, but the examination should not be painful.
- If a transvaginal scan is needed, a probe about the size of a tampon will be inserted into the vagina and moved to examine the structures that lie deep in the pelvis.
- Sometimes the position of the fetus prevents a clear view of some structures. If this is the case, you will be asked to return in 1 to 2 weeks for a limited scan of those structures.

Gender news

Medical scans are not done to determine gender. In fact, taking time to look for gender is not part of the scanning procedure. Even if technologists see the gender, they are asked to not divulge it unless they are asked to do so by the parents. Besides, ultrasound is not completely accurate in determining boys or girls, even if the picture appears convincing. There are, however, a few rare, special circumstances where knowing the gender is important. For example, some disorders only occur in one gender, and so it is important to know if the baby is at risk.

Entertainment ultrasounds

3-D and 4-D ultrasound imaging can now show the surface of the baby, producing pretty pictures of baby faces — and spawning a new entertainment industry. Ultrasound machines are being used commercially, not diagnostically, to create "baby pictures" strictly for the entertainment of parents. Such entertainment scans are not endorsed

by health authorities. Experts feel that no matter how safe ultrasound has appeared to be, it is not wise to risk exposing the fetus to sound energy when there are no expected medical benefits.

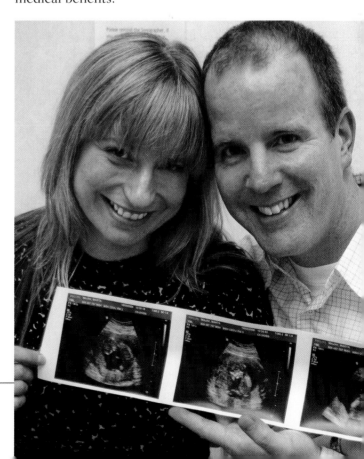

Incompetent cervix

In this unusual condition, the cervix dilates prematurely in the absence of uterine contractions and the baby can be born far too early for it to survive.

Symptoms

When you are examined vaginally, the cervix may be seen to be open, or, on an ultrasound, the cervix can be seen to be shortened. Most women will feel no symptoms, but some will experience a watery vaginal discharge, spotting, or bleeding and a vague discomfort in the abdomen or back.

Risk factors

Risk factors include previous uterine surgery, cervical surgery (removal of parts of the cervix for treatment of abnormal Pap tests), and frequent procedures that dilated the cervix. The strongest predictor of incompetent cervix is if this has happened in the past.

Treatment

If you are at high risk, transvaginal ultrasounds can be performed early in the pregnancy to see if the cervix is short. The cervix will be measured serially during the critical weeks to see if the length is shortening. If it becomes too short, you may be offered a cerclage, in which a stitch or suture is put into the cervix to help support and close it. If you have many risk factors, a cerclage may be placed at the end of the first trimester, just in case.

Incompetent Cervix with Cerclage

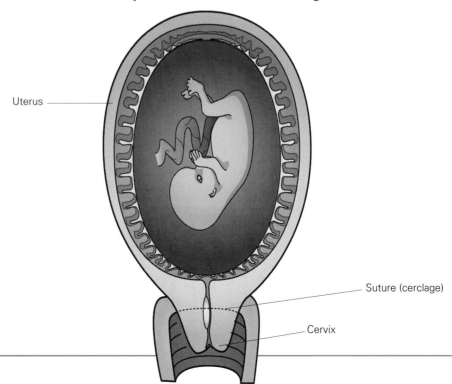

Uterus

Suture (cerclage)

Cervix

Month 6 fetal growth and development

The fetus is growing inside you, and you are growing, too. Your uterus should reach a few centimeters above your belly button by 24 weeks, and you may be gaining weight elsewhere now — on your thighs, buttocks, and upper body. You may notice that your feet are swelling a little and your shoes are tight. You're getting close to the third — and last — trimester of your pregnancy. Congratulate yourself! Consider rewarding yourself by taking some time — even a holiday — with your partner. Soon you will have trouble traveling, and it may be the last one you take without kids for a long, long time.

Pregnancy milestones

At week 24

- The fetus is 11.8 inches (30 cm) long from the top of its head to its feet and weighs 1 pound and 5 ounces (600 g).
- Fingers and toes are well developed, although still slightly webbed, and fingernails are present.
- Meconium (the first feces) is starting to form in the intestines.
- The lungs are developing alveoli, which will become air sacs when the baby is born.
- The fetus continues to swallow amniotic fluid, excreting it as urine into the amniotic fluid.
- The baby may begin to hiccup, something you may be able to feel.
- The baby has sleep and awake cycles, which you may become aware of.
- The fetus's brain is growing and growing.

At week 27

- The fetus is 15.75 inches (40 cm) long and weighs 2 pounds and 10 ounces (1.2 kg).
- The brain is developing rapidly.
- The fetus may now control some movements.
- The eyelids open and close.
- The inner ear is well developed.
- The lungs are capable of gas exchange.

Embryo at 24 Weeks

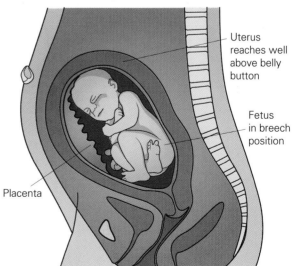

Uterus reaches well above belly button

Fetus in breech position

Placenta

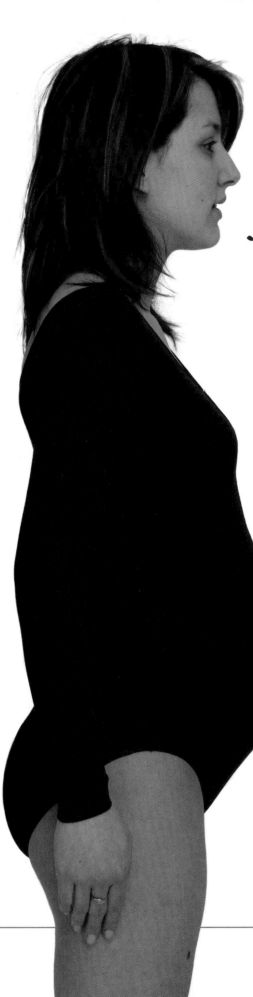

Looking and feeling pregnant

While the baby has been moving around for a while now, you may only start to feel it this month. The baby now has enough "weight" behind it that you can feel those kicks. At the beginning, you may not be certain what you are feeling — some women describe it as feeling like bubbles or little flutters. But soon enough, the movements will become more definite and you will be sure. These kicks are relatively painless, but as your belly grows, the kicks may bang into other organs in your abdomen, which may lead to some discomfort.

• You might be feeling more constipated as your bowels are compressed further.

• You might begin to have some heartburn and even acid reflux as your uterus compresses your stomach upward.

• You might have pains and aches in different places — generally a result of either the uterus or swelling tissue compressing different nerves (for example, when the sciatic nerve, running down the buttocks and the back of the thigh, is compressed, you will experience pain in that nerve, or sciatica). Other pains can be attributed to the uterus and its ligaments growing and stretching.

• You might start to have some swelling in your feet and ankles, and sometimes even in your hands and face.

• You might feel warm all the time — you will be throwing off the blankets and sweaters while your partner is piling them on.

• You might start to feel mild tightening or contractions of your uterus, called Braxton Hicks contractions, a foreshadowing of things to come.

Month 6 medical check-up

Again ... your weight, urine, and blood pressure will all be checked. Again, you will hear the heart rate and have the height of your uterus checked. Now is the time to look back at your pregnancy diary for any symptoms or problems you want to discuss with your health-care provider.

Month 6 tests

A blood sugar test for gestational diabetes mellitus is often but not always scheduled between week 24 and 28, earlier if you have any risk factors or show any symptoms. Your blood may be routinely tested for any signs of anemia.

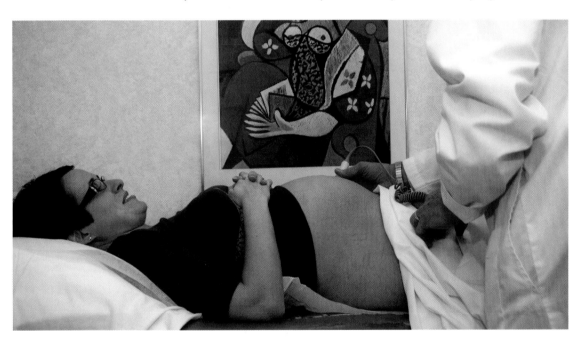

Did You Know?

Fetal movements

Sometimes, you do not feel your baby moving at this stage of development. This is not necessarily cause for concern, especially if no problems were seen in your ultrasound scans. You might have an anterior placenta, which absorbs the kicks. If the placenta is in the front of the uterus (anterior), it may act like a pillow to absorb some of the movements that the baby is making. Your uterus itself is not able to feel movement — only the muscles and skin of your abdomen can, so if the baby's kicks do not bump into the abdomen because the placenta is in the way, you may not feel as much movement. Don't worry — eventually most people with anterior placentas feel movement, too. And the baby does not harm the placenta in any way by kicking it.

Gestational diabetes mellitus

Diabetes, a metabolic disorder, results from an inability to regulate levels of sugar in the blood. One of the natural effects of pregnancy is to reduce blood sugar metabolism efficiency, causing high levels of sugar in the blood. Most women do not reach the diabetic range, but some women do develop diabetes in pregnancy, even when they do not have pre-existing diabetes. This condition is called gestational diabetes mellitus (GDM).

Screening for GDM

Screening for and treating GDM is controversial in the medical community. There are several different philosophies about screening for GDM. Some caregivers will only suggest you do a test for GDM if you have a few of the common risk factors, while others recommend screening all pregnant women, and a few recommend screening no one. In North America, more than 85% of pregnant women are tested for GDM. In Europe, far fewer women are tested. Consider discussing this with your doctor or midwife.

Test procedure

If you are tested for GDM, it will probably be between week 24 and 28. If you are at high risk of developing GDM, then it may be reasonable to consider screening earlier in the pregnancy, and then again at 24 to 28 weeks if you were negative the first time. If you have a number of risk factors, your caregiver may suggest screening for GDM in each trimester.

Risk factors for developing GDM

In North America, about 3% to 4% of pregnant women will develop GDM, although your risk may be higher if you have certain risk factors:

- GDM in a previous pregnancy
- Previous experience of glucose intolerance
- Parent or sibling with diabetes or a history of GDM
- Advanced maternal age (over 35)
- Obesity
- History of polycystic ovarian syndrome (PCOS)

- High-risk ethnic background (women of Aboriginal, African, Asian, South Asian, or Hispanic descent)
- Previous unexplained stillbirth
- Previous newborn with low blood sugars, low calcium levels, or jaundice
- Sugar repeatedly detected in urine
- Polyhydramnios (excess of amniotic fluid)
- Previous macrosomia (big baby) or suspected macrosomia

The screening test is called a glucose challenge test (GCT) and involves drinking a sweet drink containing 50 g of pure glucose (sugar), followed by a blood test 1 hour later. Remember the difference between a screening test and a diagnostic test (see page 148). The screening test identifies people at risk but generally cannot confirm a diagnosis.

If the screening test shows slightly elevated blood sugars, you will probably be asked to do a diagnostic test, called a glucose tolerance test (GTT). In this test, you will be given a drink with 75 to 100 g of glucose and have your blood drawn and tested three or four times over the next 3 hours. However, if the GCT screening test shows a very high level of glucose in your blood, then the diagnosis of GDM can be confirmed without the GTT.

GDM complications

A number of pregnancy complications are thought to be associated with GDM. However, not all complications are agreed upon in the medical community.

Macrosomia

Women with GDM have a 16% to 29% chance of having a "big baby" close to 9 pounds (4 kg), compared to only 10% for women without GDM. Macrosomia often requires an assisted delivery using forceps or a vacuum extractor. Some doctors recommend a Caesarean section.

Shoulder dystocia and birth trauma

A baby born to a mother with diabetes is more likely to have a shoulder dystocia during delivery, when the baby's shoulder gets caught behind the pubic bone. These babies are big in a different way than a big baby born to a mother without diabetes. When the mother has diabetes, the baby's weight tends to accumulate disproportionally around the torso, so that the baby's big shoulders might not deliver easily during a vaginal delivery. When this happens, the midwife or doctor needs to perform a few maneuvers to help the shoulders come out. These maneuvers can sometimes cause an injury to the baby, which is usually temporary. The most serious of these is called a brachial plexus injury, where the nerves running between the neck and arm are stretched, causing some damage to the nerves in the baby's arm. The damage is temporary in 80% to 90% of brachial plexus injuries.

■ Glucose challenge test

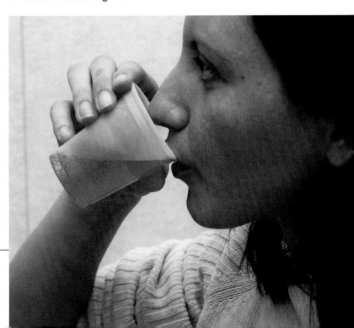

Types of diabetes

There are three basic types of diabetes: two that exist independent of pregnancy and a third that can develop during pregnancy. Type 1 and Type 2 are considered chronic diseases, whereas gestational diabetes begins in pregnancy and resolves after delivery.

Type 1 diabetes

In Type 1 diabetes (insulin dependent), the pancreas does not produce adequate insulin to metabolize your blood sugars. Many of those with Type 1 diabetes are diagnosed as children. All those with Type 1 diabetes rely on regular injections of insulin to maintain normal levels of blood sugars.

Type 2 diabetes

In Type 2 diabetes (non–insulin dependent), the insulin produced is not very efficient at metabolizing sugar. Sometimes modifying the diet and increasing exercise levels can improve the way the body uses insulin and help reduce blood sugar levels. Medications are also often used to improve the way the body produces and uses the insulin. Sometimes, the medications don't work well enough, and the person with Type 2 diabetes will need to use insulin.

Gestational diabetes

Gestational diabetes arises during pregnancy and disappears after pregnancy. Gestational diabetes is treated with a combination of diet and exercise, and, when necessary, insulin injections.

For more information on managing pre-existing chronic diabetes, see Part 13, Managing Medical and Environmental Risks (page 432).

Neonatal metabolic problems

Babies born to mothers with GDM may have problems with low blood sugars immediately after birth. Many babies born to GDM mothers will have their blood sugar tested shortly after birth in order to check for this problem. If the blood sugar is low, you will be encouraged to feed the baby, and it may even be necessary to give the baby a small amount of sugar water or formula to increase the blood sugar. This is important to prevent the seizures that can sometimes be caused by a very low level of blood sugar. Babies born to mothers with GDM also have a higher risk of jaundice in the first few days after birth. Jaundice, if recognized early, is easily treatable and has no long-lasting effect on the baby.

Perinatal mortality

In the past, a higher risk of perinatal mortality, or stillbirth, was considered one of the most important reasons to test for and treat GDM. Changes in prenatal care have made fetal stillbirth a very rare

Did You Know?

Diabetes later in life

Women who have GDM during pregnancy are at higher risk of developing diabetes in the future. The risk may vary depending upon ethnic background, so a Caucasian woman with GDM may have only a 9% risk of developing diabetes in the future, whereas the risk is 25% in Asian women, 47% in Hispanic women, and 70% in Canadian Aboriginal women.

complication of GDM, particularly if the mother's blood sugars are well controlled. While you may hear some people talk about GDM and fetal death, you can feel quite confident that the most up-to-date information does not suggest this is a significant risk.

High blood pressure

In the past, GDM was thought to put a woman at higher risk for having blood pressure problems in pregnancy, but, again, more recent research suggests that this is probably not true. It is more likely that women who are older and obese are at a greater risk for GDM, and they are also at a higher risk of blood pressure problems for the same reason.

Guide to...

Treating GDM

- **Diet and exercise:** Usually the first step in treating GDM is to meet with a dietitian to review your diet and activity level. You will be asked to reduce your intake of carbohydrates (sweets, bread, pasta, juice). You will also be asked to exercise a bit more. This might just mean going for some short walks during the day, not necessarily a full gym routine. You will probably also be taught how to test your blood sugar on a home monitor and asked to keep a record of your blood sugar levels.

- **Medications:** If your blood sugar levels remain too high despite changing your diet and exercising, you may be prescribed insulin to help your body metabolize sugar. Insulin is a drug that must be injected just under the skin, and you will be taught how

Did You Know?

Brachial plexus injury controversy

Although some medical authorities suggest GDM mothers deliver by Caesarean section when a big baby is suspected in order to prevent brachial plexus injuries, there are a few reasons why this doesn't seem like a good idea. First, most big babies will deliver vaginally without a shoulder dystocia. Second, some small babies have a shoulder dystocia, so it is very difficult to predict when it will happen. Third, statistics indicate that over 450 women with suspected big babies would be subjected to a planned Caesarean section in order to avoid one case of brachial plexus injury. Finally, one study of babies with brachial plexus injuries showed that only 6% had mothers with GDM.

to do this yourself. If you are seeing a midwife for your prenatal care, a diagnosis of GDM requiring insulin usually will lead to a consultation with an endocrinologist or obstetrician.

- **Ultrasound monitoring:** If you have GDM, especially if you need insulin, your health-care provider will probably arrange for some additional ultrasound monitoring of the fetus to ensure that it remains healthy. Many doctors arrange an ultrasound every 2 weeks until delivery.

- **Induced labor:** The usual recommendation for women with insulin-dependent GDM is to induce labor around 38 to 39 weeks. This is advised because of a fear of fetal death in the last weeks of pregnancy. If your blood sugars are well controlled without insulin, it is probably not necessary to induce your labor before your due date. Talk to your doctor or midwife about this decision.

Anemia in pregnancy

Anemia is a condition that results when there are fewer red blood cells than expected in your blood. Pregnant women normally develop some degree of anemia as a result of the expanding blood volume that happens during the first trimester, but the condition can become more severe as the pregnancy progresses.

Anemia complications

Women who have anemia may experience fatigue, decreased ability to accomplish all their normal daily tasks without feeling unwell, cardiovascular stress, or an impaired resistance to infection. Untreated anemia may lead to low maternal weight gain, preterm birth, or a low birth weight infant. Postpartum depression rates are also increased in women who have anemia during pregnancy.

Diagnosing anemia

As a part of the routine blood work done in the first trimester, your health-care provider will be checking your blood count to test for anemia. Many will also check again at the end of the second trimester. If you seem excessively fatigued or very pale, that is another reason to check for anemia.

Treating anemia

Iron-deficiency anemia can be treated by increasing your intake of dietary and supplemental iron while consuming a source of vitamin C. Be sure to consume foods that inhibit iron absorption (calcium-rich foods, tea, and coffee) at a different time. Some women will have to take a separate iron supplement in addition to the iron in their prenatal vitamin. This additional iron may cause constipation, so be certain to increase your intake of fiber and fluids if you are consuming additional iron.

Types of anemia

- **Iron-deficiency anemia:** As the blood volume increases in pregnancy, the number of red blood cells does not increase in the same proportion. Iron, an important element of hemoglobin, also needs to be increased to meet the expanding blood volume. If the iron is not increased to adequate amounts, anemia can result. Iron-deficiency anemia is the most common type of anemia seen in pregnancy.

- **Pernicious anemia:** This type of anemia is the result of a deficiency of folate or vitamin B_{12}.

- **Secondary:** Anemia may be secondary to a number of inherited conditions, such as thalassemia or sickle cell anemia.

Risk factors for iron-deficiency anemia in pregnancy

- Low dietary intake of meat, fish, and poultry
- Low dietary intake of vitamin C
- Pre-pregnancy anemia
- Multiples gestation (twins, triplets, or more)
- Frequent consumption of coffee or tea close to meal time

Rest and relaxation

Stress affects both mind and body. In pregnancy, stress can cause sleepless nights, loss of appetite, and emotional instability, all of which can have a negative impact on you and your ability to cope with your pregnancy. It's a good idea to learn ways to handle stress as early as possible in your pregnancy. The good news is that the baby is well insulated from stress. We don't know exactly how stress affects a growing baby, but there is no evidence to suggest that stress plays a negative role in fetal development.

Sleep

Start by sleeping as much as you can, especially when your body tells you to. Of course, that's easier said than done. As pregnancy progresses, poor-quality sleeping can be a problem, and stress only makes it worse. If you're having trouble sleeping, try some light exercise during the day, curb daytime naps, and don't eat too close to bedtime. Develop a relaxing nighttime routine like reading, listening to music, having a bath, or doing some yoga or relaxation routines before bed. Encourage your partner to join you in some quiet time together. Continue this habit once your baby is born.

Relaxation exercises

There is a wide array of relaxation exercises you can try, some on your own, some in classes. Give one or two a try.

Breathing exercises

Breath awareness will benefit you and the baby during pregnancy and can also help get you through the different stages of labor. During pregnancy, breathing deeply and rhythmically can ease muscle tension, lower your heart rate, and help you fall asleep faster.

It's simple: take a deep breath through your nose, then exhale slowly through your mouth, so that your lungs empty completely. Then pause, rest, and repeat.

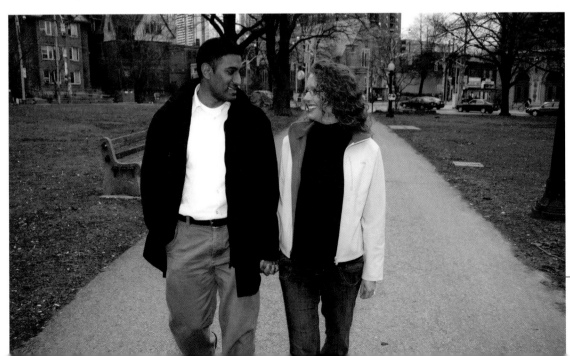

Yoga exercises

Yoga can help you relax, as well as maintain muscle tone and flexibility during pregnancy. Yoga focuses on breathing, relaxation, posture, and body awareness. It will keep you looking fit and healthy, as well as teach you useful breathing techniques to use during labor. Many gyms offer yoga and stretch classes, but take care — some yoga techniques are not safe to do during pregnancy. Make sure you sign up for a prenatal yoga class.

Muscle relaxation exercises

Lying on your bed or even on the floor, you can release tight muscles by first tensing and then completely relaxing them. Focus on one group of muscles at a time and alternate between your right and left side. For instance, start by tensing and releasing your hand and forearm muscles, followed by your biceps and triceps, face and jaw, chest and shoulders, stomach and thighs, until you reach your feet. Rotate your ankles, and squeeze and release your toes.

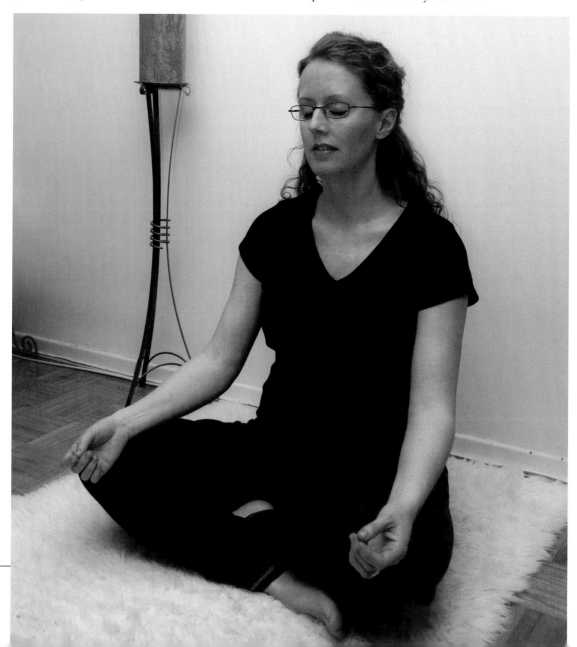

Did You Know?

Safe massage therapy in pregnancy

Massage is known to be safe during pregnancy, but you will still need to take a few basic precautions:

- Choose a licensed massage therapist with special training in prenatal massage, because knowledge of pregnancy and the anatomy of a pregnant woman is very important.

- There are parts of the pregnant woman's body that should not be massaged. Avoid the abdomen, or at least limit massaging to a very light touch.

- Experiment until you find a comfortable massage position — lying on your back or stomach will probably not work because of the increasing weight of your uterus.

Many women find it most comfortable to lie in a semi-reclining position. Your massage therapist will probably have you turn from side to side for access to your back and hips, and might also use body pillows, wedge pillows, or extra padding to increase your comfort level.

- If you would like your partner or someone else close to be able to you give you a massage, have them come with you when you have a prenatal massage by a professional massage therapist. The therapist can illustrate comfort measures that can be used at home and will also explain why some techniques might be unsafe and show the proper technique for those that are safe.

Massage

Treating yourself to a regular, relaxing massage might be just the key to reducing stress levels during pregnancy. Gentle massage techniques can reduce aches and pains, increase your mobility, and relax tense or tight muscles. Massage is one of the oldest forms of healing therapies, known to benefit the circulatory, digestive, and excretory systems. It can also help with getting a good night's sleep.

Back pain is one of the more common side effects of pregnancy — it can continue even after delivery. If you have small children and find yourself carrying them around a lot while you're pregnant, your backache may become worse. Massage can help relieve back pain and edema (swelling) by stimulating circulation throughout the body. It can reduce anxiety and help prevent pregnancy-related insomnia. Massaging different parts of the body will achieve different results. Leg massage, for example, can help reduce leg cramps and swelling.

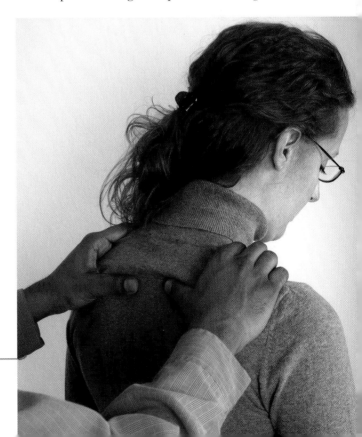

F.A.Q.

We answer many questions from pregnant women and their partners. Here are some of the most frequently asked questions. Be sure to ask your health-care providers any other questions that may arise. If they don't have the answers, they will refer you to a colleague who does.

Q: *When will I start to show?*

A: The answer is … it depends. It depends on how many times you have been pregnant. In second and third or more pregnancies, you tend to show sooner — your abdominal muscles tend to be a little more stretched and your body returns to a pregnant shape quickly. It also depends on your pre-pregnancy body weight. If you are heavier at the outset, in the early weeks your pregnancy may not be as obvious as it will be in someone who was very thin pre-pregnancy.

Q: *Is ultrasound safe for my baby?*

A: Yes. There is no evidence that ultrasound causes any harm to a fetus. Researchers have looked for evidence of increased cancers, developmental problems, and low birth weights but have not found any evidence that ultrasounds confer any harm. Still, we can never be 100% sure there is no harm. Although we believe ultrasound is safe, most of us will not recommend ultrasounds be

done without a good reason. Many women have ultrasounds to check specific problems. In these cases, the potential benefits of knowing how a fetus is coping (and the possibility of intervening to optimize health) outweigh any theoretical risks of harm to the baby.

Q: *Does a normal ultrasound examination guarantee a normal baby?*

A: No. Ultrasound is good, but it is not perfect in detecting problems. It just means that no abnormality was visible in the structures that could be seen at the time of the scan. The scan evaluates major organs only and may not detect small abnormalities in smaller structures. Even the ability to see large abnormalities depends on factors such as the position of the fetus and how large or conspicuous an abnormality is. Some abnormalities develop only in late pregnancy. These will not be present at the time of the 18- to-20 week scan. The size of the mother is becoming an increasing issue. Sound has to pass through the mother twice to see the baby. A thick or fat abdominal wall acts like fog — the thicker it is, the worse the visibility. In some women, a thick abdominal wall can prevent ultrasound evaluation of the baby.

Q: *How can I prevent stretch marks?*

A: There is very little you can do to prevent stretch marks, although there are lots of people selling creams and lotions and potions who will try to convince you that their product can do just that.

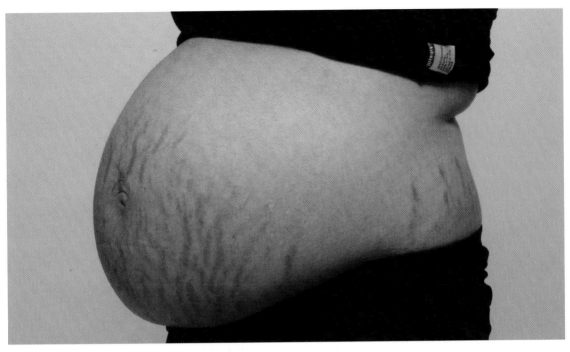

Stretch marks are pink-purple marks that can develop on the belly, breasts, and thighs, typically in month 6 or 7 of pregnancy. Unlike pigmentation changes, they won't disappear after pregnancy, although they fade to finer lines that are often very pale or silvery in color. Risk factors for developing stretch marks include a family history of stretch marks — so if your mother and sisters developed stretch marks, you may also develop them. You are also at higher risk if you are not Caucasian, if you have gained a lot of weight during pregnancy, or if you already have stretch marks on your breasts or thighs.

Q: *What do you mean when you say a woman is likely to have a "big baby?"*

A: Macrosomia, or having a big baby weighing 9 pounds (4 kg) or more, is not a problem if the baby is otherwise healthy, but a big baby can pose some difficulties during delivery. A big baby may need extra help because going through the birth canal will be a tight fit, which means a higher chance of having a vaginal delivery assisted with a vacuum or forceps. There may also be a higher Caesarean section rate. This is a controversial area. Some health-care providers will be quite worried about a big baby and may be more inclined to suggest a Caesarean section sooner when labor is not progressing well. Others will decide to wait and see.

What's next

Believe it or not, as you enter the third trimester, it's time to start planning your labor and delivery — and life with your newborn. Things go so fast now it's hard to keep up.

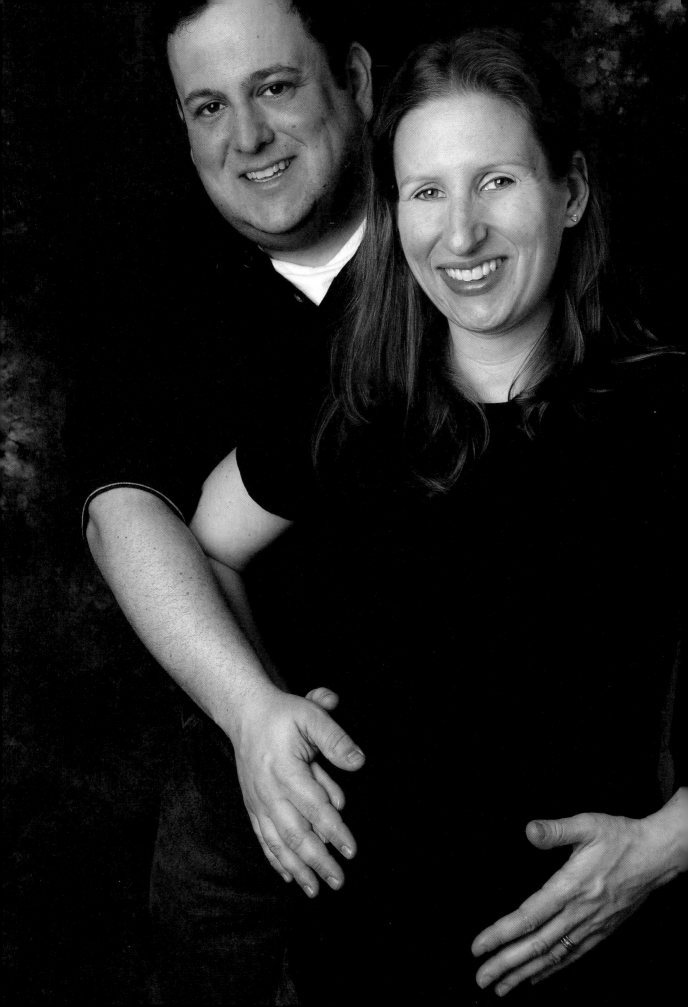

Part 7

Birth and Newborn Baby Planning

Things to do ...

Start planning for the baby's arrival in your home! You're entering your third trimester now, and time will fly. Within a few weeks, you will be pushing your baby into the world, so now is the time to draft a birth plan, furnish the nursery, and stock up on diapers, to name but a few tasks. While it is true that you don't need much more than a few diapers and sleepers at the beginning, it won't be long before your baby has more baggage than you do. And don't forget to pack your bag and set it at the door, ready for the moment when ...

Big decisions

Now is the time to make some big decisions. To breastfeed or to formula-feed ... that is one question you need to answer. Have you decided yet if you want pain medications during labor? Do you plan to "bank" your baby's umbilical cord blood at birth? If your baby is a boy, will you and your partner want him to be circumcised? Make the big decisions while you have time now, and you won't need to make them in haste later.

Ten tips for planning your labor and the care of your newborn

1. Make a birth plan and choose a birth partner now.

2. Attend your third trimester childbirth classes focused on labor and delivery.

3. Review the signs and symptoms of labor and when you need to go to the hospital or call your midwife.

4. Take a tour of the hospital so you know where to go once you are inside, even if you are planning a home birth. Things can go wrong at home, and you may need to go to the hospital.

5. Furnish the nursery — there's no time left to procrastinate — and have a car seat installed in your car. In some places, the police will install or inspect the installation, which is a great way to make sure it is done properly.

6. Use acetaminophen as the analgesic of choice for a variety of aches and pains in pregnancy. Avoid using non-steroidal anti-inflammatories (NSAIDs), including ASA (acetylsalicylic acid — widely known as Aspirin), ibuprofen, and indomethacin.

7. Discuss labor pain relief options with your health-care provider or with an anesthesiologist.

8. Organize primary care for your newborn. Your baby will need to see a doctor in the hospital for a routine newborn examination (often the doctor on call handles this) and within 3 days of leaving the hospital. You may choose your family doctor or a pediatrician to take care of your baby.

9. Plan for some help at home. Can your partner take a few days or weeks off work, or can a family member stay with you? It's nice to have not only their moral support, but also some help with meals and laundry so that you can get a little rest!

10. Go to a movie. Visit friends. On the spur of the moment. No need to book a babysitter (yet).

Birth plan

A birth plan is simply a set of written notes describing the kind of labor and delivery you would like to have and any procedures you would like to avoid. Writing a birth plan helps you focus on the different aspects of your care during labor and birth. To ensure that the expectations and wishes outlined in your birth plan can be accommodated at the place where you will be giving birth, ask your doctor or midwife to review it with you, ideally in the last month or so of pregnancy.

Flexibility

While a birth plan is an easy way of communicating your wishes to your health-care providers and others who will be attending your labor and delivery, don't think of it as a rigid set of rules. Not every labor goes according to plan. A birth plan that doesn't take a variety of possible outcomes into account can lead to feelings of disappointment and failure. You want your birth plan to be flexible enough to give your health-care providers alternative courses of action that will be in the best interests of you and your baby.

HOW TO ...
Write a birth plan

Starting on the next page is an outline of information you should include in your birth plan. Perhaps only some of these topics are really important to you, while there might be others you can think of that aren't included here. If you're having a hospital birth, bring a copy of this birth plan with you, or set it out for your midwife to review if you have chosen a home birth. Your birth partner should also have a copy handy. Spend time personalizing your birth plan and making it your own.

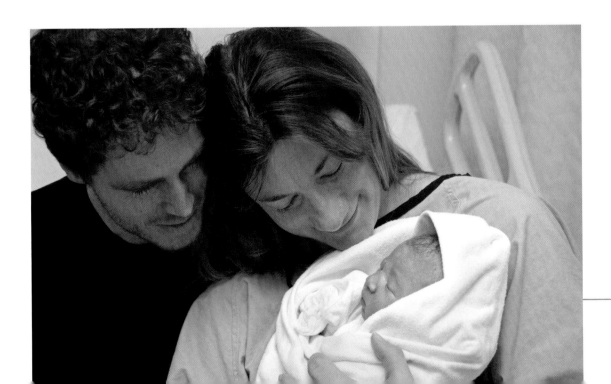

1. Labor and delivery plans

Birth setting

Specify where you want to give birth — in a hospital, birthing center, or at home. Make a list (and pack or set aside) the things you would like to have with you in the birth setting in order to make your environment more personal and comfortable — perhaps a CD or MP3 player with your favorite music, a camera, snacks, or other personal items.

. . . .

. . . .

Birth partners

Write down who will be in the labor room with you — your partner, friends, and family members, for example. Do you plan on having a doula? Are there any procedures or stages in labor during which you'd prefer that some or all of these people leave the room?

. . . .

. . . .

Positions for labor

Describe the positions you think you will prefer to use during labor. Write down how active you expect to be. For example, would you like to remain upright and mobile for as long as possible, or would you prefer to be in bed the whole time?

. . . .

. . . .

Pain management

Specify your pain management plan. What techniques do you plan to use? If you would like to avoid pain medications, such as an epidural, say so, but try to think whether there are any circumstances in which you might want one. Write down any medications that you should not have due to other health issues so everyone is clear. Brief your birth partner on this information.

. . . .

. . . .

Fetal monitoring

If the fetal heart rate is reassuring, you may have a choice regarding fetal monitoring. Specify if you would like your health-care provider to listen to your baby's heartbeat intermittently (using a hand-held device) or if you would prefer continuous fetal monitoring (using a belt strapped around your waist).

. . . .

. . . .

Cutting the umbilical cord

If you want your partner or some other family member to cut the umbilical cord, indicate this in your birth plan.

. . . .

. . . .

Interventions in labor and delivery

This is probably the trickiest part of a birth plan for everyone involved — laboring women, their families, and the health-care team. Write down how you feel about induction of labor. You might also want to express a preference for forceps or vacuum techniques if, at the end of labor, you need some assistance in delivering your baby. What are your feelings about having an episiotomy? Many women include blanket statements in their birth plan, such as "no oxytocin," or "no forceps." Instead, give some thought to circumstances in which you might consider an intervention. For example, "oxytocin only to be used if there is no change in cervical dilation in 4 hours."

. . . .

. . . .

. . . .

. . . .

. . . .

2. Newborn baby planning

Newborn baby care

Assuming your baby looks well at birth, would you like the baby placed directly on your chest to be dried off and maintain skin-to-skin contact initially? Or would you rather the baby be taken to a baby warmer to be dried off, cleaned, and wrapped up for you? Routine vitamin K injections and eye drops for the baby can be given immediately or delayed 20 to 30 minutes so you can have more uninterrupted time with your newborn.

. . . .

. . . .

Feeding your baby

Be clear about your decision to breastfeed or formula-feed your baby. Also be clear if you want your breastfed baby to be given any bottles.

. . . .

. . . .

Caring for your newborn baby

If you are giving birth in a hospital, specify if you want your newborn to stay in the hospital nursery or with you (called "rooming in") either all or part of the time.

. . . .

. . . .

Umbilical cord blood

Do you want to recover the blood from the umbilical cord to be "banked" for later use by your child, a family member, or any other person with a serious disease? Where will it be banked? Who is your contact?

. . . .

. . . .

. . . .

Circumcision

If your baby is a boy, state clearly whether you want him to be circumcised or not.

. . . .

. . . .

Special Needs

Note any special needs you may have. For instance, if you have a disability, note the kind of help you will need in labor and if there is any special equipment you need to assist you.

. . . .

. . . .

Religious beliefs and customs

If you have particular religious needs — birth rituals or dietary restrictions, for example — include these in your birth plan.

. . . .

. . . .

Other wishes

. . . .

. . . .

. . . .

. . . .

. . . .

. . . .

Antenatal record

Since your first trimester check-up, your primary care providers have been keeping a record of their findings at each prenatal appointment. In some places, the record is kept at the health-care provider's office, and in others, the pregnant woman carries the record with her. Known as the antenatal record, these notes communicate the course of your pregnancy to the doctors or midwives who will be attending the birth of your baby. If you are not carrying the antenatal record with you, it will be sent to the hospital at about 36 weeks.

Antenatal record form

The following information is typically recorded:

Due date .... based on a last menstrual period of ....

and/or an ultrasound on (date) .... with a gestational size of .... weeks.

Medications: ....

Allergies: ....

Blood tests:

Initial hemoglobin ....

Blood type: A, B, AB or 0 .... Rhesus + ...or – ....

Sickle cell screen: + ...or – ....

Chronic conditions: ....

....

Diabetes screening:

Normal .... or abnormal..................................

Genetic screening results:

Type of test: .... Result: ....normal or ....abnormal

Amnio or CVS result (if done) ....

Other: ....

Infectious disease immunity/exposures:

Rubella (German measles): + ... (immune) or – .... (not immune)

Hepatitis B: +....................................or – ....

Syphilis: +..or – ....

HIV: + ...or – ....

Varicella (chicken pox): immune ....or not immune...........
(often determined by history of infection or vaccination, not a blood test)

Other: ....

Ultrasound scans:

Date.. Gestational age......................... Finding...................................

Date.. Gestational age.........................Finding...................................

Date.. Gestational age.........................Finding...................................

Charting: On average there are 10 prenatal visits

Date	Gestational age	Weight	Blood pressure	Symphysis-fundal height	Fetal heart rate

Issues or problems arising:

....

....

....

....

Birth partner

A birth partner (also called a labor partner or labor coach) is someone who remains with you during labor and childbirth. It is often your partner, but it could also be a close friend or relative, or even a doula. It should be someone with whom you are very comfortable, because their main job will be to help you feel safe, secure, and supported during labor and delivery, providing practical assistance and, if necessary, helping you to communicate with the attending health-care providers. Make sure you inform your health-care providers who your birth partner will be so that they know who will be with you during labor.

Birth partner benefits

Medical studies have shown that the continuous presence of a labor-support person has a number of benefits for the progress of labor, including slightly reducing the need for epidural analgesia, shortening labor by up to 2 hours, and slightly reducing Caesarean section rates. In addition, women report less anxiety and usually report that having a labor-support person is very helpful. Having a birth partner will be particularly helpful if this is your first pregnancy.

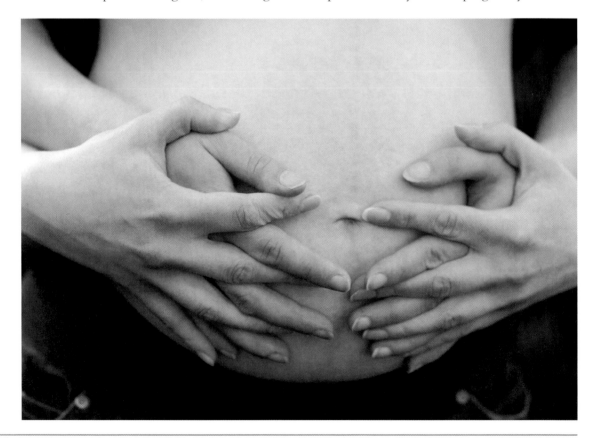

Guide to ...

Birth partner's role

Birth partners typically help you before and during labor and delivery, making sure you are ready for the occasion and attending to your needs in childbirth. Your birth partner is your assistant, your trusted collaborator, and your advocate.

Before labor and delivery

- Help you prepare your birth plan.
- Attend your medical checkups with you.
- Take childbirth classes with you and spend time reviewing what you've learned in class.
- Visit the hospital maternity area with you — birthing room, nursery, and postpartum rooms — and plan the trip to the hospital from your home — the means of transportation, the route, the travel time, the entrances to use.
- Help you pack your hospital bag with the necessary supplies for labor, birth, and homecoming.

In early labor

- Help you time your contractions in the first stages of labor.
- Support you through your contractions.
- Help you decide when to go to the hospital.
- Travel with you to the hospital.
- Help with any necessary administrative paperwork once you arrive at the hospital.

During active labor and delivery

- Fetch and carry things (ice, popsicles, warm blankets ...), contact people who are waiting for news, and sometimes ... manage your visitors!
- Help you manage your pain using whatever techniques you have planned (and perhaps practiced). If one technique is not working, your birth partner should be ready to help you consider alternatives. Your birth partner must support your pain management decisions without reservation.
- Provide undying support and comfort by:
  - Remaining calm, speaking in a relaxed, confident tone of voice
  - Staying close to you
  - Keeping eye contact with you
  - Talking to you between contractions
  - Offering encouragement as you push
  - Celebrating the birth of your baby with you!

Packing your bag

Pack you hospital bag now — no delays — but bring only what you need, nothing else. There is not usually a lot of space in hospital rooms for "stuff." Leave your valuables at home. Don't forget the camera and extra batteries! Be sure to include the following items. Check them off as they go into your bag.

Paperwork
- Health card and insurance information
- Copy of your birth plan

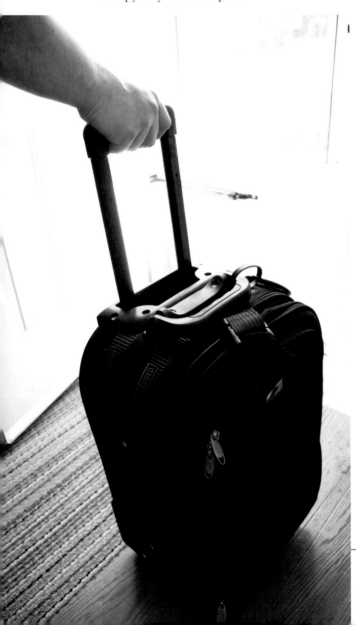

- Antenatal record, if not already sent to the hospital
- Important contact information (friends and family to notify after birth)
- Small amount of money for incidentals

Toiletries
- Toothpaste, toothbrushes, and other personal hygiene products
- Shampoo and soap
- Sanitary pads (large size)

Clothing
- Warm socks and slippers
- Dressing gown
- Nightgown or pajamas (possibly with slits for nursing)
- Outfit to wear home (soft, loose pants advised)
- Nursing bra if you are breastfeeding
- Plenty of underwear — older rather than new

Baby supplies
- Diapers: newborn size, 1 package
- Baby clothes: 1 to 2 sleepers, cotton hats, cotton mittens (to prevent scratches)
- Receiving blankets: 2 to 3
- Sweater or snowsuit for going home in cold weather
- Car seat

Other useful or comforting items
- Snacks (sandwiches, crackers, and fruit, for instance)
- Watch or clock with second hand for timing contractions
- Magazines and books (especially if you plan on having an epidural)
- CD or MP3 player
- Your own pillow

Furnishings and clothing for the newborn

Furnishing a nursery and buying clothes for your newborn do not have to be complex undertakings — nor do they have to break the bank. There are relatively few items of furniture you absolutely need to have for your newborn, the most important being a crib, a car seat, and a stroller. Borrowing items from friends and family, as well as visiting second-hand shops, is cost-effective (and good for the environment). And … your baby won't know the difference!

Newborn clothing

Keep in mind that infants are wriggly and do not like to have their clothes changed, so choose items that are easy to put on and remove. Look for things that stretch and have wide necks, as well as items that open in front and have snaps. Avoid clothes with buttons and ties, and try to pick items made of cotton, which is comfortable and easy on a baby's soft skin. Launder the baby's clothes in a mild detergent.

Babies grow out of their clothes quickly, so don't buy too much right away. Always buy according to weight, not age, and try to get enough clothing to give you some respite between loads of laundry.

Baby linens

Look for the same qualities in baby linens as in your choice of clothing.

Blankets

Swaddling blankets, or receiving blankets, are very useful for wrapping your baby, protecting the baby from cold, covering surfaces prior to laying the baby down and, yes, protecting your clothing from baby burps. At least six thin, cotton receiving blankets would be extremely useful, plus one or two thicker blankets for use outdoors.

Did You Know?

Basic baby clothes

Here's a basic list of items for your baby's wardrobe:

- 6 onesies (one-piece, undershirt-like garments with snaps at the crotch)
- 2 nightgowns
- 2 or 3 stretchy pull-on pants
- 4 to 8 pairs of socks or baby booties
- 4 to 6 T-shirts with shoulder snaps
- 1 sun hat and 1 or 2 light jackets or sweaters for mild weather
- Warm hat, mittens, and snowsuit for winter
- 5 sleepers with feet and 2 blanket sleepers
- 1 fancy outfit for special occasions and photo opportunities

Sheets

Fitted crib sheets are the safest. You will need at least two.

Bath towels

Baby towels are softer and smaller than adult ones. Optional, but very nice to have. Some baby towels have hoods to help keep the baby warm. Baby washcloths are essential, and fortunately cheap. Stock up.

Baby carriers

An infant carrier or body sling worn on the body is among the most useful items of baby gear you'll buy. That's because babies love to be held, and they love motion. Infant carriers hold the baby close and safe next to your body, leaving both of your hands free, and allow your infant to cuddle with you while feeling the rhythmic motions of your breathing and walking. Using a baby carrier can be the fastest way to soothe a fussy infant — it's even a good way to put him to sleep.

A baby carrier need not be a major purchase. In fact, you can use any sort of fabric to wrap around yourself and your baby. There are, however, many commercial choices available, from designer slings and wraps to front carriers, and even special hiking backpacks.

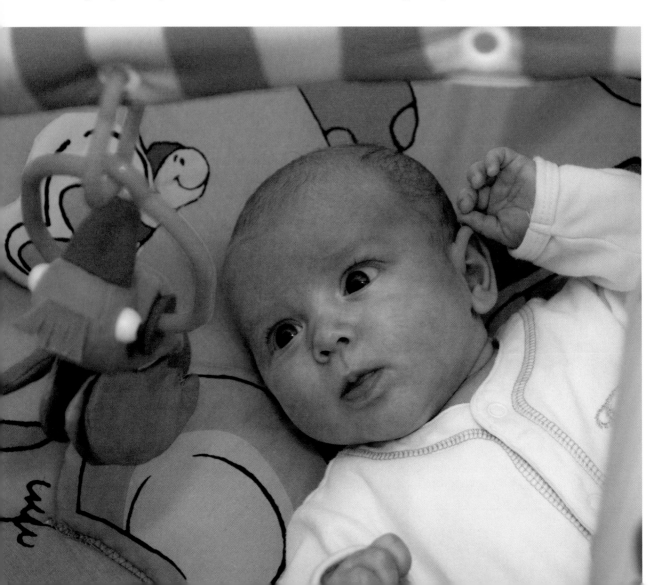

Guide to ...

Crib safety

The safest place for your baby to sleep is in a crib in your room. Follow these important safety recommendations:

- Look for a label stating that the crib conforms to American and Canadian safety standards.

- Check the space between the bars of the crib rail. The bars should be no more than $2\frac{3}{8}$ inches (6 cm) apart, so that babies can't get their heads caught between them.

- Be sure the crib mattress fits properly. An undersized mattress will leave a gap along the side or end of the crib where an infant's head can get caught. To check the fit of a crib mattress, push it to one corner. There should be no more than a $1\frac{1}{2}$-inch (4 cm) gap between it and the side or end of the crib. If you can fit more than two fingers between the mattress and the crib, the mattress is too small.

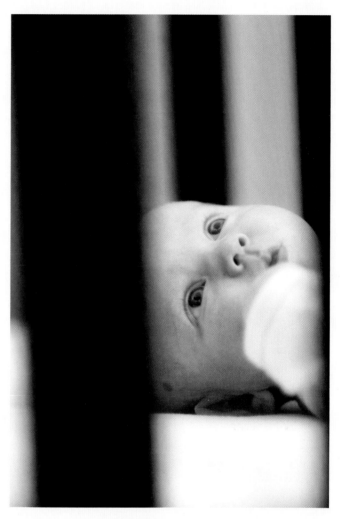

- Spread sheets smoothly and tuck them snugly under the mattress. This lessens the chance of wrinkles in the bedding obstructing your baby's breathing.

- Do not use crib bumper pads.

- Remove anything that could obstruct your baby's breathing passages — things like decorative pillows, fuzzy stuffed animals, tiny toys, and, of course, bumper pads.

- Put your baby to sleep on her back. Infants under 6 months should not sleep on their tummies unless there is a doctor-recommended reason for it. However, if a baby rolls onto her tummy on her own, you do not need to roll her back.

- Don't place the crib near a heater, against a window, near any dangling cords from blinds or draperies, or close to furniture that the baby will eventually be able to use to climb out of the crib.

- Be careful with crib toys (like mobiles) that are fastened between the side rails and hang over the crib. These toys are recommended only from birth to 5 months and should be removed when the baby is old enough to push herself up on her hands and knees.

Guide to ...

Furnishings and equipment

Bassinet, or Moses basket

A small, portable bed is perfect for babies from birth to about 4 months. The shape and size provide a "cocoon" that infants seem to find comforting. Bassinets are also quite convenient because you can easily move them from room to room, keeping the baby with you as she naps.

Crib

Shop around for a crib that meets all safety standards. Make sure the crib is sturdy and quiet as you slide the guardrails up and down. It should also be at a height that's comfortable for you to reach your baby.

Bedding

Although those bedding sets that come with crib bumpers, blankets, and pillows are very attractive, they are also a potential health hazard for your baby. Avoid any soft bedding in your baby's crib to help reduce the risk of sudden infant death syndrome (SIDS). The only bedding advised is a bottom sheet for the mattress and perhaps a light blanket.

Bathtub

You'll need a bathtub made for newborns that fits into the family bathtub or sits on a counter. Never leave your baby alone in the bathtub. Never.

Changing table

The changing table should be sturdy and have protective sides or belts so your baby

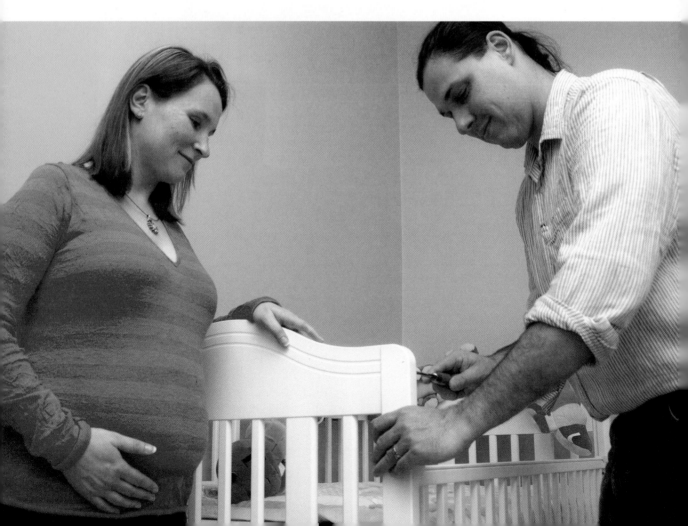

can't roll off. Be sure the table gives you easy access to all the items you need when changing the baby — diapers, powders, wipes, lotion, and a change of clothes. (Assume you'll have only one hand free to get these items.) Make sure the height is right — you don't want to have to bend over to change the baby. You will also need a diaper pail nearby.

Stroller or baby carriage

Many families splurge on a stroller or carriage. A good stroller will probably get daily use for 3 or more years. Consider a stroller that is sturdy in all kinds of weather, adaptable for use with a baby and, eventually, a toddler, and collapsible if you need to put it into a car.

Rocking chair

Some parents and their babies enjoy a rocking chair or glider, both as a place to cuddle and soothe the baby and as a place to nurse or bottle-feed.

Baby swing

Some babies love motion, and swinging can be soothing for a fussy baby, but not all babies like swings. A baby swing should be durable and comfortable.

Mobile

Colorful mobiles that hang above a crib are stimulating for infants, who can recognize things that are 8 to 10 inches (20 to 25 cm) in front of them. Some mobiles play music, which can be calming.

Baby monitor

A baby monitor is a remote intercom system that allows you to hear your infant when you're in another room. Some even have video capabilities so that you can see your baby. Choose a good-quality monitor with amplification and range that suit the size

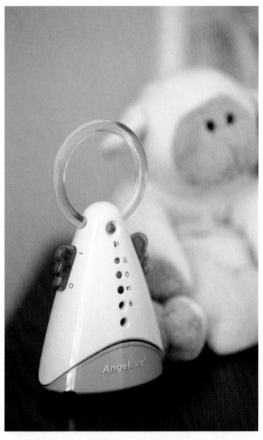

of your home. Make sure it's convenient enough to carry with you throughout the house while the baby is sleeping.

Be aware that this is a transmitting device that uses a radio frequency. You may hear sounds from your neighbor's baby if their monitor uses the same frequency as yours, or you may pick up conversations from cordless phones for the same reason. (Or you may find out that a conversation you thought was private was broadcast outside your home!)

Playpen

Not many children are dropped in a playpen just to play anymore. More often, a playpen is used as a portable bed or a place to put your baby out of harm's way, protected from other children, pets, and hazards.

Infant car seats

An infant car seat is one thing that should be on your "must-have" list. Buy one before your baby is born, so you'll be prepared right from the first car ride you take with your infant — probably the trip home from the hospital. In the event of a serious accident, a properly installed car seat can reduce the risk of serious injury or death by as much as 71%.

Car seat models

Car seats are not one-size-fits-all. They are made to accommodate three different stages of childhood: newborns and infants, toddlers, and older children. For newborns and infants, use rear-facing seats until they are at least 1 year old and have reached the seat's maximum height or weight limits. Then you will need to switch to a forward-facing seat.

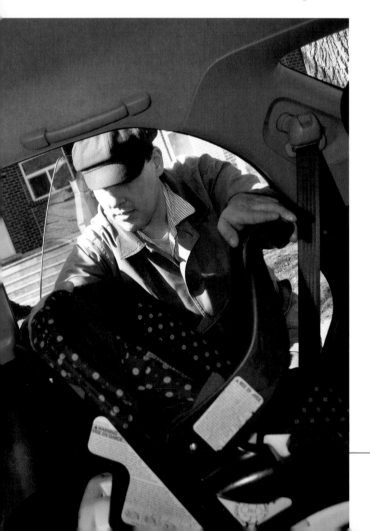

Guide to ...

Car seat safety

For rear-facing car seats for use from birth to 22 lbs (10 kg), here are some tips for making sure your newborn is protected when riding in a car:

1. Place the infant car seat on the back seat of the vehicle. Front seats are not safe for children younger than 12 years. The safest place is the middle of the back seat

2. Never install a rear-facing car seat in a seat equipped with an air bag.

3. Hold the seat in place using the car's seat belts, with the baby facing the rear of the vehicle. The seat should rest on a 45-degree angle and move no more than 1 inch (2.5 cm) side to side or forward at the base. If necessary, put a towel or piece of foam under the base of the seat to adjust the angle.

4. When tightening the vehicle seat belt, push the infant seat down and into the upholstery, and pull the belt as tight as possible. There should be very little movement.

5. Slot the harness straps at or below the baby's shoulders. You should not be able to fit more than one finger underneath the harness straps at the child's collarbone. The chest clip should be flat against the chest at armpit level.

Breastfeeding or formula-feeding

There is no doubt that breast milk is the best food for a newborn baby, and with good support, more than 95% of women are able to breastfeed successfully. Still, some women choose to formula-feed for a variety of reasons. Weigh all the factors and make this decision for yourself. Remember, your baby's nutritional and emotional needs will be met regardless of your feeding choice. Breast milk or formula both provide all the nutrition babies need until about 6 months, when they start eating solid foods. Water, juice, and other foods are usually not needed until then.

Benefits of breastfeeding

Breastfeeding has many benefits for babies, their families, and society in general. There are many medical, developmental, emotional, economic, and environmental advantages. Besides promoting bonding between mother and child, breastfeeding is free, readily available, and environmentally friendly — and it has never been recalled by the manufacturer!

Food value

Most importantly, breast milk is a living, dynamic fluid that changes from feed to feed and from day to day, during the first year, to exactly meet the demands of a growing baby. The milk of mothers of pre-term infants is even different from that of mothers of full-term infants, providing babies with more of the specific nutrients they need. Breast milk is easily digested by the baby's immature systems. Breastfed babies tend to grow more appropriately than formula-fed infants. Obesity is rare among breastfed infants — it is difficult to overfeed a breastfed infant.

Physical development

Breastfeeding helps the baby develop strong facial muscles for speech and correct teeth formation and alignment.

Did You Know?

Professional position

Most professional groups concerned with the care of newborns advocate breastfeeding exclusively for about the first 6 months. These groups include the World Health Organization (WHO), the American Pediatric Academy, and the Canadian Paediatric Society. "Exclusive breastfeeding is recommended for the first 6 months of life for healthy term infants," Health Canada recommends, "as breast milk is the best food for optimal growth. Infants should be introduced to nutrient-rich, solid foods with particular attention to iron at 6 months with continued breastfeeding for up to 2 years and beyond."

Did You Know?

Peer pressure to breastfeed

There is a great deal of pressure on new mothers to breastfeed, so much so that women who are unable or choose not to breastfeed often end up feeling guilty. For most women, this is undoubtedly a difficult decision, fraught with emotion and not lightly taken. You need support and assistance in the challenging first weeks of motherhood, not negativity. Try to move forward with your decision to formula-feed, and do not allow any judgmental commentary from the people around you to upset you.

Remember, a mother's happiness is essential to a baby's happiness. Formula-feed your baby with joy and love, and take advantage of the opportunity to allow others to share in the opportunity to enjoy feeding your baby as well.

Immunological protection

Among other things, breast milk contains white blood cells, antibodies, and immunoglobulin A (IgA), which are important for immunological protection against allergies, gastrointestinal disorders, respiratory infections, and ear infections throughout childhood and adulthood.

Recent studies have shown that breast-fed babies have significantly fewer infections in the first year of life when compared to formula-fed babies.

SIDS prevention

A number of studies have suggested an association between breastfeeding and protection against sudden infant death syndrome (SIDS). Although the exact cause of SIDS is not known, we do know that breastfed babies have a lower incidence of SIDS than formula-fed babies.

Lower risk of chronic conditions

Studies have also shown that breastfeeding may help reduce the risk of your child developing certain chronic conditions, such as asthma, allergies, and diabetes. The benefits extend beyond the infancy period, offering protection against disease onset in adulthood.

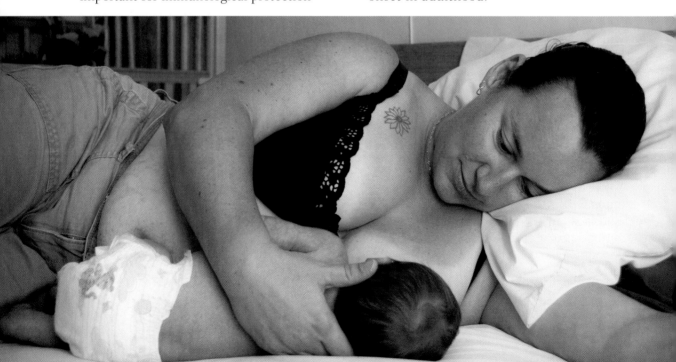

Breastfeeding challenges

Although breastfeeding is clearly beneficial for mother and baby, there are some challenges to consider:

- **Learning curve:** Breastfeeding is a learned skill, especially if this is your first baby. Even your baby needs to learn to breastfeed herself! Many women and babies are able to breastfeed easily and intuitively, but for some women and babies, it is a more difficult process.

  It is a good idea to think about where you will find breastfeeding support if you need it after the baby is born. Good options include:
  - Lactation consultants — both in hospital-based clinics and in private practice.
  - Your midwife, if you have one
  - Breastfeeding clinics. Find out what is available in your community and take down some phone numbers... just in case.

- **Maternal demands:** Breastfeeding requires a substantial commitment from you. Some women feel tied down by the constant demands of a nursing newborn. Since breast milk is easily digested, breastfed babies tend to eat more often than babies who are fed formula. This can be tiring, though before long babies feed less frequently and sleep longer at night.

- **Portability:** Some new mothers need to be away from their babies from time to time — for instance, to return to work outside the home. Some may opt for formula-feeding so that others can give the baby a bottle. Working mothers who want to continue breastfeeding can, however, use a breast pump to collect breast milk to be given in a bottle so their babies still get its benefits when they're not available to breastfeed.

- **Vitamin D supplements:** Because vitamin D is not present in breast milk in adequate amounts, breastfed infants require a supplement: 400 IU is recommended.

- **Modesty:** You might feel uncomfortable about breastfeeding in public. If you are not able to find a private place to nurse, cover yourself with a blanket so that no one is any the wiser.

- **Contraindications:** Breastfeeding should not be used by mothers with untreated, active tuberculosis, those in long-term chemotherapy treatments, those using street drugs, those who are HIV positive, or those whose infants have galactosemia (a rare genetic metabolic disorder).

Enhanced cognitive development

Although the mechanism remains unclear, studies indicate that breastfed babies score slightly higher than formula-fed babies from similar environments on cognitive development tests.

Maternal benefits

For the mother, breastfeeding has been linked with a shortened postpartum length of stay in hospital, a quicker return to pre-pregnancy weight by burning calories, and delayed menses. It also helps shrink the uterus. Extended periods of breastfeeding are also associated with a reduction in rates of breast cancer.

Formula-feeding limitations

Although some women may prefer formula-feeding, there are some limitations to consider:

- **Decreased immunity:** Your baby will not receive the immunity agents found in breast milk that protect against allergies, infections, SIDs, and other conditions that can develop during childhood and adulthood.
- **Inconvenience:** Formula-feeding can require a great deal of organization and preparation, especially for outings.
- **Costs:** Formula-feeding is more expensive than breastfeeding.

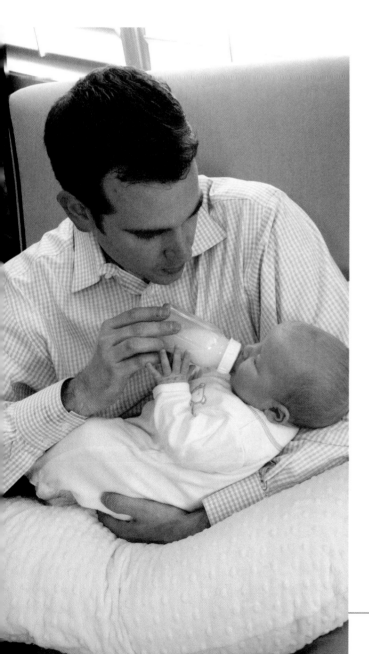

Reasons for formula-feeding

Despite the clear benefits of breastfeeding, some women may not be able to breastfeed for medical reasons, while others may choose to formula-feed for lifestyle reasons or personal preference. And sometimes, breastfeeding just does not work out; for example, sometimes there is not enough milk to support complete breastfeeding, which is most common following breast reduction surgery.

Sharing bonding

Formula-feeding allows you to share not only the work but also the pleasure of feeding your baby with your partner, your parents, your other children, and your friends, who all have a chance to bond with your baby.

Fewer feedings

Because babies digest formula more slowly than breast milk, a baby who is getting formula may need fewer feedings than one who breastfeeds.

Fortified

There is no need for nutritional supplements, because infant formula contains the right blend of vitamins, including vitamin D. Iron-fortified formula is recommended for a baby's first year (12 mg iron per quart/liter).

Pain relief in pregnancy

No question, pregnancy can be painful at times, ranging from everyday aches and complaints to the pain of labor and delivery. Many women would rather suffer pain than take a painkiller in pregnancy, fearing that the medication may harm the fetus. Fortunately, there is a wide array of pain relief strategies and safe medications available with no potential harm to your health or your baby's.

Everyday analgesics

For the backaches, the headaches, the leg pains, and more, you will want to have at hand an effective and safe pain relief medication, or analgesic. Analgesics are medications used to relieve pain. They are available for purchase over the counter or by prescription.

Multi-modal analgesia

Current approaches to pain management are known as multi-modal analgesia, where the three chief classes of analgesics are combined so that their positive effects are compounded while their negative effects are minimized because less of each is needed. All three classes of medications are taken together to decrease pain and enable an early return to normal function. The first two classes of drugs are considered opioid-sparers because they help decrease the amount of opioids that are required.

Three classes of analgesics

1. Acetaminophen
2. Non-steroidal anti-inflammatories (NSAIDs), such as ibuprofen, diclofenac, ketorolac, or indomethacin
3. Opioids, such as morphine and codeine

Safety in pregnancy

Some analgesics are safe in pregnancy, but a few should be used with caution and avoided or substituted with a safe alternative.

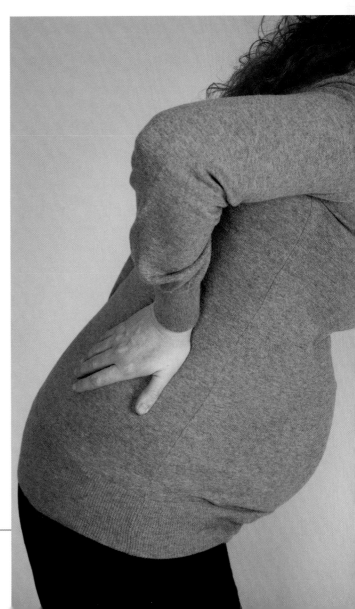

Did You Know?

Analgesic effectiveness and safety in pregnancy

Acetaminophen

Acetaminophen is widely used in pregnancy for relief of pain and fever. Acetaminophen does cross the placenta, but is considered safe in usual doses. It can be used routinely in all trimesters. It is the analgesic of choice for a variety of aches and pains in pregnancy.

Non-steroidal anti-inflammatories (NSAIDs)

NSAIDs include ASA (acetylsalicylic acid widely known as Aspirin), ibuprofen, and indomethacin. These medications also cross the placenta and should be avoided during pregnancy, particularly in the last trimester.

They can delay labor, increase the length of labor, and cause complications in the newborn baby. Aspirin can also increase the risk of bleeding in the mother and baby if taken in the third trimester. The use of NSAIDs later in the pregnancy has been associated with constriction of a major fetal blood vessel and low amniotic fluid levels. Evidence also indicates that these medicines should be avoided in the first trimester because they may increase the risk of miscarriage and fetal malformations.

Nevertheless, low doses of ASA are sometimes prescribed during pregnancy for the treatment of specific conditions.

Opioids

Many narcotic preparations for pain relief containing opioids, such as codeine, morphine, Demerol, and dihydrocodeine, cross the placenta during pregnancy, but they have not been associated with adverse fetal affects when used in standard dosages. However, if used in high doses immediately prior to the delivery of the fetus, opioids have been associated with depression of a newborn's breathing, and so they are generally avoided in laboring women, if possible. Long-term use may also cause a withdrawal syndrome in the newborn infant. If opioids are used long-term during pregnancy, this should be under the supervision of a health-care provider, and, post-delivery, a pediatrician should be informed of its use in order to look for signs of withdrawal in the newborn baby.

Local anesthetics

Local anesthetic for pain relief can be applied as a cream (such as EMLA), a gel (such as Xylocaine), or an injection administered by a health-care provider. This includes the administration of local anesthetics to provide relief of pain in preparation for dental work. All of these forms of pain relief are safe for use in pregnancy.

Pain relief in labor

There are many choices to make in the weeks leading up to your labor and delivery, none more complicated than deciding if you want to use pain relief medications. Labor pain hurts, but you can manage the pain in may different ways. Consider this issue now, prior to beginning labor — once you are in pain, it is virtually impossible to think clearly and make a decision about the different options.

"Natural" childbirth

Many people refer to a labor and delivery without the use of pain relief medications as "natural childbirth." Some women put a premium on not using pain relief medications and stigmatize others who give birth "unnaturally" by using pain relief medications. Medical professionals know this is a false dichotomy. Every woman's experience of pain is different, and every mother is entitled to deal with labor pain in the way that suits her best.

Pain relief without medications

Women have managed labor pain without medications for millennia. A recent study showed that 60% to 70% of women surveyed still use at least some traditional methods

Sources of labor pain

First stage: Originates in the uterus and cervix, which are being stretched and deprived of oxygen by uterine contractions.

Second stage: Originates in tissues of the pelvic floor, ligaments, vagina, and perineum as they are stretched by the fetus.

during their labor, either alone or in combination with medications. Few of these methods have been subjected to rigorous scientific study to test their effectiveness, but they are considered safe. The goal of most of these methods is not to eliminate the physical perception of pain, but to help you manage the pain so you are comforted and able to cope with it effectively, often by distracting your attention. The most important element of all these methods is the continued presence of a supportive and encouraging birth partner and team. Education and assistance by your health-care providers, before and during labor, will increase your sense of control and confidence, contributing to your ability to cope with labor pain.

Pain relief with medications

Labor progress and labor pains can be unpredictable, and some women change their minds about methods of pain relief during labor. You may start out convinced you do not want medications, but circumstances might dictate otherwise — for example, if your labor is particularly long, if you have back labor, if you have to have an assisted delivery by forceps, or even if the pain is simply more intense than you were anticipating. Don't judge yourself or allow yourself to be judged

Guide to ...

Non-medicated pain relief

Movement and positioning: Moving around is a great way to reduce your pain. In the first stage of labor, being upright is considered less painful than lying down. Try to walk around, sit, stand, stretch, get on your hands and knees, and change positions as you feel best. Sometimes a large exercise ball (or birthing ball) can be helpful, allowing you to sit-squat on a soft surface.

Massage: Massage of your head, back, hands, and feet during labor reduces your anxiety levels and pain. It is probably most effective in the first stages of labor.

Bathing and showering: Many women find relief by showering or bathing. A hot shower directed toward a sore back can be helpful. Immersion in a warm bath has been shown to reduce pain during labor. Keep the water temperature just above body temperature so you don't overheat. If you find it soothing, you can spend much of your labor in the water.

Heat and cold: Some women have tried using hot and cold packs on the back, lower abdomen, and groin. Be careful not to burn or freeze the skin through prolonged exposure! Heat sources can include hot water bottles, heating pads, or warm and wet cloths, while cold sources include bags filled with ice, frozen gel packs, bags of frozen vegetables, or even cold drinks in cans. Alternate the heat and cold, and keep the intervals to a few minutes at a time.

Breathing techniques: Breathing and relaxation techniques are usually taught in childbirth education classes. Although often parodied in comedies, about 50% of women in labor use breathing techniques — and most find them helpful.

Audioanalgesia: No, this is not a fancy car stereo... rather, it is the use of music or other sounds to reduce your perception of pain. Modest reductions in pain perception have been reported but it hasn't been well studied in laboring women. Using headphones may help you focus more on the music, providing a better distraction. Make your own playlist for labor!

Hypnosis: This technique involves significant pre-labor training by a hypnotherapist. Usually, the pregnant woman is taught to self-induce a hypnotic state during labor; sometimes her labor partner can be taught to help her with this process. Most studies have reported a reduction in the use of anesthesia in women who have used hypnosis. You shouldn't use this method if you have ever had a psychotic episode.

Acupuncture: Although it is unclear whether or not acupuncture reduces pain perception, it does seem to increase relaxation and lead to less use of pain medication. Acupuncture needles are placed at specific sites, depending upon the location and nature of the pain. Acupuncture must be performed by someone well trained in the procedure. There do not seem to be any risks to using acupuncture in labor. Shiatsu massage may have similar effects.

TENS: Transcutaneous electric nerve stimulation (TENS) is the use of low-voltage electrical impulses that are transmitted to the skin from a small hand-held device. The intensity of the impulses can be controlled by a dial on the machine. TENS causes a buzzing or prickling sensation that distracts you from the labor pain. TENS has a modest impact upon pain perception and is probably most effective in the earliest stages of labor. TENS units are available at health-care supply stores.

negatively for changing your mind. Your goal is a manageable and safe delivery experience for both you and your baby. If you feel pain relief medications should or could be part of the process, don't hesitate to include them.

For most women using medications for pain relief during vaginal births, an epidural is the method of choice, while spinal procedures are more commonly used in Caesarean births. Because both epidural and spinal medications are directed specifically toward the nerves in the spine, none reach the mother's bloodstream or the baby.

For those who cannot have an epidural or a spinal procedure, or prefer not to, other options are available. These options include opioid drugs, nitrous oxide, and nerve blocks. General anesthesia can be used in Caesarean births but is not commonly necessary.

Epidural procedure

Epidurals are usually given upon request and are available 24 hours a day in most intermediate and large hospitals. If you will be at a smaller hospital for your baby's birth, inquire about availability, because many rural hospitals either do not offer epidurals or provide them only at specific times.

You may request an epidural at any time after an obstetrician has determined that you are in labor, and it can be given up until it is time to deliver. Once you have requested an epidural, an anesthesiologist will see you as soon as possible. The anesthesiologist will review your medical chart and antenatal record while discussing the procedure, risks, and complications with you. Most women experience high rates of satisfaction with this form of pain relief.

Spinal procedure

A spinal is a single injection of a small amount of local anesthetic (freezing medicine) and painkillers directly into the fluid that bathes your spinal cord. It works very quickly and lasts for 2 to 3 hours. The spinal needle is very tiny and is removed immediately. Nothing is left in your back. Once the medications are delivered, you will immediately start to feel a warm and tingling sensation in your legs, which will spread up to your chest. Within minutes, you will not be able to move your legs. Although your legs will be lying straight on the table, it is common to feel as if your legs are in another position. Spinals are commonly used in planned Caesarean births, as well as Caesareans preceded by labor where no epidural was placed.

■ Spinal procedure

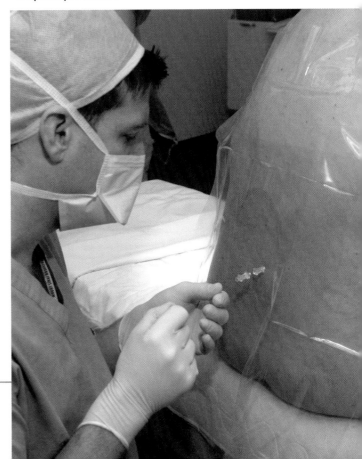

Did You Know?

Epidural procedure

1. Once you have consented to the epidural, your anesthesiologist will help place you in a sitting position or a position lying on your side, and show you how to arch your lower back to make it easier to perform the procedure. Your lower back will be cleaned with a cold solution, and a drape will be placed over the area to keep it clean.

2. An epidural delivers pain and anaesthetic medicine to the spine just outside your spinal column. The anesthesiologist will feel your back, looking for the best spot to place the epidural. He will then "freeze" the skin at that spot with a local anesthetic. You will feel a little needle prick (like a bee sting), followed by some burning when the freezing is first injected into the skin.

3. Once your skin is frozen, your anesthesiologist will insert the epidural needle, thread into place a fine plastic tube, or catheter, and then remove the needle.

4. Once the catheter is in place, anesthetic and painkillers can be delivered into the epidural space, freezing the nerves leading to the uterus the way a dentist freezes the nerves to a tooth. The catheter can be connected to a pump that delivers a constant flow of the medication to keep you comfortable. In addition, some machines have a button that you can press to obtain extra doses should you feel any discomfort. Some doctors do not use pumps and prefer to administer the medication intermittently.

5. When the catheter tube is placed, patients occasionally feel an electric shock in one of their legs (like hitting your funny bone) or an odd electrical sensation in their backs. These are brief and of no significance. Once the catheter is taped in place, you will not feel it, and you can adopt any position that is comfortable. You may feel a dull pressure in your lower back, but this should not be overly uncomfortable.

6. Occasionally, epidurals do not work the first time and need to be redone. The tip of the tube may not be in the correct location or may migrate. Fortunately, these problems are usually fixable.

Combined spinal-epidural procedure (CSE)

This procedure is a combination of the spinal and epidural techniques. A tiny needle is passed through the epidural needle directly into the water that bathes the spinal cord so that a small amount of medication can be administered there. The epidural catheter is then placed in position. Anesthesiologists vary in their opinions as to how and when to use this combined technique:

- **Early labor:** When the spinal-epidural combination is used in very early labor, many anesthesiologists put only painkillers in the spinal needle and do not use the epidural catheter until breakthrough pain (an increase in intensity) occurs. The advantage of this technique is that no freezing medication is put in, and you retain full strength and sensation in your legs. This procedure was originally known as a "walking epidural" because it allowed the patient to get up and walk around in early labor while still benefiting from pain relief.

• **Active labor:** In more active labor, a mixture of local anesthetics and painkillers is used. The advantages of the spinal-epidural method are twofold at this stage: quicker pain relief than a traditional epidural and maintenance of leg strength. Your legs will be numb, but you will still be able to move and push, if you need to, soon after the medications are given. Your anesthesiologist will control both the speed of the painkilling action and the effect on your legs by the type and amounts of local anesthetic used.

Labor pain effects

Uncontrolled labor pain can have negative effects on you during and after delivery, making the management of this pain important for the successful birth of your baby and your own well-being. These effects can include:

• Emotional distress

• Increased oxygen consumption

• Hyperventilation

• Increased blood pressure

• Reduced blood flow to the placenta

• Uncoordinated uterine contractions

• Postpartum psychological effects, including post-traumatic stress disorder

Epidural Placement

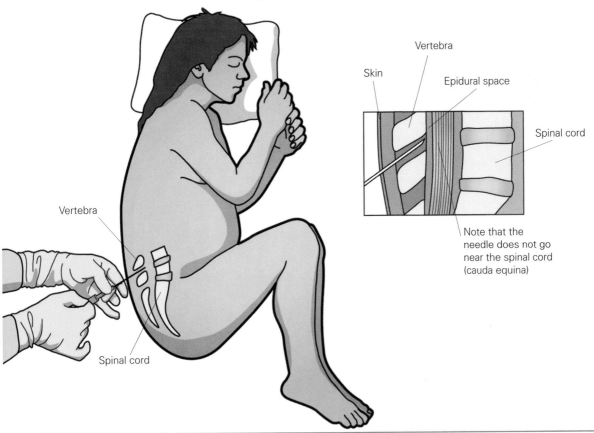

Vertebra

Skin

Epidural space

Spinal cord

Vertebra

Spinal cord

Note that the needle does not go near the spinal cord (cauda equina)

Did You Know?
Walking epidural

The original walking epidural referred to a combined spinal-epidural with no freezing medicine. During the last decade, the amount of local anesthetic used in epidurals has generally decreased to the point where most (but still not all) epidural techniques can be considered to be walking epidurals. Ultimately, whether or not you are able to walk depends on the amount of local anesthetic and your response to it. Most women feel numbness in their legs but are able to walk, at least with support.

Complications and side effects

For epidural, spinal, and CSE procedures, serious complications are extremely rare but can include nerve damage, paralysis, or toxic drug reactions that may lead to loss of consciousness or seizures. More common side effects are much less serious and easily managed:

- **Spinal headache:** Headache occurs when the spinal membrane is punctured and spinal fluid continues to leak. A special treatment, known as an epidural blood patch, usually fixes the problem. The tiny, blunt needles used for spinal anesthetics rarely cause this complication. A puncture is usually caused by larger epidural needles or sharp needles used for spinal tap procedures in other settings.
- **Itching:** Itching can occur as a reaction to the painkiller. If it is severe, there are several medications that can counteract it.
- **Temporary drop in blood pressure:** A drop in blood pressure is due to the dilation (opening up) of your blood vessels.

If your blood pressure drops, there are several medications readily available to bring it back to normal. A secondary effect of a drop in your blood pressure can be a drop in the fetal heart rate for up to a few minutes. Although this drop in the fetal heart rate will have your health-care team running to check on you and the baby, the fetal heart rate almost always returns to normal quickly, and there are no long-term consequences. In the very unusual circumstance that the fetal heart rate does not return to normal as your blood pressure rises, an emergency Caesarean section may be needed.

- **Bruising:** The epidural or spinal needle can cause bruising. Your back may be sore for a few days at the site of insertion, but there is no evidence of long-term back pain or back problems from epidurals and spinals.

Opioids

During labor, Demerol, morphine, and codeine are commonly used for pain relief, given by intermittent intravenous subcutaneous (under the skin) injection or intramuscular (deeper) injection. They can also be self-administered using a pump-and-button method known as patient-controlled analgesia (PCA). Although pain is not eliminated, most women notice an improvement, because their pain goes from severe to moderate.

If you take opioids during labor, you may feel sleepy, dizzy, nauseous, and itchy and experience urinary retention. Your baby may experience the same side effects because the delivery of opioids is not regional, like epidurals and spinals, and small amounts do cross the placenta. Although babies

Did You Know?

Laughing gas

Giving birth may be no laughing matter, but nitrous oxide (laughing gas) has been used as an anesthetic gas for more than 100 years. It has a long safety record and may be used without direct medical supervision. This gas will take away some of the pain (similar to IV painkillers) and has a mild sedative effect. Its main side effect is nausea and vomiting. The baby is minimally affected because the effects of this gas in both mother and baby are very short-lived (less than a minute) after discontinuation.

Nitrous oxide is usually self-administered and self-regulated. You hold a mask over your nose and mouth, pushing down on a valve on the gas tank and inhaling deeply when you need pain relief. If you become too sedated, you will not be able to push the valve to give yourself any more medication.

metabolize and clear these drugs, there is always a small risk that the baby will be born "narcotized" and will not want to breathe independently. As a result, whenever these drugs are used, someone able to assist the baby in breathing and administer an antidote (drug that reverses this effect) must be present during delivery. The types of drugs given by the PCA pain pump are usually cleared quickly by both mother and baby and seem to carry a lower incidence of this type of complication than the longer-acting medications given by injection.

Nerve blocks

"Nerve blocks" refers to the injection of freezing medication around a nerve other than around the spine in order to decrease sensation. An obstetrician can administer a pudendal nerve block prior to delivery to anesthetize the perineum and decrease the pain of delivery. This involves a transvaginal needle on the right and left of the perineum to freeze the nerve as it comes out under the pelvic bones. Local anesthetic for post-delivery repair of vaginal tears is also commonly used when no other methods of pain relief are being used.

Anesthesia for Caesarean section

If you are planning to undergo a Caesarean section, you may receive either a regional (spinal, epidural, or combined spinal-epidural) or general anesthetic. In most cases, regional anesthesia is used because it is felt to be better for both you and your baby.

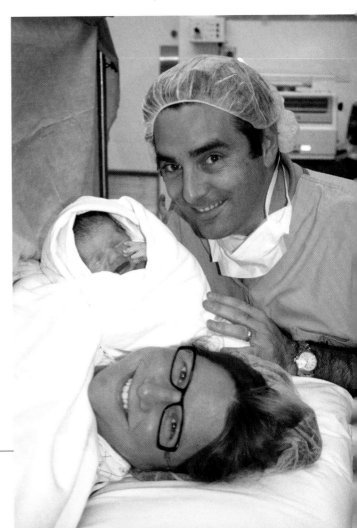

Guide to ...

General anesthesia procedure

1. You will be brought into the operating room and helped to lie down on the table. Heart monitors will be applied to your chest, and you will be asked to breathe oxygen through a plastic or rubber mask held over your nose and mouth by an anesthesia assistant. While you are doing this, the obstetrician will clean your abdomen with a cold solution and cover it with a drape to keep the area clean.

2. Once the anesthesiologist and obstetrician are ready, you will be given the medication and lose consciousness within seconds. As you are going to sleep, you may feel some pressure over your throat. This is done to prevent any contents in your stomach from coming up. Once you are asleep, a breathing tube will be inserted into your windpipe to keep the air passage clear. It is removed as you are waking up and is seldom remembered.

3. You will be kept asleep until the operation is finished and then brought to the recovery room. Your pain will be managed with intravenous painkillers, such as morphine.

4. It is very unlikely you will feel or remember anything that occurred during your operation. If you do, inform the anesthesiologist, who may be able to explain what it was that you experienced.

Regional anesthesia

Spinal anesthesia is the method most commonly used for elective, non-emergency Caesarean sections. It can also be used for those women in labor who need a Caesarean section and do not have an epidural in place. Epidurals are most commonly used for unplanned Caesarean sections where the epidural is already in place to relieve labor pains. Combined spinal-epidurals are not commonly used for planned Caesarean sections but can be used if already in place to relieve labor pains. In all cases, your freezing will be tested prior to the operation.

General anesthesia

General anesthesia is not commonly used for Caesarean section but may be needed when there are medical reasons for not using a spinal or epidural, such as bleeding tendencies or previous significant back surgery. There are also rare circumstances in which a woman in labor may need an emergency Caesarean section and there is not enough time to do a spinal or epidural. If regional anesthesia is inadequate during an operation, general anesthesia is the alternative. General anesthesia is also used if women refuse regional anesthesia.

Did You Know?

Birth partner support

Usually, your birth partner will be welcome to join you in the operating room in order to provide support and comfort to you. However, your birth partner may be asked to wait outside the operating room until the anesthetic is working well. In the unlikely event that you require a general anesthetic, your birth partner will not be invited into the operating room and will see you with your baby in the recovery room.

General anesthesia is commonly known as being "put to sleep." Medications are administered through intravenous equipment (into your vein). They work very quickly. The anesthetics used are the same as those for any other operation.

Advantages of regional anesthesia

- As safe, if not safer, than general anesthesia for both mother and baby
- No need to "wake up"
- Birth experience can be shared with birth partner
- Provides superior pain relief after the operation
- Baby is not exposed to even small amounts of general anesthetics
- Allows for early bonding and breastfeeding

Did You Know?
Mobility
In the effort to ensure safety, every hospital or birthing center has rules about how much mobility you will be allowed while under an anesthetic. Permitted mobility will vary from merely sitting up in a chair to being allowed to walk to and from the bathroom or up and down the halls. Discuss this well in advance with your obstetrician to understand what your options are and if you must be accompanied so you will be prepared. What obstetricians and anesthesiologists will or will not allow you to do once you have an epidural in place is not usually negotiable.

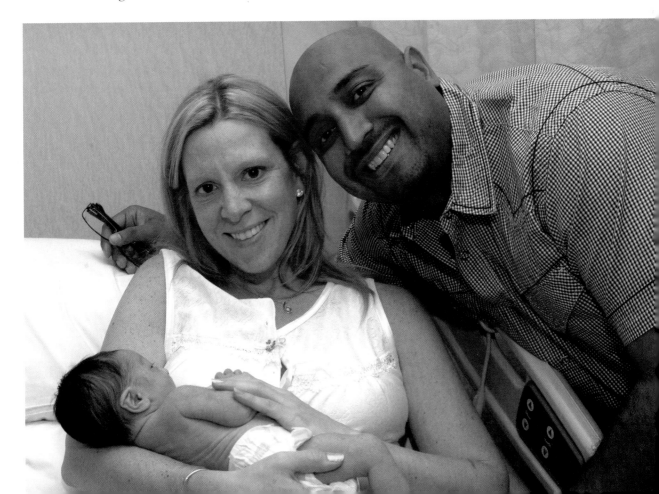

Umbilical cord blood banking

This is something relatively new to consider. You will need to decide in the third trimester if you want to bank your baby's umbilical cord blood. This blood remains in the umbilical cord and placenta after the baby is born, and can be collected painlessly and with no risk to mother or baby. It would normally be discarded but can be banked for later use in treating serious medical conditions, either in your child or in another family member.

Cord blood value

Cord blood contains stem cells that can develop into many different types of blood cells as they differentiate. Stem cells can be used to treat some types of cancer, blood diseases, and metabolic disorders.

Stem cells can be used by the individual they originated from, and sometimes by a relative or even an unrelated person. Cord blood banks have been established to store umbilical cord blood stem cells for possible future use in adult diseases, such as Alzheimer's, Parkinson's disease, and heart disease.

Cord blood banks

Cord blood can be collected at the time of birth from the umbilical cord and placenta, and then sent to a cord blood bank for processing and freezing. It is not clear yet how long cord blood samples can be stored — certainly several years, but beyond that it is not known if enough stem cells will survive to be useful.

There are two different types of banks — public and private. Public banks collect and store umbilical cord blood for the use of any individual who might need it, whereas private banks collect and store umbilical cord blood for the personal use of an individual donor child and family members.

Bank deposits

To bank your baby's cord blood, you will first need to register with a cord blood bank. The bank will provide you with a collection kit to take to the hospital to give to the delivery team. The hospital team will collect the sample for you and help you arrange its safe transfer to the cord blood bank. If you use a private bank, make sure your family physician knows that stem cells have been stored. Ask that the information (particularly the location) be recorded in the family's medical records.

Bank withdrawals

To withdraw the cord blood, notify the cord blood bank if your child becomes ill with a serious condition that can be treated by a stem cell transplant, and consult your family doctor or pediatrician. Cord blood stem cells could also be used by a child's relative who has taken ill or by a stranger whose blood is a good "match" with the baby's. In general, there are only enough stem cells in a cord blood sample to treat a child, although future research may allow transplantation into adults.

Circumcision

You and your partner should discuss circumcision now, if you haven't early in your pregnancy. Don't leave the decision until after your baby boy is born, when you're sure to have your hands full with many other things. It is best not to circumcise your baby until he is at least 24 hours old.

Optional procedure

Circumcision is a surgical procedure to remove the foreskin covering the end of the penis. The foreskin protects the end of the penis and likely contributes to sexual pleasure. Although there is no unequivocal health-related advantage to having your baby son circumcised, some research has suggested that circumcision may slightly reduce the risk of urinary tract infections and some sexually transmitted diseases, as well as penile cancer. Some parents choose to have their son circumcised based on their religious beliefs and personal preference.

Guide to ...

Circumcision procedure

- The procedure is usually performed by an obstetrician, a pediatrician, or, in the Jewish tradition, a mohel.

- Parents are often concerned about the pain their son may feel. Most doctors recommend pain control during circumcision, including sugar water (giving babies a sugar water–soaked pacifier reduces signs of distress); topical anesthetic creams, such as EMLA, applied about an hour prior to the procedure; or injections of local anesthetics (nerve blocks).

- During a circumcision, babies are restrained on a special board so that they remain still during the procedure. Clamps are used to elevate the foreskin from the rest of the penis while it is removed. The procedure should take just a few minutes.

- Afterwards, gauze soaked in petroleum jelly is placed over the penis. You should replace the gauze whenever you change his diapers for a few days.

- You will notice a crust forming, and maybe even a few drops of blood, but that is all part of the normal healing process.

- The risks are low. Although problems with too much bleeding, injury to other parts of the penis, or infection are possible, these complications are very rare.

F.A.Q.

We answer many questions from pregnant women and their partners. Here are some of the most frequently asked questions. Be sure to ask your health-care providers any other questions that may arise. If they don't have the answers, they will refer you to a colleague who does.

Q: *When should I take maternity leave from work?*

A: If you are still working and have not already done so, plan your maternity leave from work now. Check with your employer and government employment center to determine when you can take leave and for how long. You may want to and be able to work right up until you deliver the baby. Or you may want to take a few weeks off before the baby arrives, particularly if you have a physically demanding job. If you are self-employed, you will need to make arrangements with your clients. Find out what sort of paperwork needs to be completed to ensure that you receive all the benefits you are entitled to. In some jurisdictions and in some workplaces, paternity leave is also available so your partner can help out in those first few busy weeks or months.

Q: *Can my baby sleep with me when she's born?*

A: If you plan to have your baby "co-sleep" with you in your bed, use common sense. Remember that anything that could cause you to sleep more soundly than usual can affect your baby's safety. Don't sleep with your baby if you are extremely obese, are exhausted from sleep deprivation, or are under the influence of any drug (including alcohol) that could diminish sensitivity to your baby's presence. In addition, take the following precautions:

- Use a large bed (queen- or king-size).
- Place the baby between yourself and a guardrail or push the bed flush against the wall and position your baby between yourself and the wall.
- Position the baby beside you, rather than between you and your partner. Mothers seem to be physically and mentally aware of their baby's presence even while sleeping, which makes it unlikely you will roll over onto your baby.
- Do not sleep with your baby on a soft surface, such as a waterbed, beanbag, foam mat, or any other squishy surface that could obstruct breathing passages.
- Don't overheat or over-bundle the baby.
- Don't wear lingerie with string ties longer than 8 inches (20 cm).

Q: *What will I feel during a Caesarean operation?*

A: Before the operation begins, a drape is placed so that you cannot see the operation and your freezing is checked. During the operation, you will be aware that people are touching your abdomen, but you will not be able to tell what they are doing. At certain points, you will feel pushing and pulling. When the baby is delivered, you will feel a lot of pressure. It may even feel like someone is sitting on your chest. It is brief and tolerable. These sensations are normal and do not mean that your anesthesia is not working properly. You may feel light-headed or nauseous. If this happens, inform your anesthetist immediately. These side effects can be treated immediately with medications. It is common to be shivery during the operation and to feel quite tired after the baby is born. Some women also feel quite thirsty during the operation, but, unfortunately, you are not allowed anything to drink until after the operation.

What's next

While you have been making plans and more plans in these final weeks of pregnancy, your belly has been getting bigger … and bigger. There's lots of excitement as you approach your baby's birth day.

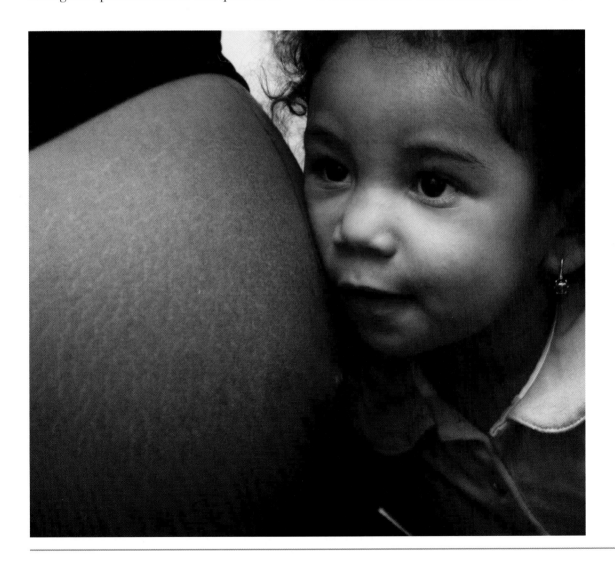

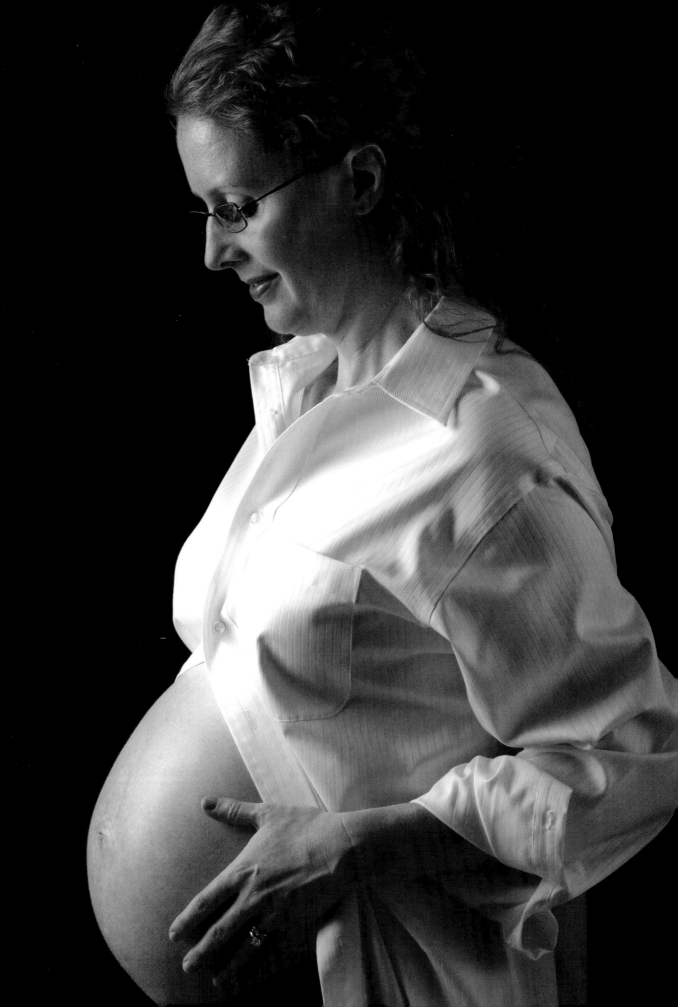

Part 8

Third Trimester Progress

Month 7 to 9 (Week 28 to 40)

Two down... one to go

As the second trimester winds to a close, you are probably excited about the next stage. Just 3 months to go until you deliver your baby. Now, that's progress! These weeks aren't all wine and roses, though. You'll be tired and ache in places you never have before. You will also be closely monitored in this trimester, with more frequent visits to your doctor or midwife.

Ten tips for a healthy pregnancy in the third trimester

1. Eat a nutritious diet, reducing portion size if necessary as your stomach becomes more compressed by the fetus.
2. Sleep as much as you can.
3. Listen to your body — if it tells you that you need to slow down, then do so.
4. Listen to your baby — pay attention to any movements. If they don't seem to be normal, then seek advice.
5. Exercise to your comfort level — sometimes this may just be a short walk.
6. Attend prenatal classes, ideally with your partner.
7. Continue to avoid alcohol, cigarettes, and any recreational drugs.
8. Prepare yourself for labor and birth by learning the signs of labor and what to expect during delivery.
9. Make plans for your baby's health and safety needs after birth.
10. Look at yourself in the mirror and admire yourself. You and your body have accomplished an amazing task!

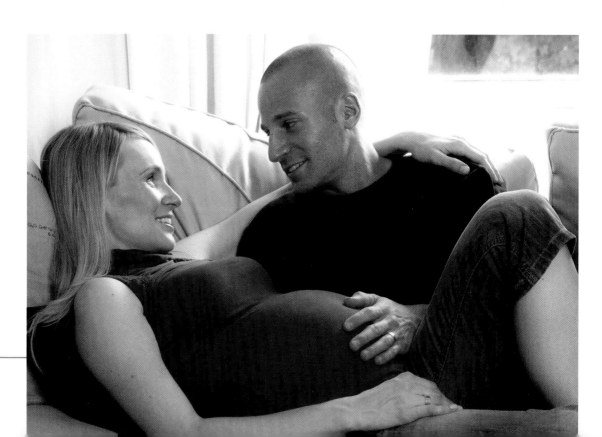

Month 7 fetal growth and development

Remarkably, if your baby was born this month, it would have a good chance of surviving outside your womb with the help of a neonatal intensive care unit.

Pregnancy milestones
At week 28

- Your baby is getting bigger and weighs about 2.5 pounds (1.0–1.3 kg).
- The lungs are still quite immature but are capable of breathing air if assisted.
- The toenails are present and growing.
- The hair is growing on the head, but the lanugo (body hair) elsewhere is starting to disappear.
- Fat starts to develop under the skin, smoothing out the previously wrinkled skin.
- Thumb sucking begins in some cases.
- The kidneys are working well, making half a quart (liter) of urine a day.
- The bone marrow is producing blood cells now.

Fetus at 28 Weeks

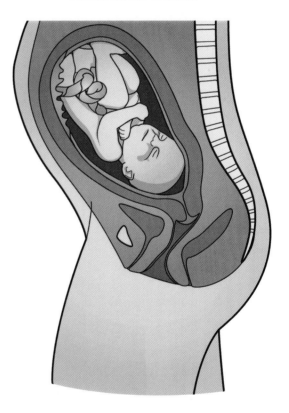

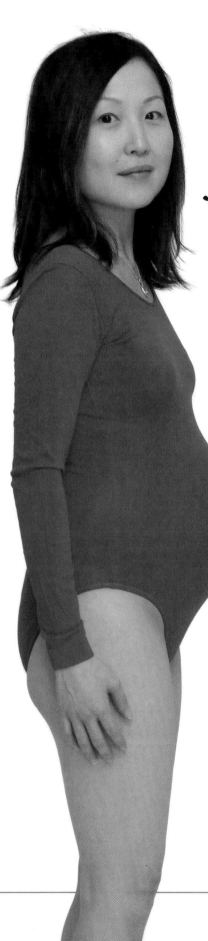

Looking and feeling pregnant

- Your belly is bigger yet!
- Your uterus and baby might be pushing in different directions, giving rise to many different aches, pains, and pressure sensations, especially in your back and perhaps under your ribs.
- Your breasts are larger.
- You might have extra weight on your buttocks and thighs as well.
- You may feel a little clumsier as you adjust to these changes.
- You might have difficulty sleeping now.
- You might feel mild, non-painful contractions of your uterus, called Braxton Hicks contractions, with your belly first getting hard and then relaxing.
  - Your breasts might begin to produce colostrum — a milky substance full of antibodies your baby will eat before your milk comes in. You might find some of this substance leaking out. Don't worry about it.
  - You might develop varicose veins as the uterus compresses the veins returning blood to your upper body, and hemorrhoids could become worse.

Did You Know?

Leg cramps

If you've awoken in the middle of the night with an unbelievable pain in your calf, you've experienced a leg cramp. They most often occur in the third trimester. The cause is not known, although it may be related to the increasing size of the baby, the stress from maternal weight gain, or changes in blood circulation. There is no proven treatment for leg cramps. Despite popular belief, increasing calcium intake through either diet or supplements will not lessen leg cramps. Magnesium may offer a marginal improvement in leg cramp pain. If a leg cramp occurs during the night, stretch the calf out by pushing your heel into the bed and flexing your foot so the toes point to the ceiling. Some women report that a light massage to the area and walking also help stop the cramp pain.

Month 7 medical check-up

This month, your blood pressure, weight, and uterine height will be measured ... as usual. You will also hear the baby's heart. At this visit, it is a good idea to review the signs and symptoms of preterm labor with your health-care provider. The signs can be subtle, so it is best to be on the look-out for them.

Month 7 tests

Back in the first trimester, at your first medical appointment, your blood was tested for the presence (positive) or absence (negative) of Rh (rhesus) factor on your red blood cells. You will be tested again this month and treated, if required. For more information on Rh disease, see page 284.

At month 7, most doctors will do a screening test for gestational diabetes mellitus and take your blood count again to make sure you do not have any signs of anemia. Some health-care providers repeat a urine culture, because pregnant women can have bladder infections and not know it. For more information on gestational diabetes and anemia in pregnancy, see Part 6, Second Trimester Progress (pages 226 and 230).

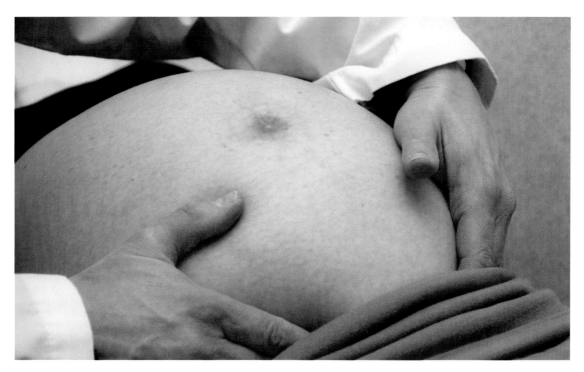

Measuring up

Many women wonder at this stage in their pregnancy if they are too large or too small — and if the fetus is over- or underweight. Your health-care providers use your belly size to estimate the growth of your uterus and the fetus, but normal variations in belly size make this an imperfect estimation.

Symphysis-fundal height

At the beginning of your pregnancy, your health-care providers will simply use their hands to feel the level of the uterus on your belly. In a normally developing pregnancy, you will not be able to feel the level of the uterus until it comes above the pubic bone.

Until this point, it is completely in the pelvis. At about 12 weeks of gestation, the top of the uterus can be felt at the level of the pubic bone. A rule of thumb is that the level of the uterus is about midway between the pubic bone and the belly button at 16 weeks. At 20 weeks, it is at the level of the belly button.

From then on, your health-care providers will start using a measuring tape to record the distance in centimeters from your pubic bone to the top of your uterus. This is called the symphysis-fundal height. It should correspond in centimeters to weeks of gestation. For example, at 28 weeks of gestation, you should measure 28 cm. This measurement is only a guide. If there is any question about the growth or size of the fetus, an ultrasound should be done.

Exceptions

This measurement includes what is in and around the uterus. For example, a woman with large fibroids will most likely measure larger. Some women have too much amniotic fluid (polyhydramnios) in the uterus, while others have too little (oligohydramnios). If you are carrying twins, your measurement will be larger than if you are carrying one baby, though it will not be double. In these cases, your must rely on an ultrasound to measure the size of the fetus.

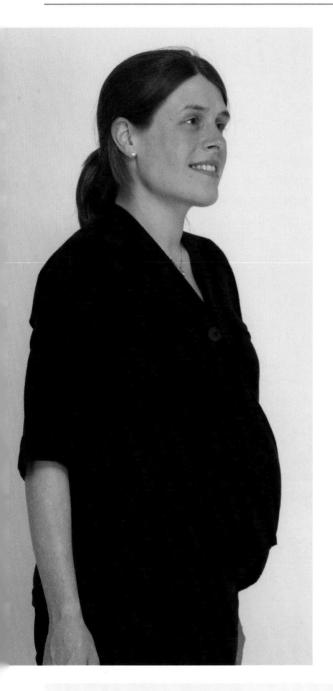

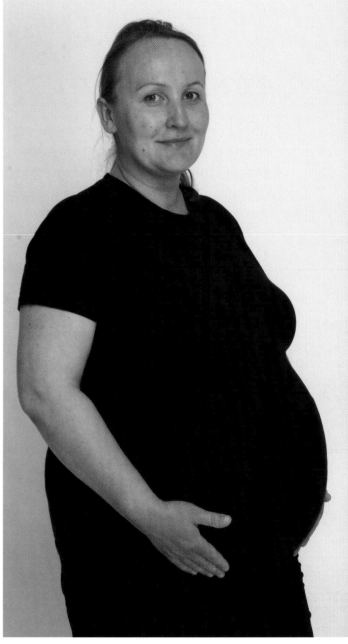

Did You Know?

Side-by-side comparisons

The shape of each pregnant woman is as unique as she is. Some expectant women have larger or rounder or more protruding bellies than others. Look at the following pictures of two women of the same gestation. You can see how different they look. Both of these women have had ultrasounds done, and their fetuses are approximately the same size at the same gestation.

Intrauterine growth restriction

During your routine medical examinations, your health-care provider may notice that the growth of your abdomen is not progressing as it should. An ultrasound may show that the growth of the fetus is behind the milestones we expect for its gestational age. This is called intrauterine growth restriction (IUGR), defined technically as "estimated fetal weight less than the 10th percentile for gestational age." This condition will be closely monitored.

Dating

Before worrying that something is wrong, check to be sure that the dating of your pregnancy is correct. The fetus may look small not because there is something wrong, but because the dates are wrong and you are not as far along as you thought you were. Review the due dates of your last menstrual period and your earliest ultrasounds.

IUGR Causes

The causes of IUGR can be subdivided into three categories: maternal causes, fetal causes, and placental causes.

Did You Know?

Growth curve percentiles

Percentiles of weight have been derived from growth curves using thousands of fetuses with known gestational ages. These weights are plotted on a graph to generate growth curves.

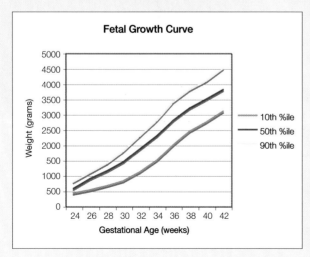

Fetal Growth Curve

This graph is used to plot the estimated weight of your particular fetus and then to make a comparison to all other fetuses of the same age. The 10th percentile means that 10% of fetuses weigh less than yours and 90% weigh more. By definition, 10% of all babies fit this definition.

Not all of the babies in the 10th percentile or less will have difficulties; in fact, studies have shown that adverse outcomes for the fetus usually do not occur until the fetus is at or below the 3rd percentile. In North America, growth curves were initially established using a mostly Caucasian population, but in many parts of the world, babies tend to be smaller and yet still perfectly healthy. Growth curves have been generated for other populations but may not be widely available.

Maternal causes

If the mother has any kind of pre-existing chronic disease, such as hypertension or diabetes, it can predispose the fetus to IUGR. If the underlying disease is quiet, it is less likely to have an impact on the fetus. Other maternal factors associated with IUGR include smoking and recreational drug use. In addition, mothers who are either very young or very old (for childbearing) have an increased risk of IUGR.

Fetal causes

Chromosomal anomalies, such as Down syndrome, have been associated with IUGR. The fetus may have other congenital disorders, such as a heart defect. Other causes can include infections that the mother can acquire and that can pass through the placenta. Twins or triplets (or more) can cause IUGR of one or all of the fetuses.

Placental causes

If the placenta has not developed properly, this can be a cause of IUGR. Even though the fetus is perfectly normal, if the placenta cannot allow adequate nourishment, the fetus will not grow properly.

Managing IUGR

The principle treatment is identifying and addressing the cause. An ultrasound is the mainstay of diagnosis and subsequent fetal monitoring. Depending upon the gestational age at which IUGR is diagnosed, your pregnancy may be considered high-risk and your care may be transferred to a high-risk center. You will be advised to rest as much as possible in order to maximize blood flow through the placenta and encourage growth. This will mean stopping work and possibly delegating your other responsibilities, such as housework and child care. You may even be admitted to hospital for daily evaluations.

Delivery

Sometimes, repeated ultrasound measurements show that the fetus is not growing any more inside your belly or is under some stress. At this point, your doctor may advise delivery, even if you are preterm. Some babies with IUGR may not be able to tolerate labor and may be delivered by Caesarean section with no attempt at labor. Depending on the gestational age, the baby may have to spend time in the neonatal intensive care unit.

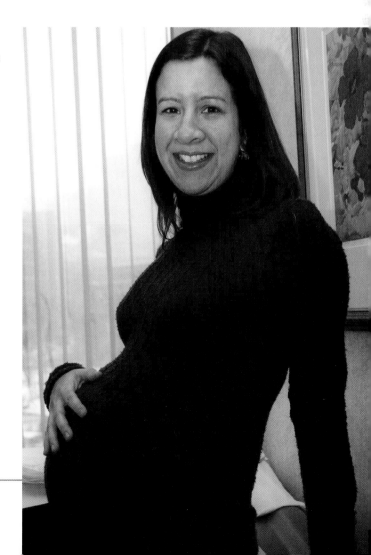

Rh disease

Rh disease is somewhat more complicated because it involves the immune system over two generations. During your first month of pregnancy or even before becoming pregnant, your health-care providers will likely have your blood tested for the presence (positive) or absence (negative) of Rh (rhesus), a protein on your red blood cells. This is the + (positive) or − (negative) associated with your blood type — perhaps you are O+ or maybe you are AB−. About 85% of the population is Rh positive.

This characteristic is determined by parental genes. If you test Rh negative and your fetus is Rh positive, there is a possibility of serious complications, not in this pregnancy but in subsequent pregnancies. Fortunately, these complications can be prevented.

Rh genetics

You have two genes for Rh factor (one you inherited from your mother, one from your father), and there is the possibility for each gene to be either positive or negative. Any positive gene leads to Rh factor being on your blood cells, regardless of whether you have one or two positive genes. If both of the genes are negative, your blood cells will not carry the Rh factor and your blood will be Rh negative.

Your baby also has two Rh genes, inheriting one from you and one from its father. This makes it possible for your baby to have a different Rh type than you do. If your baby's father is also Rh−, then the baby will be Rh− too.

Antibodies

Our immune systems form antibodies against things that are foreign to them, which is very helpful when directed against bacteria and viruses that have entered the body, but it is the source of the problem in Rh disease. Most of the time, fetal red blood cells do not cross the placenta joining mother and fetus, so the mother's immune system is not exposed to fetal red blood cells, but, at certain times, the placental barrier can be disrupted, and the Rh+ fetal blood cells will enter the Rh− mother's bloodstream.

The immune system of an Rh− mother will "see" these Rh+ blood cells as foreign and form antibodies against the Rh factor. In the current pregnancy, those antibodies will be relatively harmless and will not hurt the fetus. However, in a subsequent pregnancy, if the next fetus is also Rh+, those antibodies can multiply, cross the placenta, and attack the fetal red blood cells. This attack will destroy the fetal red blood cells, leading to very significant anemia, and, if unrecognized, potentially fetal death.

Rh sensitization

In an Rh− woman who has already made antibodies against Rh, there is no way to prevent those antibodies from crossing the placenta. The amount of antibody in maternal blood will be monitored regularly, and if the levels begin to rise, the risk that they will cross the placenta increases. The fetus will be monitored closely for signs of fetal anemia with ultrasounds.

If the fetus is thought to be anemic, a fetal blood transfusion can be given via the umbilical cord. These babies may need preterm delivery and specialized care after birth, with exchange transfusion, in which their blood is removed and replaced with blood containing no harmful antibodies.

Barrier breakdown

The placental barrier may break down at certain times in a pregnancy, allowing fetal blood cells to enter the maternal bloodstream. These times include:

- At the time of a miscarriage
- At the time of an ectopic pregnancy
- At the time of an abortion
- At the time there is bleeding in a pregnancy
- At the time of delivery
- At the time of an amniocentesis (when the amniotic fluid is tested)

All Rh– women need preventive measures at these times.

Prevention

Fortunately, very effective prevention for Rh disease is now available. An Rh– woman is given Rh antibodies at specific times in pregnancy (12 weeks, 28 weeks, and after delivery) to "soak up" any fetal Rh+ cells that may have entered her bloodstream. Rh antibodies are also given if there is a known or suspected episode of placental barrier breakdown. This will prevent her immune system from recognizing these Rh cells, and her body will not make antibodies against Rh factor, protecting her subsequent pregnancies. Rh antibodies are called RhIg and are made from the blood of Rh– people who have been exposed to Rh antibodies. Although RhIg is a blood product, it is highly purified and there is no risk of infection.

If you are 100% certain that the baby's father is Rh–, then you can be sure the baby is Rh– and you don't need RhIg.

Managing Rh disease in pregnancy

- Your blood will be tested for Rh factor and antibodies at your first visit to your health-care provider during your first month of pregnancy at about 12 weeks. If you are identified as Rh–, and you have no antibodies, you will be given RhIg if you have any unexpected bleeding.

- You will be tested again at 28 weeks. If you still have no antibodies, you will be given an injection of RhIg as a preventive measure to ensure that in the third trimester you will not make antibodies against Rh factor.

- After birth, your baby will be tested for Rh factor. If the baby is Rh+, you will receive another dose of RhIg. If the baby is Rh–, you do not need RhIg.

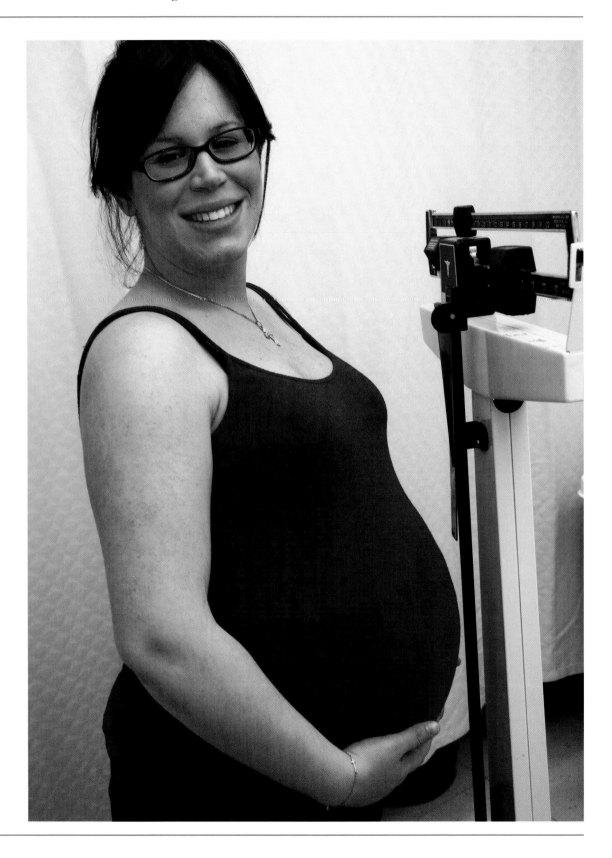

Month 8 fetal growth and development

If your baby was born now, he would likely need some help from a ventilator to keep breathing and some help with feeding, but otherwise, healthy babies born at this gestational age are likely to survive and do well in the long term. Still, you are the best incubator for the baby for a little while longer.

Pregnancy milestones

At week 32

- The fetus is still pretty slim with not much extra fat. The average weight is 3 to 4 pounds (1.8 kg).
- The arms and legs are now in proportion to the rest of the body.
- The fetus is very active. Sometimes, the kicks and punches from your baby can hurt.
- Soon, the amount of space around the baby will start to decrease and the movements will change from big kicks to smaller wriggles and turns, which may be more comfortable for you.
- The lungs are continuing to grow and develop but are still not yet totally mature.

Fetus at 32 Weeks

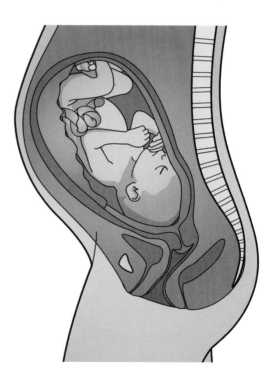

Looking and feeling pregnant

- Your belly is big, reaching at least halfway between your belly button and your breastbone. It may not seem possible for it to get bigger ... but it will!

- You may begin to feel more tired as your belly grows. Sometimes, just performing your daily routine can be exhausting.

- You may have some swelling in your feet and legs. Your swollen feet can make it difficult to wear your old shoes.

- You may have noticed that the weight you have gained is distributed around the rest of your body, even on your face.

- You may have trouble moving fast because you become short of breath when you do.

- The pressure of your baby on your back or ribs or pelvis can start to become quite uncomfortable.

- You may have heartburn.

- You might start to have trouble sleeping because you cannot find a comfortable position.

- You may feel anxious about the looming arrival of your baby. Perhaps you are worried about the delivery, or perhaps you are worried about how the baby is going to change your life and how you will care for him.

- You may be irritated with all the people who are giving you advice and asking to touch your belly.

- Or maybe you feel fantastic, and none of these things are bothering you!

Month 8 medical check-ups

Your appointments will increase in frequency to every 2 weeks in this month, and you will be given lots of time to ask questions as you get closer to your due date. Start talking to your doctor or midwife about labor and delivery. Time is flying.

Month 8 tests

As always, your weight and urine will be checked, along with the growth of your uterus and the fetal heart. Your health-care provider may advise you to have another ultrasound in the third trimester to check on fetal growth and well-being, but if your belly is growing well and there are no signs of concerns, it is not strictly necessary.

At about 36 weeks, you will have a vaginal-rectal swab to screen for group B streptococcus (GBS) bacteria. Many women naturally harbor GBS in their vagina. It does have some implications for fetal health, so testing for GBS and treating it at the time of delivery is important.

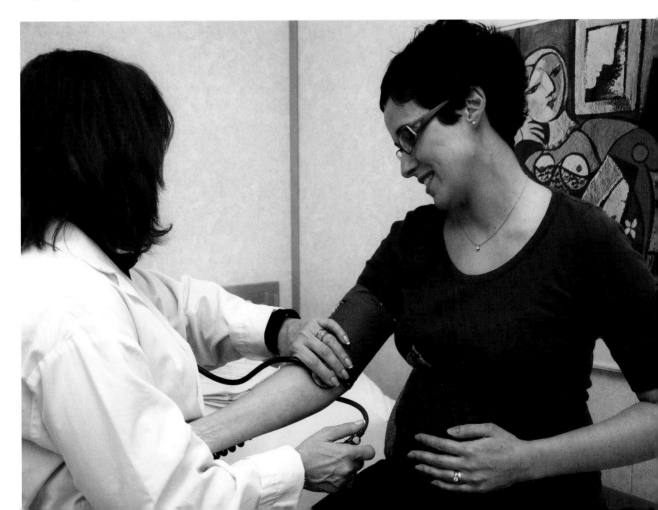

Group B streptococcus

Group B streptococcus is found in the vagina, bladder, and rectum of many women. Approximately one-third of women are carriers of GBS, which means they carry the bacteria in small amounts but not enough to cause an infection. GBS poses no risk to the mother, but it poses a risk to the baby as it passes through the vagina during birth. In the absence of antibiotics, approximately 40% to 70% of colonized mothers pass the bacteria on to their babies, but only 1% of full-term babies born to these women are actually infected. A newborn baby does not have a well-developed immune system, and any infection in the first 2 weeks of life can be very serious. Because the infection in a new baby can be so severe, it is considered worthwhile giving antibiotics to all women in labor who are carrying GBS, even though very few of their babies will actually become ill from GBS.

Testing for GBS

Universal screening for GBS takes place in the last month of pregnancy. Obstetric and pediatric societies in North America currently recommend that all pregnant women be screened for GBS near their pregnancy's term. Screening is simple; a small cotton swab is placed in the vagina and then onto the perineal skin toward the rectum. The swab is then sent to the laboratory and incubated to see if GBS grows. If you test positive for GBS, you will be advised to have antibiotics while in labor. If you are having a planned Caesarean section with no labor, it is still advisable to screen for GBS just in case your membranes rupture or you go into labor before your scheduled Caesarean date.

Treating GBS

GBS is not treated until labor. Although it seems like a good idea to treat GBS prior to labor, if GBS is eradicated even just 4 weeks prior to labor, it can come back. GBS disease in newborns can be divided into early onset and late onset disease. Antibiotics in labor reduce the risk of early onset disease by approximately 70%, but so far, we don't seem able to prevent late onset disease, which is very uncommon, so you should not be unduly anxious about it.

The preferred antibiotic is penicillin G, given intravenously every 4 hours in labor until delivery so the vagina is sterilized as the baby passes through it. If you are allergic to penicillin, your health-care provider will prescribe another antibiotic.

Did You Know?
Bacterial colonization and infection
There is a difference between being colonized by a bacteria and having an infection. Being colonized means you are a carrier. The bacteria live on or in you but cause you no harm. In fact, certain bacteria, like the ones that aid digestion, are good for you. Perfectly healthy human beings are colonized by millions and millions of bacteria. An infection results when a specific bacteria causes an illness of some kind, either because the type or the location of the bacteria causes disease.

Gestational hypertension and pre-eclampsia

Hypertension (elevated blood pressure) is common in pregnancy, complicating 10% to 20% of all pregnancies. Hypertension is similar to diabetes in that it can be a pre-existing condition (chronic hypertension) or can develop during pregnancy. If it develops during pregnancy, it is called gestational hypertension, or pregnancy-induced hypertension (PIH). Pre-eclampsia progresses from PIH or develops spontaneously in women with no history of blood pressure problems.

Gestational hypertension

While chronic hypertension is defined as an elevated blood pressure of greater than or equal to 140/90 either before pregnancy or before week 20, gestational hypertension is defined as an elevated blood pressure of 140/90 or more occurring *after* week 20 of pregnancy, with no signs of pre-eclampsia and complete resolution of the hypertension by 12 weeks postpartum. For more information on chronic hypertension, see Part 13, Managing Medical and Environmental Risks (page 435).

Fetal complications

The risk of fetal complications increases as the blood pressure becomes more elevated. Mild gestational hypertension (140/90 to 159/99) poses few fetal risks, but the risk of placental abruption, preterm delivery, and growth-restricted babies goes up with more severe gestational hypertension (BP greater than 160/100). There is a chance that women with gestational hypertension will go on to develop pre-eclampsia or chronic hypertension if their blood pressure doesn't normalize postpartum.

If your blood pressure remains mildly elevated and you don't develop any complications, you should be able to deliver at term. If you develop complications because of the hypertension, it may be necessary to deliver your baby early, both for the sake of your health and the baby's well-being.

Risk factors for gestational hypertension in pregnancy

- First pregnancy (excluding miscarriages)
- Being overweight
- Multiple gestation — twins, triplets, or more
- Under 20 years old
- Over 35 to 40 years old
- Diabetes
- Previous blood pressure problems — either in or between pregnancies
- Family history of pre-eclampsia in sister or mother
- Kidney disease
- Lupus

Guide to...

Managing gestational hypertension

- **Extra fetal monitoring:** Because of the risk of growth restriction, fetal growth will be monitored frequently using ultrasound scans, usually once a month from week 24 to delivery, or more often if a concern is identified. Closer to term, you may have weekly ultrasound scans and non-stress tests. You need to be especially aware of fetal movements and notify your doctor if they seem abnormal or reduced.

- **Reducing maternal activity:** If your blood pressure is going higher and higher, your doctor may advise you to limit your activity, including stopping work, to eliminate sources of stress and exertion that may elevate your blood pressure. You may need to reduce your other activities, such as housework, shopping excursions, and child care. Some doctors will advise at least partial bed rest in some circumstances. The goal of these recommendations is to keep your blood pressure lower, increase blood flow to the placenta and baby, and prolong the pregnancy as long as possible.

- **Medications:** If your condition is severe, your doctor may prescribe safe medications to help lower your blood pressure.

- **Pre-eclampsia testing:** You will be assessed for symptoms of pre-eclampsia and asked to look out for them yourself.

Did You Know?

Measuring blood pressure

Your blood pressure reading reflects the pressure your blood exerts on the walls of your blood vessels (veins and arteries). What causes the pressure? Your heart contracts, squeezing blood into your arteries (which brings fresh oxygen to your body), and, after it contracts, your heart relaxes for a fraction of a second to allow blood from your veins to fill the heart again, just before it squeezes the blood out again.

When your blood pressure (BP) is measured, two numbers are recorded, for example, 120/80. The first number in the blood pressure reading represents the pressure exerted by your blood on the walls of your arteries when your heart contracts, forcing blood to circulate through them. It is called the systolic blood pressure and is measured in millimeters of mercury (or mmHg). The second number is the diastolic pressure, which is the pressure exerted on your artery walls at the end of the relaxation phase of the heart cycle.

A normal BP is considered to be 120/80 or lower. Many healthy women have blood pressures that are much lower, perhaps 90/60. BP generally drops in pregnancy, reaching its lowest point at about 20 weeks gestation before creeping up again to normal levels by the end of pregnancy.

Pre-eclampsia

Pre-eclampsia, sometimes called toxemia, is a condition unique to pregnancy, characterized by elevated blood pressure (higher than 140/90) and protein in the urine. It can affect almost every organ system in the mother's body. It occurs in up to 14% of pregnancies worldwide and up to 8% of pregnancies in North America.

Onset

The chances of developing pre-eclampsia depend on when the elevated blood pressure is first diagnosed. If it is diagnosed after 36 weeks, the chances of developing pre-eclampsia are low (10%). If the elevated blood pressure is first diagnosed between 20 and 30 weeks gestation, the chances of developing pre-eclampsia are much higher (42%). About 25% of cases of pre-eclampsia are severe.

Signs and symptoms of severe pre-eclampsia

If you experience these symptoms, seek medical attention immediately:

- Blood pressure greater than 160/110
- Severe headache
- Visual changes (blurred or double vision, spots, floaters)
- Pain under the ribs on the right side under the liver
- Nausea or vomiting
- Shortness of breath
- Vaginal bleeding
- Uterine pain
- Significant swelling of face and hands
- Large jumps in weight (indicating water retention)

Did You Know?

Seizures (eclampsia)

The "pre" part of the word pre-eclampsia indicates that this is a condition occurring before "eclampsia," which means seizures. Most women diagnosed and treated for pre-eclampsia will not go on to have a seizure, but, left untreated, this is quite possible (as are the other complications listed below). The condition can also have serious consequences for the fetus.

Pre-eclampsia can begin anytime after week 20 of pregnancy, but it is much more common in the third trimester. Only about 10% of cases of pre-eclampsia occur before 34 weeks gestation. The only cure for pre-eclampsia is delivery. Sometimes, this means that a baby must be delivered prematurely to protect the health of both the baby and the mother. The level of prematurity needs to be weighed against the severity of the pre-eclampsia.

Potential consequences of severe pre-eclampsia

Maternal consequences	Fetal consequences
Seizure (eclampsia)	Poor fetal growth
Stroke	Fetal distress
Heart failure	Decreased amniotic fluid
Liver disease and liver rupture	Decreased placental blood flow
Kidney failure	Placental abruption
Blood clotting abnormalities	Preterm birth

Did You Know?

Managing pre-eclampsia

- If you have mild pre-eclampsia, how your health-care provider chooses to manage your care will depend on your gestational age.

- If you are at term (37 weeks or more), there is generally no advantage in continuing the pregnancy. Induction of labor is probably the most appropriate course of action. During your labor, you will be monitored for signs of severe pre-eclampsia.

- If you are preterm (30 weeks or less), managing pre-eclampsia becomes a balancing act between your health and your baby's prematurity.

- If you are very ill, there is no doubt that you will need to deliver the baby regardless of gestational age.

- If you are not yet very ill, sometimes there is enough time to give you an injection of steroids (Celestone) to help the baby's lungs mature. Two injections are given 24 hours apart. In addition, you may need to be transferred to a hospital that is able to look after a premature baby.

- If your pre-eclampsia is not too severe, you may be monitored in the hospital over a period of days or more, and if your condition or the baby's condition show signs of deteriorating, delivery can be arranged quickly.

- If your pre-eclampsia is severe, medications will be given intravenously to stabilize your blood pressure. You may also be given magnesium sulfate to prevent seizures. Magnesium sulfate is usually continued for 24 to 48 hours after delivery, and while you are on this drug, you will be carefully monitored.

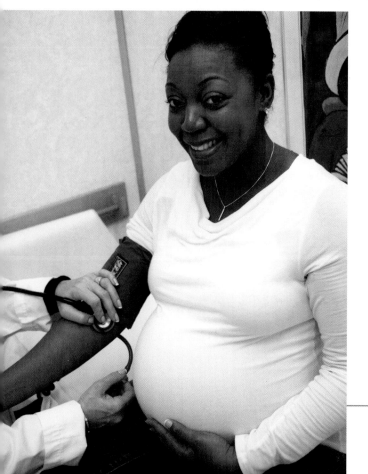

Monitoring for pre-eclampsia

Because there are often no physical symptoms in low-risk populations, health-care providers cannot predict reliably who will develop pre-eclampsia or test for it ahead of time. In high-risk populations, ultrasound assessment of uterine artery blood flow can be useful in predicting risk. The only reliable way to detect pre-eclampsia is to measure blood pressure and check for urine protein regularly, especially in the late second trimester and the third trimester. To compound this problem, women with severe pre-eclampsia can become very sick quite quickly and sometimes show no symptoms at all before the condition escalates.

Be aware of the warning signs. It is always better to be checked immediately and not wait until your next scheduled medical visit.

Month 9 fetal growth and development

Your baby is getting bigger, and during this month starts to gain some fat, almost ready to be born.

Pregnancy milestones
At week 36

- The fetus is big — an average of 5.5 pounds (2.5 kg).
- The fingernails are getting long.
- In boys, the testes are descending into the scrotum.
- The circumference of the head and the abdomen are about the same.
- The fetus is still moving, but the space is getting tighter. There should be less kick-boxing, but more wriggling and turning.
- The baby has periods of sleeping and wakefulness.
- The baby's brain is developing quickly during this time.

Fetus at 36 Weeks

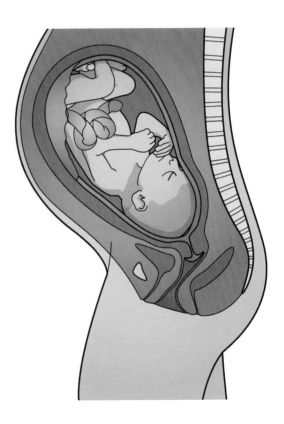

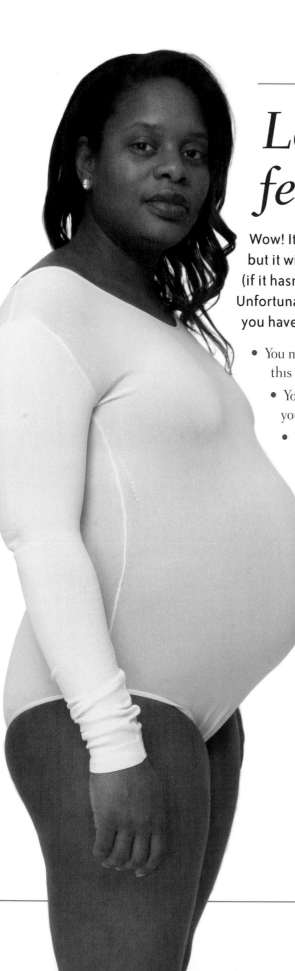

Looking and feeling pregnant

Wow! It doesn't seem like your belly can get any bigger ... but it will! Your belly button may be poking outwards (if it hasn't happened earlier) or just stretched really flat. Unfortunately ... some of the other symptoms you have felt in pregnancy may now be worse.

- You may feel big, ungainly, and awkward beginning around this time as your centre of gravity continues to change.
  - You may start to feel a lot of downward pressure in your pelvis.
    - You may be feeling a lot more Braxton Hicks contractions.
      - You may be fed up and feel ready to reclaim your pre-pregnant body, or maybe you are quite content, enjoying the last few weeks of pregnancy.

Did You Know?

Pubic symphysis separation pain

In this last month, you may develop a significant amount of pain over the pubic bone, sometimes even limiting your ability to walk well. The pubic bone is not actually one bone but two bones that meet in the middle. During pregnancy, your body makes a hormone called relaxin, which loosens your joints and ligaments to make room for the baby, particularly at birth. This can lead to some separation of the two sides of your pubic bone, called diastasis (or separation) of the pubic symphysis.

A physiotherapist may be able to help you with exercises and maneuvers to reduce your discomfort. You can also try using acetaminophen.

Month 9 medical check-ups

You will probably see your health-care provider every week at this stage. The appointment will include the usual assessment of weight, urine, and blood pressure, as well as listening for the fetal heart beat. At this stage, it is also important to know which way the baby is lying — head down, breech (head up), or transverse (sideways). If the baby is breech or transverse, an external cephalic version or Caesarean section may need to be scheduled. For more information on fetal lies, see Part 9, High-Risk Pregnancies (page 317).

Month 9 tests

If you haven't already had a vaginal-rectal swab to screen for group B streptococcus, your health-care provider will advise one now. If you or the fetus are considered to be at risk for any problem, an ultrasound may be done.

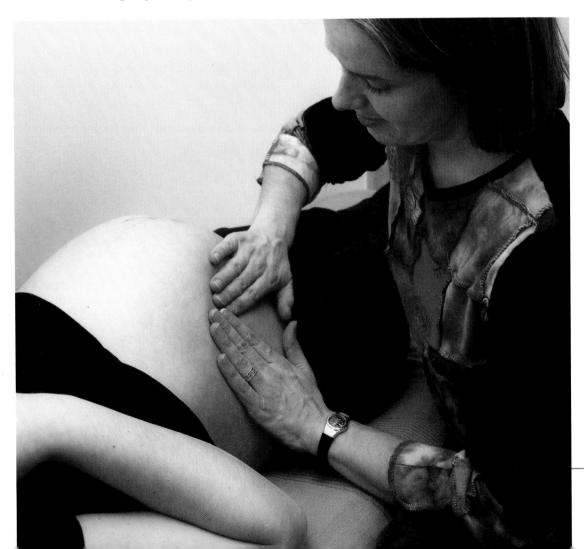

Placenta previa

In placenta previa, the placenta has attached to the uterine wall close to or covering the cervix. Problems secondary to placenta previa can arise in the latter part of the first trimester, but are more common during the second or third trimester. This abnormal placental development can lead to many other problems, including fetal growth restriction, pre-eclampsia, and premature delivery.

Placenta previa symptoms

If previous tests have indicated that you have a placenta previa, keep on the look-out for vaginal bleeding, especially in the third trimester. Bleeding from a placenta previa is typically painless (not associated with any cramping or signs of labor), but there can be a lot of blood.

The bleeding can vary from just some spotting to soaking a pad or two and, much more rarely, to significant hemorrhage. You need to get to the hospital quickly, especially if the bleeding is continuing. You and the fetus both need monitoring. If there is too much blood loss, it may be necessary to proceed with delivery and for you to have a blood transfusion. However, in many cases of placenta previa, there is no bleeding.

It is not uncommon for women with a placenta previa to bleed a few times in a pregnancy. If you do and the situation stabilizes after a first bleed, you may be asked to rest, either at home or in hospital. A second bleed is sometimes bigger than a first bleed. Each episode of bleeding requires that you and the baby be monitored.

Three Types of Placenta Previa

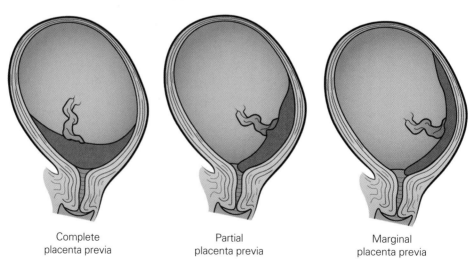

Complete
placenta previa

Partial
placenta previa

Marginal
placenta previa

Risk factors

- Multiples (twins or triplets). The more placentas you have, the more likely it is that at least one will come close to or cover the cervix. The incidence of placenta previa is doubled with twins.
- Previous multiple pregnancies.
- Previous Caesarean sections that have resulted in scarring in the lining of the uterus. The more Caesareans you have had, the greater the risk.

Treating placenta previa

The diagnosis is typically made by ultrasound during the anatomical scan performed between 18 and 20 weeks gestation. The most important principle of care with a placenta previa is to ensure that nothing is placed high in the vagina that may touch the cervix, disrupting the placenta and causing bleeding. Practically speaking, this means:

- No sexual intercourse
- No internal examinations with a hand; speculum exams are okay because they don't touch the cervix
- No tampons
- No douches

A transvaginal ultrasound is allowed because the probe only enters the lower part of the vagina, well away from the cervix. A transvaginal ultrasound can help define more clearly if the placenta is truly covering the cervix or not.

If you have had some bleeding, you may be asked to stay off your feet to reduce the chances of further bleeding. This may mean stopping work, stopping exercise, and delegating your household obligations to someone else.

Delivery

With a complete previa, the delivery method must be a Caesarean section, because any dilation of the cervix will lead to significant bleeding. If the placenta is low-lying (close to the cervix) or a marginal previa, you can consider a vaginal delivery. In this case, you (and your health-care providers) must monitor the baby carefully and be prepared to deal with bleeding and a Caesarean section if the bleeding becomes too heavy. On occasion a preterm delivery is necessary if the bleeding is significant.

Types of placenta previa

- **Complete:** The placenta completely covers the cervix, making vaginal delivery impossible.
- **Partial:** The cervical opening is partially covered by the placenta.
- **Marginal:** The placental edge lies $\frac{1}{2}$ inch (1 cm) from the cervix. Often, a placenta that is marginally previa at 20 weeks will not be previa by term because the uterus grows and lifts the placenta up and off the cervix. Vaginal delivery is possible.

Full-term fetal growth and development

Although your due date was calculated to 40 weeks, anytime after 37 weeks is considered full term. That means that by 37 weeks, your baby is fully developed and ready to be born. Most babies are born between 39 and 41 weeks, but you should be prepared to deliver your baby any day now!

Pregnancy milestones

At week 40

- The average weight of a baby at term is 7.5 pounds (3.5 kg), but anywhere between 5.5 pounds (2.5 kg) and 9 pounds (4 kg) is considered normal.
- In these last few weeks of pregnancy, your baby is continuing to put on fat, increasing in weight by about 8 ounces (250 g) per week.
- The skin is much less wrinkled, and the lanugo has disappeared, although some vernix remains.
- The baby is curled into a tight ball and has less and less room to move around. The amount of amniotic fluid around the baby may start to decrease. Because of these factors, the movements you feel may be quite different from what you felt earlier in the pregnancy — more wriggling and less kicking and punching — but you should still feel movement every single day.
- The organs are fully formed and working as they will once the baby is born — with the exception of the lungs.

- In the uterus, the baby is obviously not breathing air, but the muscles are practicing breathing and amniotic fluid moves in and out of the lungs. With your baby's first gasp after delivery, the lungs will fill up with air, and all of a sudden she — or he — will be breathing for real.

Did You Know?

Just-in-time breathing

Almost all babies have fully functional lungs by 37 weeks, but some do not. If this is the case when you go into labor, your baby will produce steroids to help the lungs mature, and excess fluid would be squeezed out of the lungs as the baby passes through the birth canal at delivery, leading to a rapid, just-in-time lung maturation. Babies without fully functional lungs who are born by planned Caesarean section do not have the benefit of labor (and therefore no steroid production and no squeezing) and may have a little trouble breathing if the delivery is scheduled too early. That is one of the reasons why your doctor will probably wait until 38½ or 39 weeks to perform an elective Caesarean section, unless there is a good reason to go ahead earlier.

Fetus at Full Term

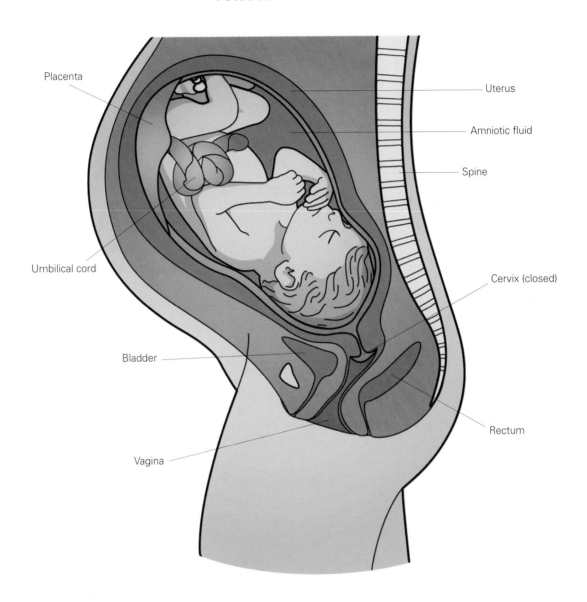

Placenta

Umbilical cord

Bladder

Vagina

Uterus

Amniotic fluid

Spine

Cervix (closed)

Rectum

Looking and feeling pregnant

This is it — your belly is as big as it's going to get! But at this size, it will affect all your activities and make them a lot more difficult. You may be happy to hear that your weight has probably stabilized — you may even lose a few pounds. Apart from the symptoms you have felt all along the way, you may begin to feel some signs that your body is preparing for labor.

- You might feel more frequent and more intense Braxton Hicks contractions and menstrual-like cramping. These contractions come and go frequently for a period of a few hours, and then disappear altogether.
- You might see light vaginal bleeding or spotting, which occurs as your cervix opens up a little bit in preparation for labor. This bleeding should be quite light — if it is not, discuss it with your health-care provider immediately.
- You might lose your mucus plug — a pinkish, clear-colored, mucus-like vaginal discharge that formed a protective barrier at the opening of the cervix.
- Your back might be more sore than it has been.
- You might feel the pressure in your pelvis becoming increasingly intense, and it may feel as if the baby is going to fall out. (It won't.)

Did You Know?

Engaged

You may notice that you have a little more breathing room up top and more pelvic pressure down below. This is often a sign that the baby has "dropped," or become engaged lower in your pelvis. The head is engaged when the largest diameter of the baby's head is below the pelvic brim. It is an early sign of your body getting ready for labor.

Full-term medical check-ups

At full term, you will see your health-care provider every week. Apart from the usual check of your blood pressure, urine, and the fetal heart rate, your health-care provider will verify the position of the baby.

Stripping your membranes

At full term, your doctor or midwife may check your cervix for two purposes: first, to see if there are any cervical changes to suggest that labor is imminent, and, second, to strip your membranes. Stripping the membranes means running a finger between the cervix and the amniotic sac in order to stimulate the release of prostaglandins, which are chemicals that help your cervix get ready for labor.

Why? There is some evidence that stripping the membranes can reduce the number of pregnancies going post-term because the procedure releases hormones that may initiate labor within the next 48 hours. So, if you have big weekend plans ... ask your doctor to wait until next week!

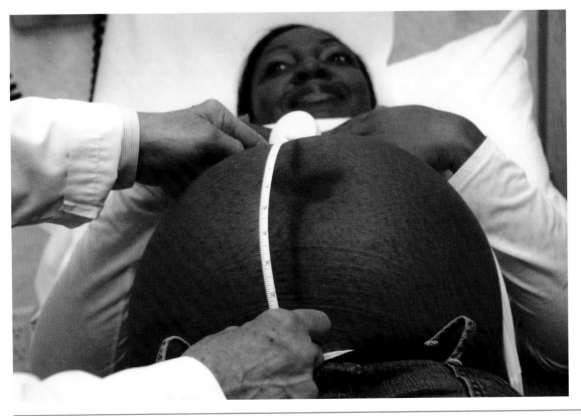

F.A.Q.

We answer many questions from pregnant women and their partners. Here are some of the most frequently asked questions. Be sure to ask your health-care providers any other questions that may arise. If they don't have the answers, they will refer you to a colleague who does.

Q: What can I do for hemorrhoids in pregnancy?

A: You're not alone — about a quarter of new mothers will have them. Hemorrhoids are enlarged varicose veins in the rectum that may protrude through the anal sphincter. They often occur in the third trimester, with additional pressure on the rectum as a result of the growing baby. Straining during bowel movements can cause hemorrhoids to appear or worsen. Hemorrhoids that develop during pregnancy will often worsen from all the pressure associated with your efforts to push your baby out, and more so if you have a larger infant. Preventing constipation is the best way to prevent hemorrhoids. You can also apply hemorrhoid creams to the area for relief. Most are available without a prescription (Anusol and Proctosedyl, for example). Sometimes blood inside the hemorrhoid can form a blood clot, causing considerable pain. If necessary, this clot can be removed by using a local anesthetic and incising the wall of the vein.

Q: What if I go into labor and my GBS status is unknown?

A: If your gestational age is less than 37 weeks, you should receive antibiotics. If you have other risk factors, such as a previous child affected by GBS, a history of GBS in your urine in this pregnancy, or a fever, you should also receive antibiotics. Otherwise, it is probably reasonable not to receive antibiotics.

Q: Does pre-eclampsia carry on after my baby is born?

A: Remarkably, pre-eclampsia resolves within a week or two of delivery. Sometimes, your blood pressure may remain elevated for a period of time, and you may need to take oral blood pressure pills for a few weeks, but eventually you should be able to stop them. Occasionally, women develop pre-eclampsia and even eclampsia in the days after delivery. If this happens, the treatment is the same — blood pressure control and seizure prevention with magnesium sulfate — but by a few weeks after delivery, the elevated blood pressure and risk of pre-eclampsia resolve.

Q: Should I be doing perineal massage?

A: Perineal massage involves stretching your vagina with your fingers to increase (theoretically) the elasticity and flexibility of your vaginal tissues, enabling an easier delivery. Unfortunately, studies have shown that perineal massage has no impact on delivery.

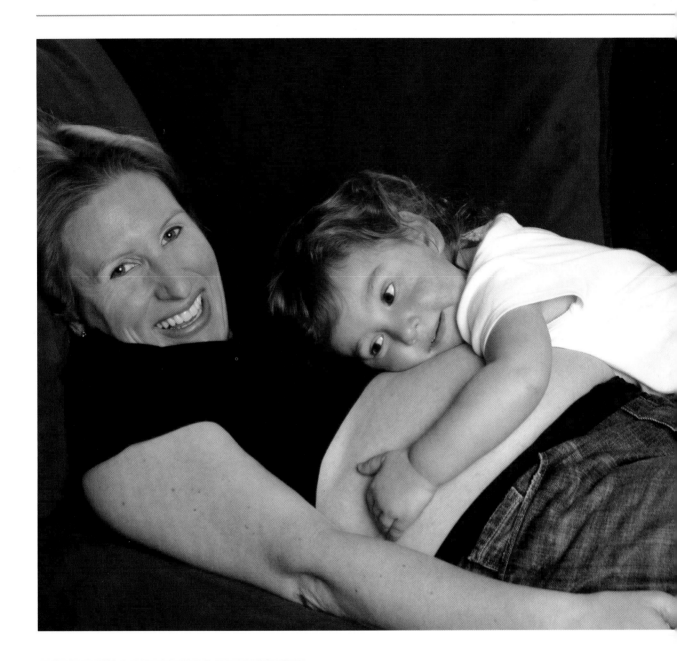

What's next

Your baby — that's what! After 40 or so weeks of planning and anticipation, the joy of your life will arrive, sometimes placidly on time, sometimes early or late, kicking and screaming.

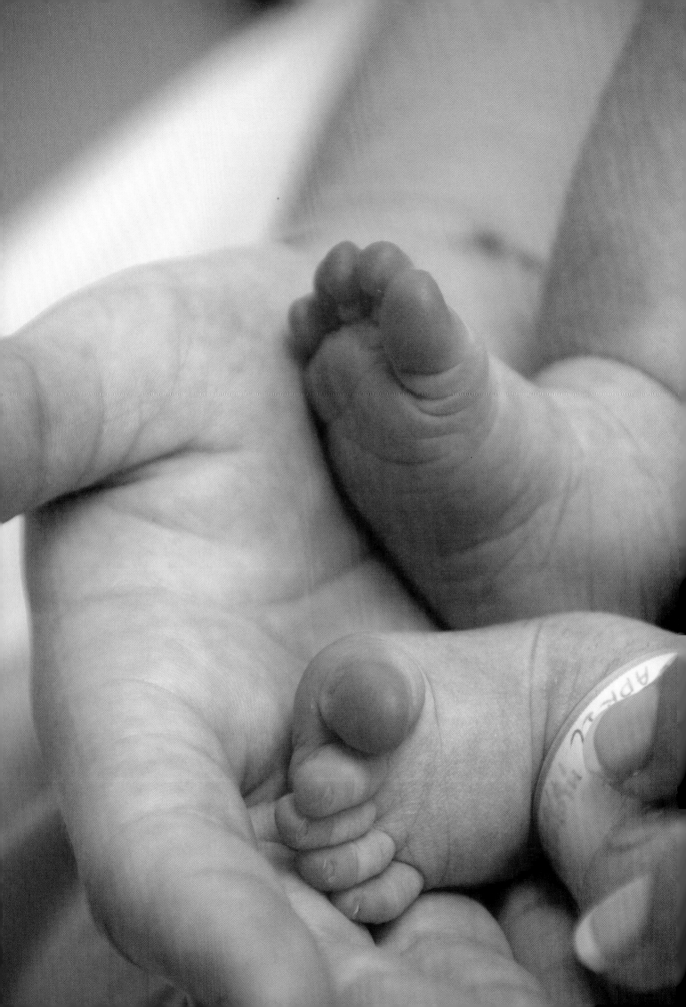

Part 9

High-Risk Pregnancies

At risk

Sometimes early, sometimes late, sometimes head first, sometimes feet first, sometimes one at a time, sometimes two or more — there are many variations on a "normal" labor and delivery that present higher risks to the mother and baby. While it's likely your pregnancy will proceed on course, it's worthwhile to be prepared for a few detours.

Ten tips for managing high-risk pregnancies

1. Be prepared for the unexpected. Not everything goes according to plan, but most things work out in the end.

2. Be alert to the symptoms of preterm labor you discussed with your doctor or midwife at your last check-up.

3. Don't get upset if you need to be admitted to or transferred to a hospital with facilities available to care for a premature baby.

4. Check out the neonatal intensive care unit (NICU) at your hospital sometime in the third trimester. It's a remarkably sophisticated yet compassionate place.

5. If your membranes rupture prematurely, go to the hospital for an assessment of your pregnancy.

6. If your baby is in the breech position, don't give up hope for an unassisted birth. The baby could flip around and turn into a head-down position anytime.

7. If you see or feel a shiny, wet cord between your legs, call 911 immediately.

8. If you are post-term, keep track of fetal movements. Fewer than six movements in 2 hours is a red flag.

9. Be open to an assisted birth even if your mind was set on a spontaneous labor and delivery.

10. Remember, most preterm babies grow into normal, healthy children.

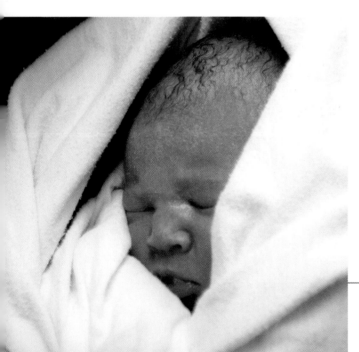

Terminology

- **Full term:** Most pregnancies end around 40 weeks, although babies born after 37 weeks are considered to be full term.

- **Preterm:** Babies born before 37 weeks are considered to be preterm, or premature.
  - *Very preterm:* Before 32 weeks.
  - *Extremely preterm:* Before 28 weeks.

- **Post-term pregnancy:** Pregnancies lasting 42 weeks (294 days) or more are called post-term.

Preterm birth

Preterm pregnancies are not uncommon — 5% to 10% of babies in North America are born prematurely. Despite advances in medical knowledge, this number has not changed significantly during the last century. However, care of premature babies has advanced, so there are fewer infant complications and deaths.

Preterm birth complications

Although a significant number of premature babies grow into normal, healthy children, some are at risk for serious health problems. Those born the earliest are at greatest risk because their organs will be less developed and more complications can occur.

Preterm birth categories

Preterm births are classified into two categories, iatrogenic and spontaneous.

Iatrogenic

In this case, the baby is delivered early to protect the health of the mother or the baby. For example, the mother has severe pre-eclampsia and must be delivered for the sake of her health. Iatrogenic prematurity accounts for 20% of cases of preterm birth.

Spontaneous

In this case, your body decides to deliver the baby early. There are three situations that can lead directly to spontaneous preterm birth:

1. **Preterm labor:** Uterine contractions begin too early, and this causes the cervix to open and the baby to deliver.
2. **Preterm premature rupture of the membranes (PPROM):** The sac of amniotic fluid around the fetus breaks.
3. **Cervical incompetence:** The cervix opens without uterine contractions. Unfortunately, this often occurs early in the pregnancy (usually around 20 weeks), so the baby will not be able to survive if born.

Risk factors

We don't understand the exact mechanism that starts labor, but there are some common maternal, fetal, and placental factors associated with preterm labor. Sometimes, preterm delivery is induced because maternal or fetal problems require it.

Did You Know?

Survival at 24 weeks

In general, 24 weeks is considered to be the youngest age at which a baby can survive outside the uterus. Actual chances for survival at any given gestational age will depend upon many factors, including other health problems the baby may have. Very premature and very sick babies are at risk of long-lasting problems, such as developmental delay, physical handicaps, lung and gastrointestinal problems, and vision and hearing loss. The risk of these problems generally decreases as the gestational age advances.

Risk factors associated with preterm birth

Category	Risk factors
Maternal	Previous preterm deliveries Certain illnesses, such as high blood pressure and diabetes Infections in the uterus, cervix, or vagina Surgery Trauma, especially to the abdomen Domestic violence Lack of social supports Short time between pregnancies Smoking, alcohol abuse, or illegal drug use Poor nutrition Abnormally shaped uterus Fibroids in certain locations Damage to the cervix from previous surgery
Fetal	Twins or triplets pregnancy Growth restriction Polyhydramnios (too much amniotic fluid) Oligohydramnios (too little amniotic fluid) Breech presentation Birth defects and chromosome abnormalities
Placental	Placenta has not grown properly, resulting in a poor blood supply to fetus Placenta previa (with bleeding) Placental abruption Cord prolapse

Stopping contractions

Medications called tocolytics can be used to stop contractions long enough to allow for hospital transfer and for two doses of Celestone to be administered. Celestone is a steroid used to mature the fetal lungs. However, there are circumstances when it is not advisable to stop the labor; for example, if there is suspected fetal abnormality, or if there is a suspected infection in the fluid and membranes surrounding the baby.

Did You Know?

Predicting preterm labor

In some hospitals and clinics, a test called fetal fibronectin (FFN) can be done with a vaginal swab. If this test is negative, there is a high likelihood you will not deliver the baby in the next week. A positive test means you have an elevated risk of preterm birth and you should be watched closely.

Neonatal care

Preterm babies must stay in a neonatal intensive care unit (NICU), which has special equipment and staff trained to deal with the multiple problems associated with premature babies. If your local hospital does not have an NICU, you may be transferred to another hospital. If possible, it is best to transfer a baby in utero.

Guide to...

Preterm labor procedures

- You may be admitted to or transferred to a hospital with facilities available to care for a premature baby.

- If you are suspected of being in preterm labor, your contractions will be monitored and your cervix assessed every 2 to 3 hours to see if it is changing.

- You will be asked to rest completely. Reducing your activity is believed to help your uterus relax. If the contractions settle down in hospital, you may be sent home to rest.

- Your blood will be tested, and a swab for group B streptoccocus will be taken. A urine culture is also advisable.

- You will most likely also be offered two injections of a medication called Celestone, or beta-methasone. This steroid helps a baby's immature lungs develop more quickly. Celestone has been proven to be effective for babies between 24 and 34 weeks gestational age.

If it is not safe to transfer you (for example, if preterm labor is moving too rapidly or the baby is in distress), you will be delivered at your own hospital and then a neonatal transfer team will travel to wherever you are to help stabilize and transfer your baby to the hospital that will provide appropriate care. The most important factor is the specialized pediatric care available for your baby, once born.

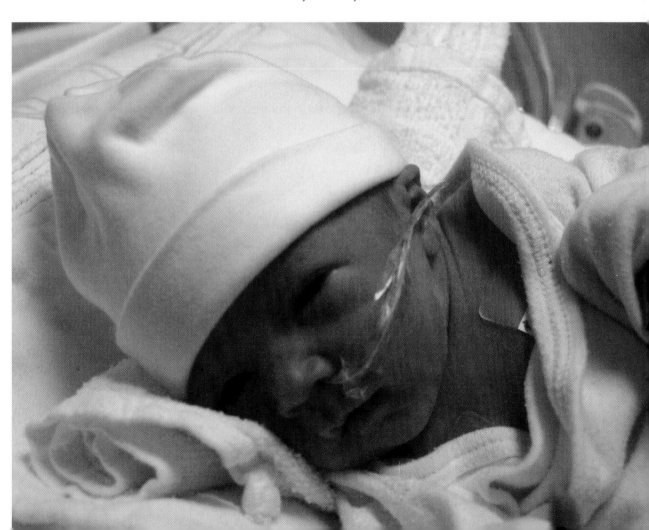

Amniotic fluid complications

Problems with your amniotic fluid can also lead to preterm birth. Believe it or not, amniotic fluid is produced by the fetus and the placenta. In the third trimester, the most important components of amniotic fluid are fetal urine and fetal lung fluid. The fetus swallows amniotic fluid, while the placenta absorbs amniotic fluid across its surface through tiny blood vessels. The fetus floats within the amniotic fluid in the uterus.

Functions of amniotic fluid

Amniotic fluid is present in the uterus from the first trimester and has numerous functions:

- Cushions the fetus from the outside world, so if the mother bumps her belly (and uterus), the fetus is protected
- Protects the umbilical cord from being compressed by the baby
- Offers some antibacterial properties
- Provides a source of nutrients and fluid for the fetus
- Plays an important role in normal development of the lungs, muscles, and gastrointestinal system

Polyhydramnios

"Polyhydramnios" means too much amniotic fluid, a condition that affects about 1% of pregnancies. Most cases of polyhydramnios are considered mild, without any significant fetal complications. More severe cases of polyhydramnios may be associated with fetal problems.

Consequences of polyhydramnios

The increased amniotic fluid can over-distend the uterus, leading to a few problems. The maternal lungs can be compressed even more by the very large uterus, making it hard for the mother to breathe. The fetus can move around very easily, even into a breech or transverse position. A cord prolapse is more likely if the membranes rupture. The over-distension of the uterus can trigger preterm labor. Bleeding after delivery may be more severe, with a risk of hemorrhage.

Treating polyhydramnios

Polyhydramnios may be suspected if your belly is bigger than anticipated. If suspected, you need an ultrasound to assess how much amniotic fluid is present and see if there is any sign of a fetal problem. If the polyhydramnios is mild, no specific treatment is warranted. Very rarely, if the condition is very severe and you are very symptomatic, an obstetrician might advise removing some of the amniotic fluid with a procedure called an amnioreduction.

Oligohydramnios

Oligohydramnios is the opposite of polyhydramnios — instead of too much amniotic fluid, there is too little fluid. Sometimes, this condition is suspected if the uterine size seems a little smaller than expected on examination. An ultrasound will confirm the diagnosis.

Fetal complications

The impact of oligohydramnios depends on how early in the pregnancy the condition appears and how severe it is. Oligohydramnios in the first or second trimester is often a poor sign, suggesting that there is a significant problem, perhaps with the fetal kidneys or with the placenta. In the third trimester, as long as no serious cause of the oligohydramnios is identified, outcomes are usually good, although labor can be complicated. Without the cushioning effect of a big waterbath, the umbilical cord can be more easily compressed between the fetus and the wall of the uterus as the uterus contracts during labor. This can lead to abnormalities of the fetal heart rate and a higher risk of Caesarean section.

Treating oligohydramnios

The underlying cause of the oligohydramnios determines the treatment. Once the cause has been established, you will be watched closely, with ultrasounds and fetal heart rate monitoring (non-stress test) weekly until delivery.

Mothers who drink lots of fluids have been shown to increase the amount of amniotic fluid around the fetus, at least temporarily, if the fluid levels are a bit low. Alternatively, some health-care providers would consider inducing labor at term (usually a bit before 40 weeks). Certainly, if the cause is thought to be related to being post-term, an induction of labor will usually be arranged almost right away.

Causes of low amniotic fluid

- Ruptured membranes (so all the fluid has leaked out)
- Fetal urine production and excretion problems (for example, blockage in the urinary system)
- Medications that affect the fetal kidneys
- Reduced blood flow to the placenta and uterus, often seen when the mother has elevated blood pressure. In these cases, the baby preferentially directs blood flow to the most important organ, the brain, and away from less important organs, such as the kidneys.
- Abnormalities of the fetal kidney
- Poor fetal growth
- Placental problems, such as an abruption or blood clots
- Chromosomal problems
- Post-term pregnancy

Premature rupture of membranes

The membranes surrounding the fetus (water sac) usually rupture prior to the onset of labor or in labor, releasing amniotic fluid. If it happens before 37 weeks of gestation, it is considered "preterm" premature rupture of membranes (PPROM), but after 37 weeks it is called premature rupture of the membranes (PROM). It happens in approximately 10% of all pregnancies. No one knows why this happens, but it can cause complications in the pregnancy if it is preterm.

PROM signs and symptoms

If your membranes break, you will feel a gush of fluid from the vagina. This will be distinct from urination, although sometimes women do wonder if they have lost control of their bladders when their waters break. The difference is that the water will continue to leak from the vagina, and you will have no control over it. The volume might be small or copious. If you suspect your membranes have ruptured prematurely, go to the hospital immediately for evaluation.

Diagnosing PROM

The fluid leaking from your vagina needs to be assessed, usually with a speculum exam and a few simple tests to confirm that it is amniotic fluid. A visual inspection of your cervix will give some indication about its length and dilation. A check of your cervix by hand will be avoided, if possible, until you are in labor, to reduce the risk of infection. In addition, your health-care provider may perform an ultrasound examination to look at the amount of fluid. They may also check for "ferning" (dried fluid looks like fronds of a fern under a microscope), and for vaginal pH (litmus paper turns bright blue if

Did You Know?
Surviving PPROM

How can the baby survive without amniotic fluid? Most babies do surprisingly well. The amniotic membranes may have a leak in them, but the fluid is being made continuously by the fetus. However, a few babies born following very prolonged periods of reduced amniotic fluid volume (AFV) when the waters break at less than 24 weeks can have poor lung development and limb contractures. In the uterus, babies "breathe" amniotic fluid in and out, which encourages lung development. In the absence of amniotic fluid, the lungs may not grow normally. Without adequate amniotic fluid, the arms and legs may not have room to stretch out and may become stiff and contracted in a flexed position.

Ruptured membranes red flags

If you have the following symptoms of premature rupture of the membranes, go to your local hospital for assessment of your pregnancy:

- You are not totally sure if your membranes have ruptured.
- You are not full term (37 weeks or more).
- The fluid you see is green, brown, or very bloody.
- The fetus is not moving.
- Your GBS swab is positive.
- You are having strong labor pains.
- Your baby is believed to be in the breech position.
- You are planning a Caesarean delivery.
- You see or feel something coming out of your vagina that looks like a loop of umbilical cord.

membranes have ruptured). If PPROM is confirmed, what happens next depends upon your baby's gestational age.

"Expectantly"

If your membranes break before 32 weeks, you will probably be managed "expectantly," that is, nothing will be done to intervene if there are no signs of infection. You will be given antibiotics to reduce the risk of infection and increase the length of your pregnancy so the fetus can continue to develop. Sometimes, your doctor will advise you to remain in hospital for the rest of your pregnancy. If you return home, you will have regular telephone check-ins with a nurse to monitor your temperature. You will be asked to rest at home. No working! No housework!

Induction

Although there is evidence that a short course of antibiotics can prolong your pregnancy, if your membranes break after 34 weeks, your labor may be induced. If you are near term or at term, the baby is fully developed and you are only waiting for the onset of labor. It is better to be induced than have a baby with an infection.

Risk factors for PPROM

- Maternal infection (urinary tract infection, lower-genital-tract infection, or sexually transmitted diseases)
- Too much amniotic fluid (polyhydramnios)
- Incompetent cervix
- Multiples (twins, triplets, or more)

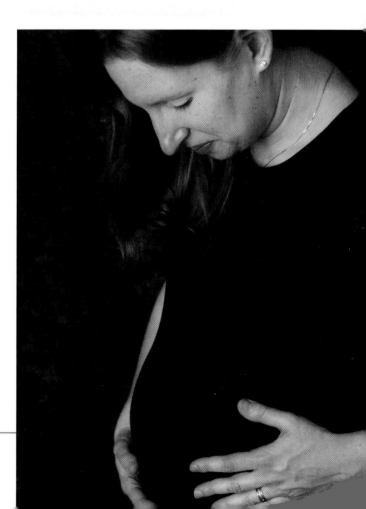

Breech presentation

Breech presentation, or lie, means that the fetus is positioned in your uterus with its head up and its bottom or feet down. If you went into labor, the first part of the baby to come through your cervix would be the feet or buttocks. If your baby is breech, your health-care provider may advise you, for the sake of your health and your baby's health, to have a Caesarean section before labor, at about week 39.

Breech symptoms

Determining the position the baby is lying in is one of the important objectives during your prenatal visits in the last several weeks of pregnancy.

- You may feel the baby kicking down low, near your bladder instead of under your ribs or on your side.
- Some women can also feel the head up near the top of the uterus — it often feels like a firm, hard ball, about the size of a grapefruit.

Your health-care provider will touch your abdomen to feel where the head is — up or down — but it can be hard to be certain. An ultrasound will quickly reveal which way your baby is lying.

Sometimes, the diagnosis of breech is not made until labor, when the examiner feels a bum instead of a head on vaginal exam. Either the fetus has been fooling everyone for a while, or it recently turned!

Best fit

The fetus floats around inside the uterus in amniotic fluid. As the space inside the uterus becomes more constricted for the growing fetus, most babies will squirm around until they find the position that is the best fit — usually head down. Some babies never quite manage this — sometimes for no good reason, and sometimes because there is some reason why the best fit for this baby might actually be in the breech position.

Did You Know?

Proper positioning

The position of the baby's head prior to labor doesn't matter very much for delivery, so don't worry about it if someone suggests your baby is OP (occiput posterior) before labor begins. Many babies in OP or OT (occiput transverse) positions will turn at the onset of (or even during) labor to a more favorable position.

During labor, once your cervix is open, it is possible for the doctor to feel the scalp bones and the soft spots on the baby's head and determine the way the baby is facing. Sometimes, the doctor can hold the baby's head and try to encourage the head to turn to a better position. Sometimes, a baby is turned at the time of delivery with forceps, in a procedure called a rotation. And sometimes, rotation is not necessary and the baby is born OP anyway! This is more likely if the pelvis is roomy and the baby is small.

Did You Know?

Fetal lies and positions

Lies
The "lie" describes the way the fetus lies in your abdomen. Is the fetus head down (vertex), head up (breech), or lying sideways (transverse)?

Positions
The "position" describes the way the fetus is facing. So a fetus in the head-down lie might face the front of your body, the back of your body, or the side of your body. These positions are given anatomic names — occiput anterior, occiput posterior, and occiput transverse. "Occiput" means "head."

Occiput anterior
In the occiput anterior (or OA) position, the fetus faces backwards, with the back of her head near the front (anterior) of the mother's body. The OA position is usually the best fit between the mother's pelvis and the baby's head. This is considered to be the easiest position in which to deliver a head-down baby.

Occiput posterior
In the occiput posterior (OP) position, the head is near the back (posterior) of the mother's body. In this position, the fetus exerts considerable pressure on the mother's spine and nerves, resulting in back pain. This is sometimes called back labor. OP can be a difficult position because there may not be as good a fit between the baby's head and the pelvis. It is more common for a baby in this position to experience a slow or arrested labor.

Occiput transverse
In the occiput transverse (OT) position, the head is near the side of the mother's body. This is a very challenging position for delivery because the fit between the pelvis and the shape of the head can be poor. These babies will either rotate prior to delivery or not descend in the pelvis.

Breech Positions
Three different breech positions are commonly distinguished: frank breech, complete breech and footling breech.

Three Fetal Lies

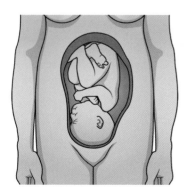

Head-down lie

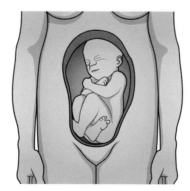

Breech lie

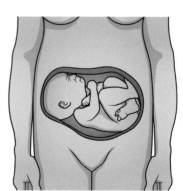

Transverse lie

Three Breech Positions

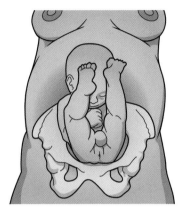

Frank breech

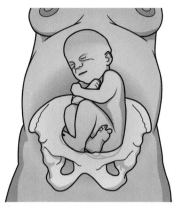

Complete breech

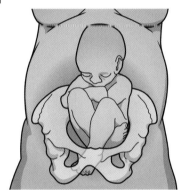

Footling breech

Breech positions

- **Frank breech:** The buttocks are lowest, the legs are bent at the hips, and the knees are straight — as if the baby is doing a "pike" dive.
- **Complete breech:** The buttocks are lowest, and the legs are bent at the hips and at the knees, as if the baby is doing a "cannonball" jump.
- **Footling breech:** The feet are the lowest and are going to come out before the buttocks.

Cord prolapse

The most serious risk with a breech presentation is called cord prolapse — the membranes rupture and the umbilical cord falls through the cervix opening. While this can happen with a baby in the head-down position, it is more likely to happen in a breech (especially a footling breech) because the baby's head is not there to act as a cork and prevent smaller parts (such as the cord) from falling down. A cord prolapse is an obstetric emergency. If the cord is compressed by a fetal part coming down upon it, this can interrupt the oxygen supply to the fetus. An emergency Caesarean section will be required.

Guide to...
Emergency response to cord prolapse
- If you see or feel a shiny, wet cord between your legs, call 911 immediately.
- Get on your hands and knees, with your head lower than your pelvis. This will help gravity pull the weight of the baby off the cord.

- Be prepared for the emergency response team to check your cervix to see how dilated you are and leave a hand inside your vagina and cervix to push the baby up and off the cord. Ideally, the person who is holding the baby up will keep his or her hand in your vagina until a Caesarean section is well underway and the baby is delivered through your abdomen. Yes, the whole way in the ambulance and right into the operating room. Not a glamorous picture, but definitely a lifesaving one.

Causes of breech presentations
There is no dominant cause of breech positioning. Most factors are natural consequences of the pregnancy:
- The shape of the space inside the uterus could suit a breech presentation more than a head-down presentation. For example, a heart-shaped uterus could have a ridge of tissue at the top, so that movement inside the uterus may be constricted.
- The placenta could be very low (placenta previa), leaving less room for the head.
- The umbilical cord could be very short, making it hard for a baby to flip.
- The mother might have given birth before, stretching her uterus so that it is less constricting to the fetus.
- If your previous baby was breech, there is a higher chance (about 10%) your second baby will also be breech.
- There could be a lot of amniotic fluid, so the baby can move around quite easily, or there could be very little amniotic fluid, so the baby cannot move out of a breech position.

- The mother could have fibroids that take up space inside the uterus and constrict the baby's movements and position.
- The baby could be one of twins (or triplets or more), making it hard to move around because space is constricted.

Spontaneous flipping
Although early in pregnancy many babies are in the breech presentation, the closer you get to your due date, the greater the chance that the baby will flip around and turn into a head-down (vertex) position. By week 32, about 15% of babies are still breech, but by full term, less than 5% of babies are breech.

Turning your baby
An external cephalic version (ECV) procedure can be used to turn your baby in some cases. If you have a heart-shaped uterus or big fibroids, the chances of success will be low and many doctors will not attempt it. If the baby has a suspected health problem, it should not be attempted.

During an ECV, the obstetrician places pressure on your belly to encourage the baby to do a somersault and turn head down. The pressure required is often quite firm, so be prepared. Sometimes, an anesthesiologist will be present to give you medication to help you relax, to prevent your uterus from contracting, and, if necessary, for pain. The changing position of the fetus and heart will be monitored with an ultrasound.

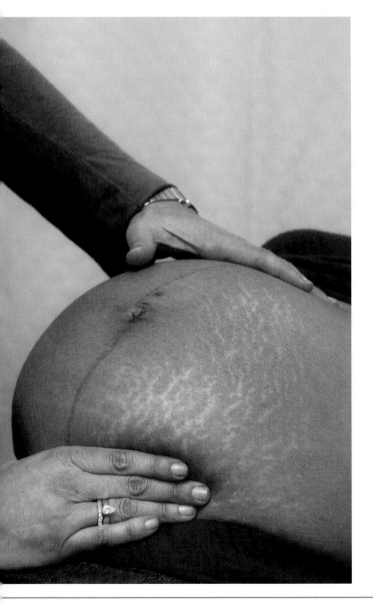

Did You Know?

Postpartum breech legs

It's true — sometimes babies who have been in the breech position seem to want to stick their legs right up around their ears for a while. Don't worry. They will relax their legs in a day or two!

ECV outcomes

If the ECV is successful and the baby turns, the next step depends on your baby's gestational age. You may be sent home to await the onset of spontaneous labor, knowing that there is a chance the baby may flip back to breech. However, if you are very close to your due date, labor might be induced right away, before the fetus has a chance to flip back to breech. If the ECV is unsuccessful, a Caesarean section is usually scheduled.

Caesarean safety

If your baby persists in the breech position right up until full term, your doctors will discuss delivery options with you. Traditionally, many breech babies were born vaginally, but this practice changed in 2000 following the publication of a large international study that concluded a Caesarean section was safer for a breech baby than a vaginal delivery. Now, most breech babies are born by Caesarean section. An exception to this common practice is a breech second twin who follows a first twin who came out head down.

Multiples complications

As the number of babies one carries in pregnancy goes up, so does the risk for major complications. The chief complication of multiple gestations is preterm birth. Although multiple births account for only 3% of births, they account for 17% of preterm births before 37 weeks, 23% of preterm births before 32 weeks, and 24% of babies weighing less than 5.5 pounds(2.5 kg). Suffice it to say that the greater the number of fetuses, the greater the risk of complications. For more information on unassisted delivery of multiples without complications, see Part 10, Spontaneous Labor and Delivery (page 353).

Preterm labor

The average length of a twins gestation is 36 to 37 weeks. For triplets, it is 34 to 35 weeks. The good news is that fetal lung maturity also comes sooner in multiples gestations. Babies born between 34 and 37 weeks usually have little or no long-term morbidity.

The earlier the babies deliver, the more likely the risk of complications. Before 34 weeks, respiratory distress syndrome, intracranial hemorrhage, and necrotizing enterocolitis can be complications of extreme prematurity. These premature infants require time in a neonatal intensive care unit (NICU) to support them until their organ systems mature. About 25% of twins and 75% of triplets require care in an NICU.

Cerclage

Although preterm labor cannot usually be stopped, it can sometimes be delayed long enough, by using antibiotics, to allow for the administration of corticosteroids to assist in maturation of the fetal lungs. Very early on in the gestation, when cervical incompetency has been diagnosed, a cerclage, or stitch, can be used to partly close the cervix. However,

there are no data to support routine use of a cerclage in multiples to prevent preterm labor. For more information on incompetent cervix treatments, see Part 6, Second Trimester Progress (page 222).

Premature rupture of the membranes

As is the case with singletons, if your water breaks prematurely after week 34, you will likely have labor induced as soon as possible. Studies have shown that induction of labor shortly after premature rupture of membranes can reduce the risk of infections in the fluid and membranes around the baby (chorioamnionitis) and in your uterus after the baby is born (endometritis). Both of these infections need to be treated with

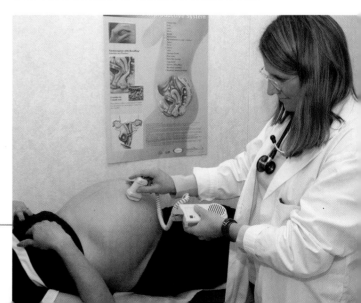

antibiotics if they occur. If you are group B streptococcus (GBS) positive, then it is best to receive antibiotics right away to help prevent transmission of GBS to your baby in delivery. For more information on GBS, see Part 8, Third Trimester Progress (page 290).

One argument against inducing women who have ruptured membranes but no labor has been a concern that this will increase the risk of Caesarean section. However, studies have shown that the Caesarean section rates do not differ between women induced within several hours of membrane rupture and women who wait for spontaneous labor.

Other pregnancy-related complications

Other complications of multiples pregnancies include gestational diabetes mellitus, placental abruption (the placenta separates from the uterine wall prematurely), and low birth weight infants. Multiples babies are smaller than a corresponding singleton baby of the same gestational age. Smaller babies may have difficulties at birth with breathing, feeding, and maintaining body temperature. Other complications that we see more often in women carrying multiples include deep vein thrombophlebitis and pulmonary embolism (blood clots in the veins and lungs, respectively) and acute fatty liver of pregnancy (a serious form of liver failure). Of special concern for the mother is an increased risk for gestational hypertension and pre-eclampsia. For certain types of identical twin fetuses, there is the unique risk of twin-to-twin transfusion.

Gestational hypertension and pre-eclampsia

The incidence of pre-eclampsia is 2.6 times higher in twins gestations than singletons and accordingly higher in triplets than in twins. When gestational hypertension, or pregnancy induced hypertension (PIH), occurs, it is likely to come sooner in multiples and in a more severe form. Multiples gestations as a result of assisted reproductive technologies, such as in vitro fertilization (IVF), are also at increased risk to develop PIH over their naturally occurring counterparts. Severe forms of PIH may lead to preterm delivery. For more information on gestational hypertension and pre-eclampsia, see Part 8, Third Trimester Progress (page 291).

HELLP Syndrome

In this more severe form of gestational hypertension, liver enzyme levels may be found to be very high, a condition called HELLP (hemolytic anemia, elevated liver enzymes, low platelet count) syndrome. The only treatment is stabilization of the mother with medications, which will include antihypertensives, and preterm delivery of the babies. In milder forms, and in cases where the babies are extremely premature, some temporization may take place to allow for the babies to mature a little more. Admission to hospital and more intense fetal and maternal surveillance is usually required, with possible induction or Caesarean section, as indicated.

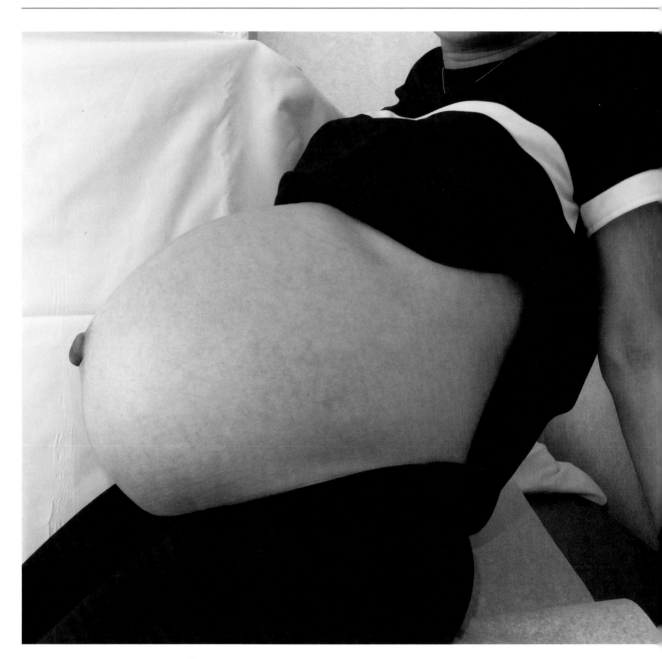

Twin-to-twin transfusion

This is an uncommon but serious complication in twins and higher multiples. In this condition, there is communication between the circulations in the placentae in identical (monoamniotic) twins. Blood flows preferentially from one twin to the other, creating a dangerous situation for both. This may occur in 15% of identical twins. Treatment involves laser surgery to the placenta to obliterate the communication between the two circulations.

Overdue

As pregnancy progresses beyond 40 weeks, there is an increased possibility that placental function may decline. This leads to decreased placental blood flow with decreased delivery of oxygen and nutrients to the fetus. In turn, this may cause reduced amniotic fluid as the fetus maximizes blood flow to critical organs, such as the brain and heart, instead of the kidneys, which produce some of the amniotic fluid. The risk of stillbirth is twice as high at more than 42 weeks and six times as high at 43 weeks when compared to delivery at 39 to 40 weeks.

Accurate dating

Confirming your due date at the time of first trimester screening and having a dating ultrasound between week 11 and 14 are the most important things you can do to prevent inaccurate dating. If the gestational age according to your last menstrual period and the dating ultrasound are within 7 days of each other, then the due date is confirmed. Interestingly, the simple act of confirming dates by ultrasound prior to 20 weeks reduces the incidence of induction for post-term pregnancy by more than 30%.

Defining overdue

There are several categories of post-term pregnancy, with slightly different terms:

- **Post-dates pregnancy:** Often refers to a pregnancy that has gone 10 days beyond the due date (40 weeks or 280 days).

- **Prolonged pregnancy:** Defined as a pregnancy that lasts until 41 weeks (287 days).

- **Post-term pregnancy:** Defined as a pregnancy that has lasted 42 weeks (294 days) or more.

Fetal surveillance

Fetal well-being is checked in a number of ways, including fetal movement counts and a biophysical profile (BPP) with non-stress testing (NST). If any of these test results are not reassuring, immediate induction of labor will be planned.

Fetal movement count

Generally speaking, daily fetal movement counts are advised from week 40 to 41 on, and even earlier in high-risk situations (for example, hypertension, diabetes, or advanced maternal age).

A fetal movement count of six movements in 2 hours is considered normal and reassuring. Ideally, you are lying down and concentrating on feeling movements. If you do not feel six movements within 2 hours, you should seek further reassurance of fetal well-being by having a biophysical profile with or without a non-stress test at your hospital.

Post-term pregnancy risks

- Fetal feces (meconium) could be drawn into the baby's lungs
- Fetal distress, as shown by abnormal fetal heart rate patterns
- Less oxygen in the newborn baby's blood because the placenta is becoming less efficient
- Continued fetal growth with macrosomia ("big baby") and birth weight over 9 pounds (4 kg), associated with difficult labors and vaginal deliveries
- Caesarean section
- Stillbirth or neonatal death

Biophysical profile

A biophysical profile (BPP) can demonstrate fetal well-being in an objective fashion. A reassuring BPP has been correlated with a low risk of fetal problems, such as distress or stillbirth, in the ensuing 48 hours.

In its classic form, a BPP has two components: an ultrasound and a non-stress test. Sometimes only one component is done.

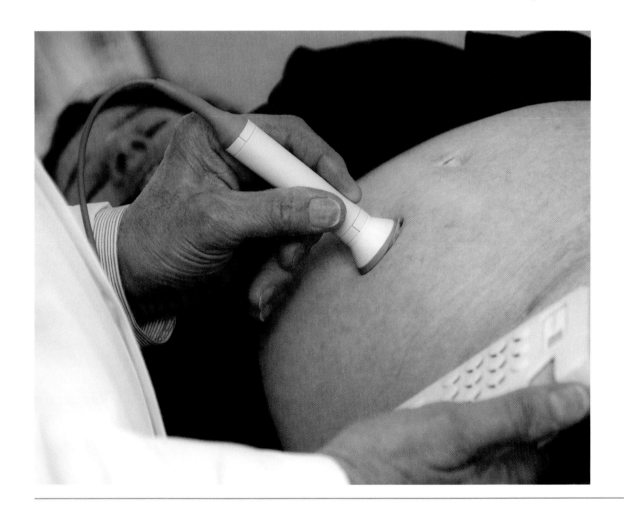

Guide to...

Biophysical profiling

Ultrasound parameters

Each of four elements of the ultrasound is scored out of 2 — 0 if absent, 2 if present. A score of 1 does not exist! Thus, a perfect ultrasound score is 8/8.

1. *Amniotic fluid volume (AVF).* An adequate amount of amniotic fluid is a reasonable indicator that the placenta is continuing to function well.

2. *Fetal breathing movements.* Babies near and at term practice breathing, expanding their chest wells and filling their lungs — except they fill their lungs with amniotic fluid, not air.

3. *Fetal movement.* Healthy babies move around inside the uterus. Even though there is not much space left at term, they should be wiggling a little bit.

4. *Fetal tone.* This refers to muscle tone. Good tone is demonstrated if the baby is seen to be sucking or moving her mouth and lips, or if the baby extends and flexes an arm or leg or opens and closes her hand.

Non-stress test

A non-stress test (NST) is also scored out of 2. Combining the ultrasound and the non-stress test, the BPP is scored out of 10.

A non-stress test looks at the fetal heart rate over a period of 20 minutes using a fetal heart rate monitor attached to the mother's belly. A reassuring fetal heart rate pattern will show some elevations of the fetal heart rate and no drops in the fetal heart rate in the 20-minute period.

BPP score results

A reassuring BPP is a score of 8 to 10 out of 10.

Action taken

If the NST is not reassuring, immediate induction of labor is usually recommended. Reduced amniotic fluid volume needs to be carefully monitored, perhaps daily, unless induction is planned in the next 24 to 48 hours. The decision to induce labor for the absence of breathing, movement, or tone will be based on discussions with your health-care provider in the context of your entire pregnancy and the remainder of the BPP parameters.

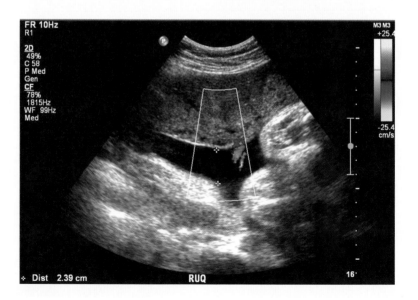

Induced labor

Labor is induced when continuing a pregnancy poses greater risks to the mother or fetus than the risks of delivery. If the cervix is already "ripe" — soft, shortened, and a little bit open — a successful vaginal delivery is possible. If the cervix is long, closed, and posterior, the induction may take longer and is less likely to be successful. By itself, induction of labor does not increase the risk of Caesarean section.

Slow process

If you do not go into labor spontaneously by about $40\frac{1}{2}$ weeks, an induction of labor will probably be arranged in the next few days, provided the fetus remains healthy. An induction of labor can be a slow process, especially with prostaglandins. Be prepared for an induction to take up to or more than 24 hours, particularly if this is your first baby. Sometimes, you will be sent home or out to walk for several hours to await the onset of labor. Other times, your doctor may prefer you stay in the hospital. Once you are in active labor, events usually unfold as they would have had you come into labor spontaneously.

Guide to...
Methods of inducing labor

Three different methods are used to induce labor. In all methods, you and your baby will be monitored before the procedure is begun and periodically while you await the onset of labor.

1. **Rupturing the membranes:** If the cervix is favorable, labor can be induced by artificial rupture of membranes. This sometimes causes the release of the hormone prostaglandin, which will stimulate uterine contractions. In some women, particularly second- and third- (or more) time mothers, this can work very well.

2. **Oxytocin:** To stimulate uterine contractions, a synthetic version of the hormone oxytocin can be given intravenously. This tends to work best in women who have a favorable cervix or who have had a baby before. It can also be used when prostaglandins should not be used; for example, in a woman with serious asthma.

3. **Prostaglandins:** A number of different formulations of prostaglandins are available that can induce labor. Vaginal administration is most common.

F.A.Q.

We answer many questions from pregnant women and their partners. Here are some of the most frequently asked questions. Be sure to ask your health-care providers any other questions that may arise. If they don't have the answers, they will refer you to a colleague who does.

Q: Can I avoid artificial induction of labor if I'm post-term by somehow putting myself into labor?

A: This is a common question toward the end of pregnancy. Many women want to know how they can put themselves into labor. Although there are three commonly suggested techniques, none are terribly practical, nor is there any evidence to suggest a benefit with any of these techniques:

1. Repeated sexual intercourse is sometimes suggested. Just once probably won't do it. The theory is that having sex will cause the release of prostaglandins from your cervix, leading to uterine contractions. In all, this seems like a benign way of inducing labor, if it works, though some couples have very little interest in sex at this stage of the pregnancy.

2. Nipple stimulation will lead to the release of oxytocin, a natural hormone that can stimulate uterine contractions. Oxytocin is the same hormone used to stimulate labor medically. You would have to do a lot of nipple stimulation, by mouth or mechanically with a breast pump, to express enough oxytocin to get labor started.

3. Castor oil is an old trick. It causes bowel symptoms, such as bloating, gas, and diarrhea, which may irritate the uterus into labor. All in all, a somewhat unappealing way of stimulating labor. Some doctors are also concerned about higher rates of meconium passage in babies when the mother uses castor oil.

Q: What is the latest point at which a breech baby can turn?

A: There is no absolute limit. The baby can turn anytime prior to birth. We are often asked whether or not the baby will turn. Experience has taught us to expect anything. Babies have been known to turn at 41 or more weeks. At our hospital, we once had a baby turn from vertex (head down) to breech in labor. This was distinctly unusual, but taught us all to be humble. The babies are in charge! Before a scheduled Caesarean section for breech presentation, a quick ultrasound should be done to confirm the position of the baby.

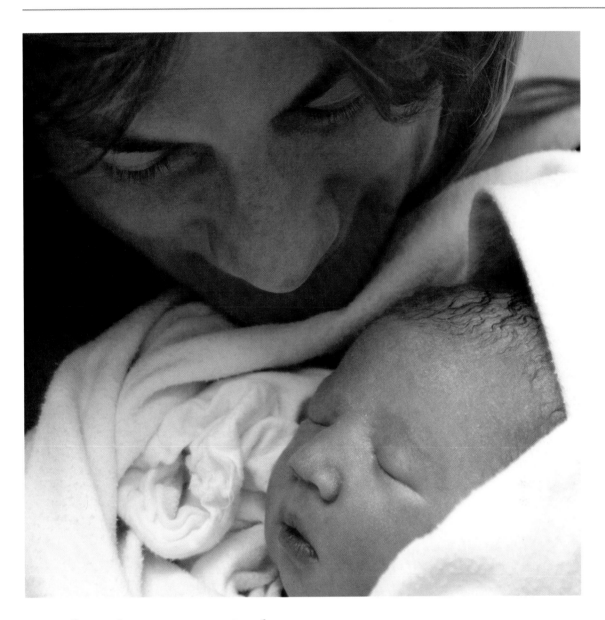

Q: *What if I want a vaginal delivery of my breech baby?*

A: You will need to discuss this thoroughly with your doctor. Make sure you understand the risks and benefits of vaginal delivery vs. Caesarean section. Also make sure that your caregiver is experienced at breech births. Most doctors trained in the last 10 years will have very little experience with vaginal breech birth because of the change in clinical practice that advises Caesarean section in these cases.

What's next

Spontaneous labor and delivery — the combined effort of your contractions and pushing.

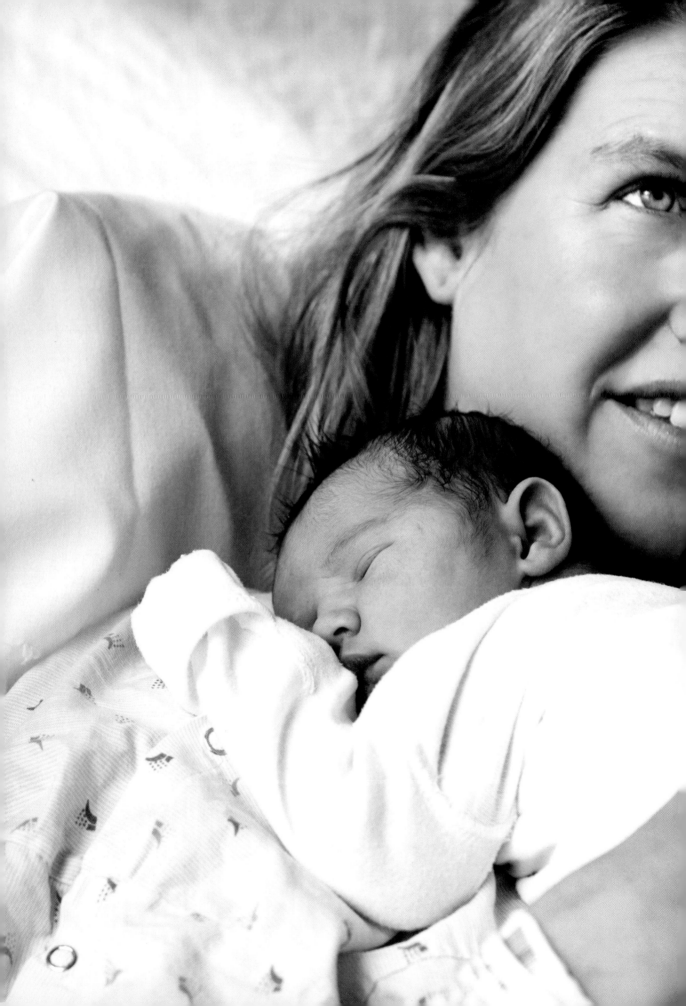

Part 10

Spontaneous Labor and Delivery

Birth day party

Your pregnancy has been focused on growing the healthiest baby possible and, after a long gestation, it's finally time for your baby to come out of hiding! While you and your family are excited to meet the new baby, like many women, you may be thinking of labor and delivery with some trepidation. This part of the book will give you some hard facts and gentle advice about the expected course of events.

Spontaneous outcomes

Like most women, you may be anticipating a spontaneous vaginal delivery, in which your baby is delivered by a combination of uterine contractions and your pushing efforts. This delivery is associated with the best outcomes and lowest risk for you and your baby. In North America, about 70% of births are vaginal. For the remaining 30%, a spontaneous vaginal delivery is not possible or safe and some assistance will be needed. For information on assisted labor and delivery, including the use of vacuum, forceps, and Caesarean section, see Part 11, Assisted Labor and Delivery (page 359). Throughout your labor and delivery, just remember that everyone shares the same goal — a healthy mother and baby. Happy *birth* day!

Ten tips for healthy spontaneous labor and delivery

1. Review the signs of labor discussed with your doctor or midwife and at your childbirth classes.
2. Be patient, especially in early labor, if things stop. Contractions will begin, we assure you, and your cervix will dilate.
3. Brace yourself for some pain and ensure your pain management strategy is ready to go.
4. Try to stay active in early labor.
5. Stay hydrated and urinate. A full bladder will prevent the baby's head from settling low into the pelvis. Think of it as a water balloon blocking the path.
6. Rely on your birth partners for support.
7. Find the best position for you to push.
8. Push and push again.
9. Look down and watch as your baby is born.
10. Celebrate the birth of your baby! Hug him to your chest.

Stages of Delivery

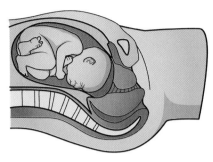

1. Head floating, before engagement

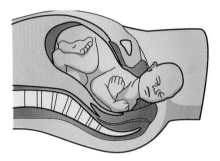

5. Complete extension

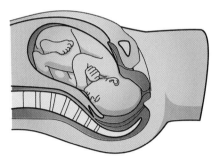

2. Engagement, descent, flexion of head

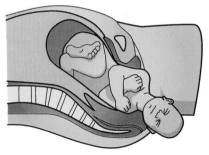

6. Restitution, (head rotates to side in alignment with shoulders)

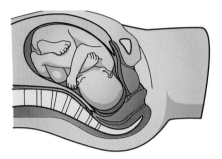

3. Further descent, head rotates to face spine

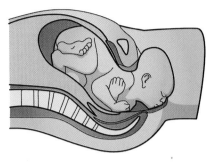

7. Delivery of anterior shoulder

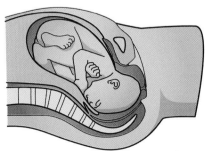

4. Complete rotation, beginning extension of neck

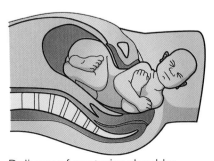

8. Delivery of posterior shoulder

Labor signs

How do you know if you are in labor? Friends and family who have had a baby will give a simple answer: "Don't worry — you'll know!" That may be so, but for the first-time mother, there are a host of early and imminent signs to tip you off.

First indications

In the week or so prior to your labor and delivery, you may notice some of the following signs. Note that none of these are suggestive of delivery tomorrow, or even the next day, just "soon"!

These first signs of early labor can be variable:

- Braxton Hicks contractions increase in number.
- Fetus "drops," or sinks deeper into your pelvis, causing increased pressure sensations in your pelvis while easing pressure at the top of your abdomen and giving you more room for breathing and eating.
- Vaginal discharge increases.
- The mucus plug, the sticky blob of mucus that has acted as a seal between your vagina and uterus, drops out.
- "Bloody show," or light vaginal bleeding, appears as your cervix starts to open up.

If you have any concerns about these signs, call or visit your doctor or midwife.

Imminent indications

The two most common events that send women and their partners out the door and

Did You Know?

True or false contractions

Sometimes, it's not easy to determine if you are in "true" labor when Braxton Hicks contractions and "false" labor symptoms can get your hopes up. You will know a true contraction primarily by its intensity.

False labor contractions

False labor is characterized by Braxton Hicks contractions (named after Dr. John Braxton Hicks). These contractions can occur as early as the second trimester. The uterus typically tightens softly for about 30 to 60 seconds in irregular intervals, but these contractions do not increase in intensity or frequency. They simply stop without progressing. Although Braxton Hicks contractions are not meant to hurt, sometimes they do, and this can be confusing.

True labor contractions

The uterus tightens hard for about 30 to 60 seconds in regular intervals, at 20 to 30 minutes to start and progressing to 5-minute intervals. At this stage, you should head to the hospital or call your midwife, because you are well into labor. As the interval decreases, the contractions increase in intensity and frequency. They are regular and typically progress to delivery. Pain usually begins in the lower back and radiates to the abdomen, becoming more intense as labor progresses and the contractions come harder and closer together and last longer.

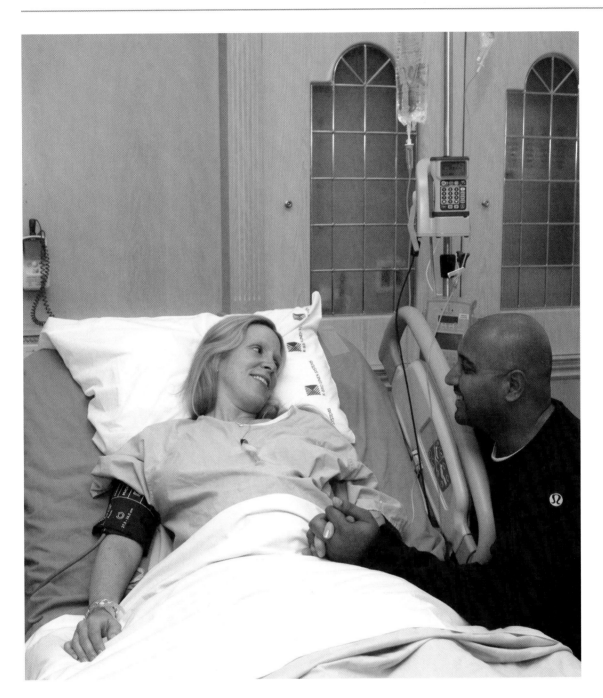

on their way to the hospital (or trigger a telephone call to the midwife) are labor pains and ruptured membranes.

Labor pains may take the form of any one of the following:

- Back pain, either constant or intermittent

- Abdominal cramping, sometimes like menstrual cramps
- Abdominal pain
- Contractions, in which the uterus becomes hard and tight in a rhythmic fashion

Labor Decision Tree

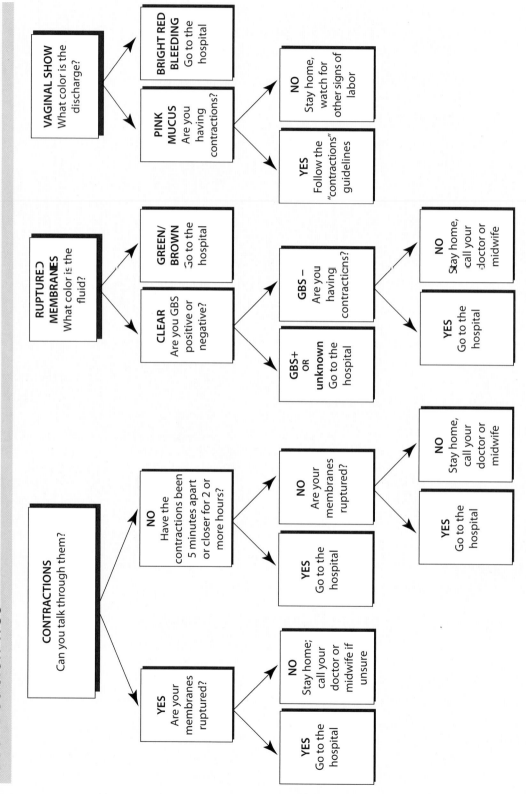

Stages of labor and delivery

Labor is traditionally divided into three stages: first, second, and third. The first stage is defined as the onset of contractions and lasts until the cervix is fully dilated. The second stage runs from full dilation until delivery. (A further "transition" stage is sometimes identified near the end of the second stage.) The third stage begins with delivery of the baby and ends with delivery of the placenta.

First stage

The first stage is further divided into two phases, latent (or early) labor and active labor. Latent labor runs from the onset of contractions until the cervix is about 3 to 4 cm dilated, while active labor runs until the cervix is fully dilated (10 cm). In labor, cervical dilation is measured in centimeters.

Latent labor

During latent labor the cervix typically dilates slowly, at less than 1 cm per hour. The length of the latent labor period is highly variable and averages 6.4 hours in a first-time mother, but it can last up to 20 hours. For a woman who has given birth previously, the average latent labor phase lasts 4.8 hours, but it can last up to 14 hours.

When you first start latent labor, your cervix will likely be only 1 to 2 cm dilated, your contractions more than 5 minutes apart (or 5 minutes apart but not seem very strong), and your baby's heart rate will likely be normal.

Risk signs during early labor

Regardless of the frequency or duration of your contractions, if you experience any of the following situations, consult your doctor or midwife, or go to the hospital immediately:

- You cannot feel any fetal movement.
- You are bleeding heavily (soaking a pad or more).
- You have had fast deliveries in previous pregnancies.
- You are preterm (before 37 weeks) and are having regular or increasing contractions.
- Your membranes have ruptured.

Ruptured membranes

In 8% of labors, the waters will break before the onset of labor. If you think your waters have broken, but you are not having any labor pains yet, call your doctor, your midwife, or the labor room nurses at the hospital for advice. There are some circumstances when you should go to the hospital straight away, but in most cases, you don't have to rush in. You can wait a couple of hours to see if you go into labor.

HOW TO…
Cope with latent labor pains

Most women cope well with the latent stage of labor at home, where they can be more mobile in surroundings that are familiar. Being active in early labor encourages the progression of labor. As long as you are coping with the pain well, and you can still feel your baby moving, use some of these strategies at home:

- Go for a walk.
- Have a hot shower.
- If your membranes haven't ruptured, have a hot bath.
- Have your birth partner massage your back or apply steady pressure to it.
- Place a heating pad on your back.

If these strategies are not helping, it's time to go to the hospital or call your midwife.

Most women at full term will go into labor spontaneously within 12 to 24 hours of having their waters break: 70% will go into labor by 24 hours after the membranes rupture, 85% by 48 hours, and 95% by 72 hours, although health-care providers don't usually wait that long anymore.

If you don't go into labor within a short period of time, most health-care providers will recommend that your labor be induced to minimize the risk of infection in your uterus. If you are group B streptococcus positive, you should go to the hospital to start your antibiotics. Your caregiver will probably recommend induction to decrease the risk of infection in the baby. You should also go to the hospital immediately if you cannot feel your baby moving, your baby is known to be breech, or the amniotic fluid is anything but clear in color (for example, green, brown, or red).

Meconium aspiration

If the amniotic fluid is greenish in color, it is a sign that the baby has passed meconium (or stool) inside your uterus. Fetal and newborn stool is dark green, so it can color the amniotic fluid. Sometimes, but not always, this is thought to be a marker of fetal distress, either now or at some time in the past. Because of this concern, the baby should be monitored closely during labor. The meconium in the amniotic fluid can be "thin" or "thick" — depending on how much it has been diluted by amniotic fluid.

Meconium aspiration is a condition that affects a small number of newborns exposed to thick meconium. The meconium can end up in the baby's lungs, leading to some short-term breathing problems. If there seems to be a risk of meconium aspiration, your newborn-care team may try to suction any thick fluid and meconium from the baby's lungs before his first gasp.

Did You Know?
5 minutes apart
Go to the hospital when your contractions are about 5 minutes apart, last a minute or so, and are strong enough to take your breath away — that is, you can't talk or do anything during the contraction and you have to stop what you are doing and focus on your breathing in order to get through the contraction.

Labor assessment

When you arrive at the hospital, you will be seen by the nurses or doctors to confirm the stage of your labor and to rule out any problems.

Antenatal record

Your baby's gestational age will be verified and your medical history reviewed, including the progress of this and any previous pregnancies, using the antenatal record you are carrying or your doctor sent ahead to the hospital. Now would be a good time for you and your birth partner to review your birth plan with the attending labor and delivery team.

Physical exams

At this point in your labor, you will undergo a series of physical examinations to determine your progress and the health of your fetus:

- **Fetal heart rate:** The fetal heart rate will be measured for at least 20 minutes by a monitor held in place with stretchy straps.
- **Uterine contractions:** Your uterine contractions will be timed by a pressure transducer also strapped to your abdomen, and their strength will be assessed by feeling how firm your uterus gets during a contraction.
- **Head position:** Your abdomen will be examined by hand to ensure the baby is lying head down.
- **Vaginal speculum exam:** Your vagina may be examined for "pooling" of fluids and tested for the presence of amniotic fluid.
- **Cervical dilation:** Your cervix will be examined to assess its dilation, effacement, consistency, and position. (See below for a definition of any unfamiliar terms.)

Planning the next step

Once the assessment is complete, the doctor or midwife will discuss the exam results with you and your birth partner and map out a plan for your labor. Your physical exam will reveal how your labor is progressing and if any special procedures will be required:

Cervical exam terms

A number of specialized terms, mostly to do with your cervix, are used to indicate the progress of your labor:

- *Dilation.* This means how open the cervix is. A cervix can range from "closed" (0 cm) to "fully dilated" (10 cm).
- *Effacement.* This refers to the length of the cervix. Before labor, a normal cervix is about 3 to 4 cm long. During labor, the cervix shortens until it is paper-thin. This is measured in percentages. A cervix that is about 2 cm long is called 50%

effaced. When the cervix is paper-thin, it is 100% effaced. A cervix will usually efface almost totally before it dilates significantly.

- *Consistency.* An unripe cervix is firm, like the tip of your nose, but when a cervix is ready for labor, it is much softer.
- *Position.* In the preparation for labor, your cervix moves from a position at the back of your vagina (posterior) to the front of your vagina (anterior).

- If there is no sign of ruptured membranes + the fetal heartbeat is reassuring + your contractions have slowed down ... you will probably be asked to return home.
- If your membranes have ruptured + the fluid was clear + your contractions have slowed down + the baby is head down + the fetal heart rate is normal + you are GBS negative ... you will likely be asked to wait several hours, often at home, to see if labor intensifies spontaneously.
- If the amniotic fluid is green ... you will be admitted for fetal monitoring and induction of labor; if the fluid is red ... you will be admitted for an induction.

- If the fetal heart rate is not reassuring ... you will be admitted for fetal monitoring prior to an induction.
- If the baby is not head down ... you will likely be admitted for a Caesarean section to be performed within a couple of hours. A transverse baby (sideways) cannot be delivered vaginally, and while a breech baby (head up) can be delivered vaginally sometimes, it is safer if it is born by Caesarean section.
- If your contractions and cervical dilation indicate you are now in active labor ... you will be admitted directly to a labor room.

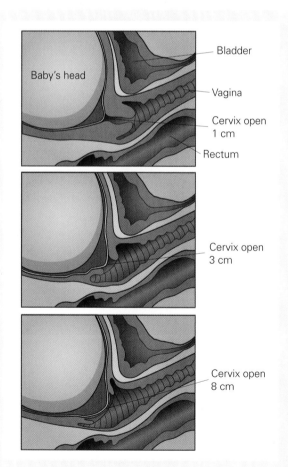

Baby's head

Bladder

Vagina

Cervix open 1 cm

Rectum

Cervix open 3 cm

Cervix open 8 cm

Did You Know?

Cervical dilation

Measuring cervical dilation is done with an examiner's index and ring finger. The two fingers open to touch either side of the cervical opening, and by practice and experience, the examiner can determine how open the cervix is.

- 1 cm: single digit inside cervical opening
- 3 cm: two fingers fit side by side
- 5 cm: two fingers separated
- 8 cm: about a ½-inch (1 cm) rim of cervix felt all around
- 10 cm: fully dilated with no cervix detected

Did You Know?

Partogram

Most caregivers will examine your cervix approximately every 2 to 3 hours to assess changes. Once you are in active labor, a doctor is looking for your cervix to dilate about 1 cm per hour, although it might dilate a little more slowly if this is your first baby. The rate of cervical change can be charted on a graph called a partogram. A partogram makes it very easy to see if the cervix is dilating at the usual rate.

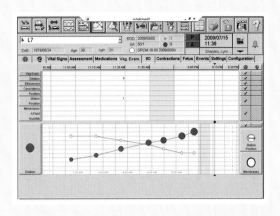

Back home again

Since women in early labor usually have better outcomes if they are active and mobile, you may be encouraged to return home for a little while longer, to go out for a walk, or to stay nearby in an early labor lounge that some hospitals have for their patients.

Try not to be too frustrated or discouraged if this happens to you. Early labor is an important part of labor, but it can take a long time. Try to stay mobile, have a light snack, and even rest a little bit when you can. Then return for another assessment when your labor pains get stronger and more frequent.

If you are exhausted or cannot cope with the pain any longer using the measures you have tried so far, discuss this with your doctor. Sometimes, women are admitted to the labor floor in early labor for these reasons.

Active labor

At the start of active labor, your cervix will be dilated 3 to 4 cm, and your contractions will be strong, occurring at least every 5 minutes.

During active labor, your contractions will increase to approximately three to five contractions in 10 minutes. The cervix will dilate more rapidly now, about 1 cm per hour. In one study of women with low-risk pregnancies, delivering without epidurals or oxytocin, the average duration of the active phase of labor was 7.7 hours for a first-time mother and 5.6 hours for subsequent babies, with a range of up to 17.5 hours and 13.8 hours, respectively.

In addition to measuring your cervix, the depth of your baby's head relative to your perineum will be measured during each vaginal exam in order to trace its descent. Your baby's head needs to descend into your pelvis, moving closer and closer to your vagina.

Labor room assessment

By now, you are probably in a labor room, having been welcomed by a nurse and encouraged to change into something comfortable — usually but not necessarily a hospital gown. The nurse will listen to the baby's heart rate again and assess your contractions. Your vital signs (heart rate,

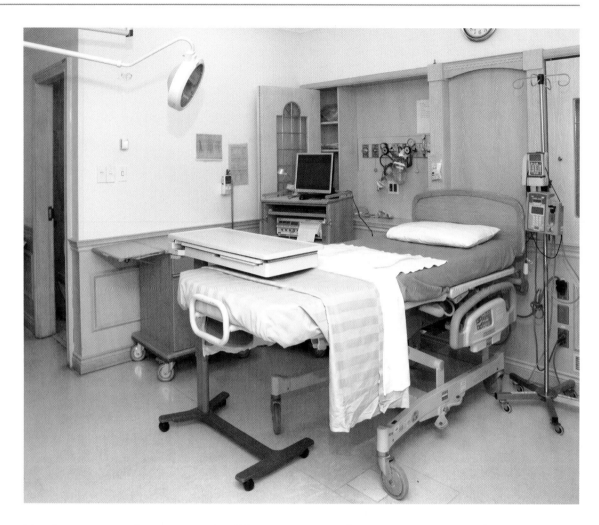

blood pressure, and temperature) will be measured. Your urine will be checked for protein. Depending on hospital policies, blood may be drawn at this time to check your CBC (complete blood count) and to provide the lab with a sample of blood to confirm blood typing. If you are GBS positive, an intravenous line will be placed in your arm and you will be given intravenous antibiotics.

Fetal well-being

The best way to assess fetal well-being is to listen to the fetal heart rate. This can be done in two ways: intermittent auscultation or continuous fetal heart rate monitoring

Intermittent auscultation is the periodic assessment of the baby's heart rate during labor, usually every 15 to 30 minutes in the active phase, for at least a minute before and a minute after a contraction, using a hand-held doptone machine (like the one used in your medical check-ups) or a fetal monitor. This is the preferred method of fetal monitoring in low-risk labors, because studies have shown that it leads to fewer interventions than continuous fetal heart rate monitoring, and the neonatal

Did You Know?

Contraction frequency and strength

- *Frequency:* The frequency of the contractions can be determined by timing them (from the beginning of one contraction to the start of the next). If you don't have an epidural and can feel them, your labor coach can help you time them. If you do have an epidural in place and can't really feel your contractions well, they can be assessed by a hand examination of your uterus (it will get hard as it contracts) or by using a contraction monitor belt, which measures pressure and shows the frequency rate on the fetal heart rate monitor.

- *Strength:* Judging the strength of your contractions is subjective. You will definitely feel them get stronger. If you are not feeling them well because you have an epidural in place, the nurses and doctors (or midwife) can feel how strong they are with their hands. In general, a mild contraction means the uterus can be indented with pressure from the examiner's hand during a contraction, and if they are strong, the uterus resists being indented with the same external pressure.

outcomes are the same as for continuous monitoring.

Continuous fetal heart rate monitoring involves placing a fetal monitor onto the mother's belly and holding it in place with belts. Alternatively, an electrode can be placed directly on the baby's head to monitor the heart rate. The monitor runs continuously, producing a graph, known as a tracing, of the fetal heart rate that is used to assess the baby's well-being.

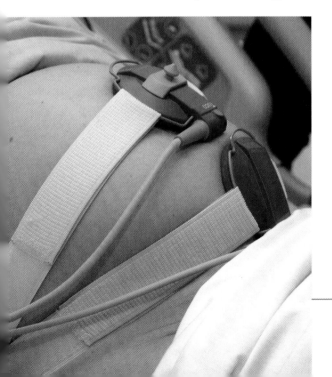

Continuous fetal heart rate monitoring is advised for women who have had a complication in pregnancy or labor.

Fetal scalp electrodes

A fetal scalp electrode can be placed on the baby's head, but only after the cervix is open and the membranes are ruptured. A wire leads from the electrode out of your vagina to your leg and then to the fetal heart rate monitor. Fetal scalp electrodes are not used routinely, but they are particularly useful if the external fetal heart rate monitor is picking up a pattern that is slightly abnormal. They are also useful if the baby's heart rate is difficult to pick up externally for technical reasons.

Maternal well-being

While you are in labor, your vital signs will be checked periodically for signs of high blood pressure and fever. Your hydration status will also be monitored. You may not want to eat much, but it is a good idea to stay hydrated. Your ability to empty your bladder will also be monitored.

Did You Know?
Fetal heart rate tracings
The important elements of a normal fetal heart rate tracing are:

- *Rate:* The baseline fetal heart rate is normally between 120 and 160 beats per minute (bpm).

- *Variability:* Fetal hearts rates vary from minute to minute, ideally changing at least 5 bpm within a minute.

- *Presence of accelerations:* The heart rate increases over baseline by at least 15 bpm for at least 15 seconds at least twice in 20 minutes.

- *Absence of decelerations:* Decelerations are drops in the fetal heart rate below baseline. They are sometimes, but not always, signs that the fetus is not coping well with labor.

- *Contraction pattern:* Contractions are monitored at the same time, and their frequency can be assessed, as well as their timing in relationship to fetal heart rate patterns.

Sometimes, it is hard for women who have had an epidural to urinate properly, and if that is the case with you, your bladder can be emptied with a small catheter. A full bladder will prevent the baby's head from settling low into the pelvis.

Pain management
One of the most important elements of monitoring your well-being is assessing how well you are coping with the pain of labor. Different women experience pain, and especially labor pain, in very different ways. Some request pain relief medications; others do not.

If you are coping well, keep up the pace. If you're feeling a bit uncomfortable, you might try switching gears and trying a different position. If you need help with pain, now is the time to ask. There are several procedures available, including epidurals, for administering pain medication. For more information on pain management options, see Part 7, Birth and Newborn Planning (page 261).

Assessing progress
In the active phase of labor, your health care team will be monitoring you for specific signs of progress:

1. **Cervical dilation and effacement:** Your cervix will be examined by your nurse, doctor, or midwife at regular intervals, usually every 2 to 3 hours. The dilation and effacement of your cervix will be assessed. The descent of the head and position of the head can also be assessed. Ideally, your cervix will be more dilated and more effaced with each examination, and the head will be lower.

2. **Vaginal and rectal pressure:** As you near full dilation, you may begin to feel an intense pressure deep in your vagina and rectum. Some women report that they feel constipated or as if they need to have a bowel movement. This pressure is usually a sign that the head is descending lower and lower. Some women feel this, even with an epidural, while others do not. Don't worry if you do not.

Transition stage

This is a stage of labor frequently discussed by nurses, midwives, and mothers themselves, but not much by doctors, because it is based on how a laboring woman feels, without any objective findings. When the term is used, it refers to a time near the end of first stage labor, between about 7 cm dilation and full dilation. It tends to last 30 to 60 minutes. With good support, you will get through transition and into the next stage — delivery!

Transition signs

- Increased frequency and intensity of contractions
- Increased rectal pressure as the head descends
- Nausea and vomiting
- Shaking of legs and body
- Alternating sweats and chills
- Increased irritability
- Sense of hopelessness, as if you cannot continue

Some of these symptoms may be absent if you have an epidural in place during transition.

Second stage

In a study of women with low-risk pregnancies, the average duration of the second stage of labor in first-time mothers was 54 minutes, and in subsequent pregnancies, 18 (but can last up to 2.5 hours and 1 hour, respectively). These times may be longer if an epidural is used, if the baby is big, or if the mother is small.

Progress

What happens next? Simply stated, your contractions persist and the baby's head moves lower and lower with the force of the contractions, combined with your pushing efforts. Labor progress is assessed by determining how low in the birth canal the head descends over time. Ideally, the head descends a little bit with each contraction and each push until it reaches your perineum. Then, with continued contractions and pushing, the head will crown, deliver, and the rest of the body will follow. During this second stage of labor, your delivery team will continuously assess both fetal and maternal well-being.

Pushing, pushing

During the second stage, you begin to push the baby out, aiding the uterine contractions in the delivery of the baby. How you will feel at this point will depend a lot on whether or not you have an epidural.

If you do not have an epidural, you may begin to feel (if you haven't already) a lot of pressure in your vagina and rectum and an increasing need to bear down. If so, it is time to start pushing. Many women report that pushing seems to lessen the pain and it is a tremendous relief to be able to use the pain of labor to push the baby out.

If you do have an epidural, your sensation may be lessened, and you may

HOW TO...

Push

You may receive a lot or a little coaching from your birthing partner and delivery team in how to push. At that point, you may be less than receptive to advice, so here's some in advance:

1. When you have a contraction, put your hands behind your thighs and pull them toward your chest, curling your spine forward so it makes a letter "C," and bring your chin to your chest.

2. Take a big breath, close your mouth, and push down into your bottom, holding the downward pressure as long as you can.

3. Take another big breath, and push again.

4. Try to get three or four good pushes in with each contraction, then lie back, close your eyes, relax, slow your breathing, and wait for the next contraction.

5. Try counting out each push with your partner. Some women find it focuses their pushing if their birth partners guide them verbally by counting out with each push — for example, saying, "Okay, now take a big breath in, push down and hold it for 10, one, two, three, four... nine, ten. Great — now take a big breath, close your mouth, and push again for 10, one, two..." Other women find it annoying and would rather just push without the counting. Let your team know what is helpful and not helpful for you.

Did You Know?

Pushing positions

There are three positions commonly used for pushing:

1. *Semi-reclined:* Semi-reclined on a labor bed, with the head of your bed elevated to at least 45 degrees. If you have an epidural, your legs are probably very heavy and will need support. They can be held by your labor team (one on each side), by foot pedals on the side of the bed, or, less commonly, in stirrups. If you do not have an epidural, you may feel strong enough to support your legs yourself with a hand under each knee.

2. *Side lying:* Lying on your side, with your lower leg bent and your upper leg also bent but elevated and supported in the air by an assistant.

3. *Squatting:* If your legs are strong, a squatting support bar can be added to your labor bed and you can pull yourself forward, lean on it, and bear down with your contractions while you are pushing, but for delivery you may have to recline.

not feel much pressure. Or you might. It is a little hard to predict. If you are not feeling much pressure, it is useful for the examiner to assess how high the head is in your pelvis. If the head remains high, it is usual to wait 1 or 2 hours before beginning to push. This allows the head to come down a little further so you don't have to push so hard and long, and it also allows some time for the epidural analgesia to wear off so that you have a little more sensation, which aids in the pushing effort.

Episiotomy

As the head of the baby comes through the opening of the vagina during delivery, the skin and underlying muscles of the pelvic floor are being stretched. Despite this stretching, the baby's head is sometimes too large to fit through, and there is spontaneous and natural tearing of the tissue at the opening of the vagina and the muscles underneath. Sometimes this tearing can extend into the anal sphincter or the rectal tissue.

An episiotomy involves surgical cutting of the vaginal tissue and muscles to allow the baby's head to emerge more easily and to enable a neat stitching of the clean cut. There are two kinds of episiotomy: medial, where the skin is cut from the opening of the vagina straight down; and mediolateral, where the skin of the vagina is cut to the side. A mediolateral episiotomy prevents the incision from extending further into the rectum, although it tends to be associated with more pain during healing.

Crowning

Once your cervix has reached 10 cm, you are fully dilated. You are almost there!

As the baby's head begins to stretch your perineum, it is beginning to "crown." You may feel an intense burning as the head stretches the perineum. With each push, the head will stretch your perineum a little bit more, until the widest diameter of the head is delivered.

At this point, you may be told to breathe slowly, and not to push, or to push very gently.

Episiotomies

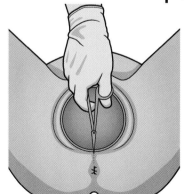

Medial

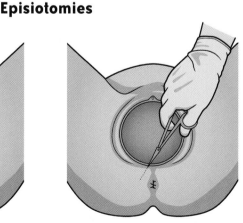

Mediolateral

The goal is to allow the head to stretch the perineum gently and perhaps minimize any tearing. With the next one to two pushes, the head will usually deliver.

Then, you will be asked to give a big push to help the shoulders deliver. Once the shoulders have delivered, the rest of the baby will follow easily.

Congratulations! Your baby is born! Your birth partner or a delivery team member may now clamp and cut the umbilical cord.

Guide to...

Episiotomies

Re-evaluation

At one time, doctors thought that an episiotomy had several benefits aside from controlling tearing. It was thought to prevent pelvic relaxation or prolapse later in life because the muscles would not get stretched out during the pushing stage of the delivery. Decreasing the time that the baby's head pushed at the opening of the vagina was thought to be less traumatic for the baby. This was particularly true in preterm deliveries, because it was felt that the premature baby would be more prone to skull damage.

Since that time, there have been many randomized, controlled trials that dispelled the idea that an episiotomy is better than a natural tear. Studies showed that tearing resulted in less pain and fewer complications with recovery than routine episiotomy. The majority of practitioners providing obstetrical care no longer routinely perform episiotomies.

When an episiotomy is advised

There are still some occasions when an episiotomy is advised:

• If you are having an assisted delivery with forceps, your caregiver may choose to perform an episiotomy. The delivery of the baby is being expedited during this procedure, and there is no time to slowly stretch the muscles of the pelvic floor. In this case, it may be better to make a cut to prevent extensive tearing.

• If you have a very short perineum (the distance between the opening of the vagina and the anus) and the tissue is not stretching well, the tear could easily extend into the rectum. Studies have shown that some patients with a tear of the anal sphincter or rectum or both may have prolonged difficulty with uncontrollable passing of gas or stool.

• If your vaginal tissues are not stretching well when you are pushing, this tissue can become very swollen. In these cases, the vagina can tear very badly. This can be difficult to repair and can result in greater postpartum bleeding and pain. It is hard to predict ahead of time if your perineum will stretch well or not; it may be related to genetic factors determining the proportions of collagen and elastin in your skin.

• If the baby's head is pushing against your urethra and clitoris, you can develop tearing in the tissue around these structures, which can cause pain postpartum. Sometimes, if it seems as if there will be extensive tearing in the front of the vagina, a small episiotomy at the back of the vagina will minimize tearing in these tender areas.

• If the only obstacle to delivery seems to be a tight perineum, a small episiotomy can hasten delivery — sometimes a welcome option!

Vaginal birth

■ The perineum is bulging as the baby's head becomes visible between the labia. The doctor's hand supports the perineum.

■ The head crowns while the doctor's hand prevents the head from "popping" out. A slow, controlled delivery is ideal for minimizing tearing.

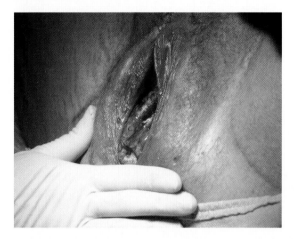

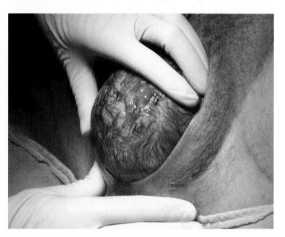

■ The face and chin are delivered.

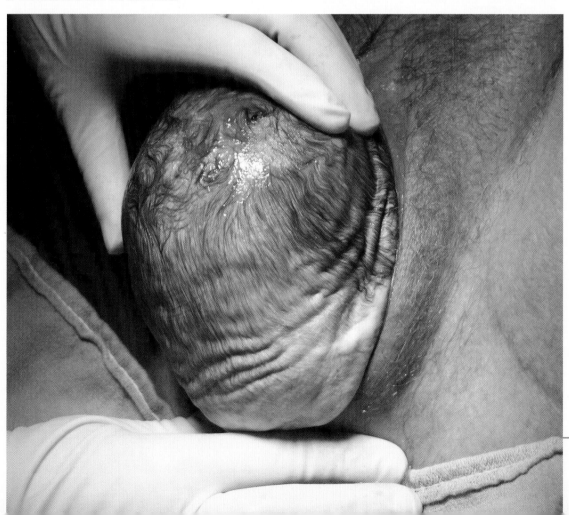

■ The face rotates to the side while the doctor makes sure there is not a loop of cord around the neck.

■ The doctor guides the baby upward to allow the shoulders and arms to be delivered.

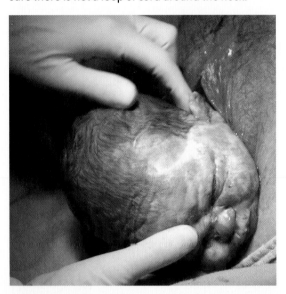

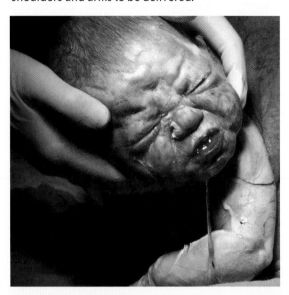

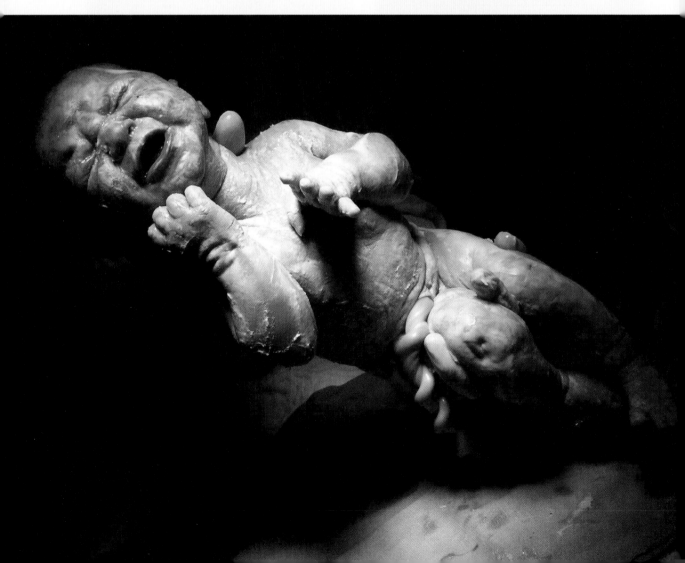

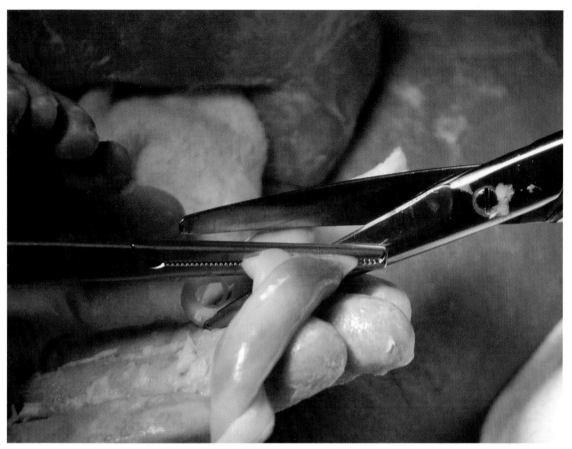

■ The umbilical cord is clamped and cut.

Immediate postpartum

If your baby looks well, he can be put on your chest immediately after delivery. All amniotic fluid and blood will be dried off so that he is warm and dry, and if your baby begins to breathe easily, he can remain with you, naked chest to naked chest.

Delayed umbilical cord clamping

In the past, the umbilical cord was cut and clamped fairly quickly after delivery, for convenience. More recently, some studies have suggested that delaying cord clamping and holding the baby below the level of the placenta until the cord stops pulsating, or

for about 1 minute, may increase the amount of blood that goes to the baby, preventing anemia and low iron levels. This may be particularly important if the mother is iron deficient.

However, this procedure can result in some babies developing "polycythemia," a condition associated with too many red blood cells, and, rarely, jaundice as those red blood cells are broken down. In a full-term infant, neither anemia nor polycythemia is particularly likely, but this may be an important issue in smaller or preterm infants.

If you have a strong feeling that you would like cord clamping delayed, make sure you let the delivery room staff know.

Third stage

You are not finished yet! It is time for the placenta to be delivered. This stage can last up to 30 minutes. The placenta will separate from the wall of the uterus and usually come away with a gush of blood. Once the gush of blood is seen, the doctor may put one hand on your lower abdomen and use the other hand to pull down gently on the umbilical cord, encouraging the placenta to come loose. You may be asked to help push the placenta out — but don't worry. It's not as big (or bony!) as the baby.

Oxytocin

Once the placenta is delivered, you will receive oxytocin to help your uterus contract. If you have an intravenous in place, it will be given intravenously; otherwise, you will get an injection in your thigh. By helping the uterus to contract firmly, oxytocin reduces postpartum bleeding significantly.

Suturing

Once your uterus is firm and the bleeding slows down, your perineum will be examined for any tears. If an episiotomy was made, or if there are any tears in your vagina and perineum, they will be repaired now. These sutures are absorbable, meaning that they will dissolve by themselves in a week or two —

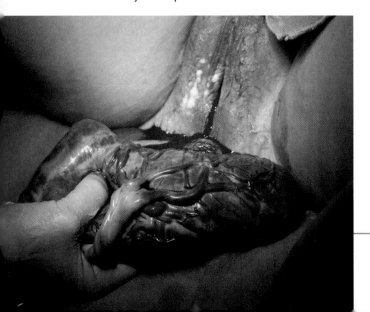

■ Delivery of the placenta

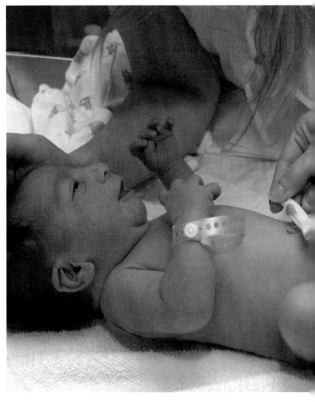

there is no need to have them removed. (That's good news.) If you need pain control for the stitches, some local anesthetic can be used. Sometimes, if you have an epidural, you don't need any local anesthetic, and sometimes you do. After delivery, if your perineum is swollen, some ice can be applied for the next several hours to help reduce the swelling and the pain.

Multiples labor and delivery

Twins can be born through a spontaneous labor and delivery, but higher-order multiples (triplets, quadruplets, or more) are almost always delivered by Caesarean section. While the labor and delivery for twins is not unlike the process for singletons, there are important differences. The average length of gestation for twins is between 37 and 38 weeks. For higher multiples, labor ensues somewhat earlier. Doctors define term for twins as 38 weeks and will often consider induction of labor in an uncomplicated twins gestation by this time if conditions are suitable. In the case of a twins gestation with medical complications, an induction may be planned earlier than term. For more information on multiples risks, see Part 9, High-Risk Pregnancies (page 321).

Conduct of labor

Labor for multiples is considered a high-risk situation and should take place in a hospital under the supervision of a doctor with considerable experience in delivering twins.

Fetal monitoring

Electronic fetal monitoring (EFM) is the most effective way of monitoring the two fetal hearts during labor, allowing for continuous surveillance during the course of these high-risk deliveries. Initially, the monitoring can be external, with two monitors held on the mother's belly with belts. Sometimes, it can be challenging to differentiate between the two fetal heart rates using this method, so once the membranes surrounding the leading twin have ruptured, a fetal scalp electrode is applied to the first twin and an external fetal heart rate monitor is applied to the abdomen of the mother to monitor the second twin. Once the first twin has been delivered, a fetal scalp electrode is applied to the second twin to monitor its heart rate until delivery. Intermittent auscultation is not reliable for distinguishing one twin heart beat from another and cannot be used when monitoring twins.

Pain relief

Early on in labor, injectable opioid narcotics are a good choice for pain relief. Once labor is established, epidural anesthesia is the preferred method for pain relief. An epidural is advised, not only for good pain relief in labor, but also so that you are ready (from an anesthetic point of view) to face any possible outcome in labor, including intrauterine manipulation for delivery of the second twin, an operative vaginal delivery of either twin, or an emergency Caesarean section for either the first or the second twin. Having an epidural in place allows the obstetrician to move quickly to delivery if either twin shows signs of distress.

Guide to...

Twins delivery possibilities

The planned method for delivering your twins will depend on how they lie:

- *Both are head down:* Roughly 42% of twins will present with both heads down. In this case, they are usually delivered vaginally. Elective Caesarean section is not recommended for twins where the leading twin is head down unless there are complicating circumstances. Sometimes a vaginal delivery is planned, but during the course of the labor a Caesarean section is advised due to circumstances that arise in the labor (10% to 30% of cases).

- *Leading twin is not head down:* Roughly 20% of twins will present with the leading twin not being in the head-down lie. These twins will, in most cases, be delivered by Caesarean section.

- *Leading twin is head down, second twin is not:* Some studies favor Caesarean section, while others favor vaginal birth. Currently, many doctors would advise you to plan a vaginal delivery in this circumstance.

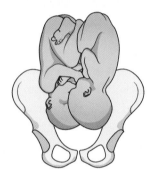
Two vertexes

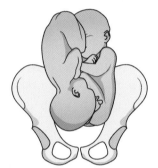
Vertex and breech

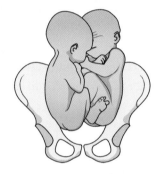
Two breeches

Twins delivery

If the leading twin is head down, a vaginal birth is often anticipated. Once pushing has commenced for the leading twin, the mother is often transferred to an operating room for the delivery. Although this is not mandatory, it is often done in case there are difficulties in delivering the first or second twin and an emergency Caesarean section is required. In the room, your obstetrician and an anesthesiologist are present, along with a respiratory technologist or neonatologist (experts in neonatal resuscitation) and an extra delivery room nurse.

Twin A

Although it is preferred that twin A be delivered by spontaneous vaginal delivery, it is possible that an assisted vaginal delivery using a vacuum extractor or forceps will be required. Oxytocin might also be required to augment labor before delivery of twin A. The delivery of twin A should proceed much as it would for a singleton. Once the first twin is delivered, his umbilical cord is clamped and cut, and the baby is handed to other members of the delivery team. You will see the baby, but probably will not hold him immediately, because your attention is required to deliver twin B!

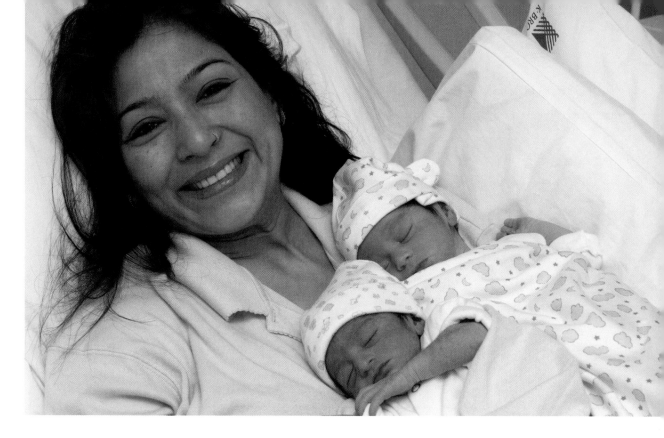

Twin B

Your contractions should persist, but sometimes oxytocin is required to make sure they do.

If the second twin is also head down, the head is guided toward the cervix and vagina as the contractions push the head lower. When the head is low enough, the membranes for twin B are ruptured. Provided that the heart rate of twin B is reassuring, you will deliver your second twin spontaneously, with only your pushing efforts.

Complications

- If the fetal heart rate pattern is not normal and there is a concern that twin B may be in distress, an assisted vaginal birth may be performed with either forceps or vacuum extractor.
- If the second twin is not head down, either a breech extraction or an internal podalic version may be performed. In a breech extraction, the obstetrician reaches into the uterus and searches for the baby's feet and pulls them gently down into the vagina, and ultimately, out. The doctor's hands then move to the baby's buttocks, continuing to pull down, delivering the chest. The arms are delivered, and finally — the head! In an internal podalic version, the obstetrician puts a hand into your uterus and coaxes the baby to turn into a head-down position, allowing for a normal vaginal delivery of the second twin.
- If the heart rate of the second twin is not reassuring or the second twin fails to descend, a Caesarean section may be required for the second twin, which is the case in 6% to 25% of these births.

Did You Know?

Twins timing

The ideal delivery interval between twin A and B is under 30 minutes, although in the presence of a reassuring fetal heart rate, a doctor may allow a longer interval if the second twin is descending lower in the pelvis and the labor is progressing well.

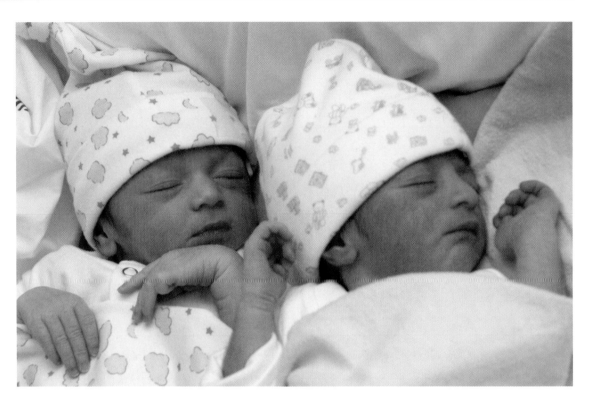

F.A.Q.

We answer many questions from pregnant women and their partners. Here are some of the most frequently asked questions. Be sure to ask your health-care providers any other questions that may arise. If they don't have the answers, they will refer you to a colleague who does.

Q: How do I know if my membranes have ruptured?

A: Sometimes it is very obvious, and sometimes it is not. If there is copious fluid flowing from your vagina, and you can't control it the way you can control urine, then your membranes have likely ruptured. Sometimes, you may just have a sensation of wetness or dampness and wonder if maybe ruptured membranes are the cause. If this is the case, then see your health-care provider or go to the hospital. It is better to do this sooner rather than later, because if you just have a fluid leak, you want the diagnosis made while the wetness is still there, not tomorrow morning, when it may have settled down.

Q: Why is labor induced after ruptured membranes?

A: It has been shown that induction of labor after ruptured membranes leads to a lower chance of maternal and neonatal infection, and a lower chance of the baby needing special care in an NICU after birth.

In addition, the Caesarean section rate is not increased, nor is the chance of needing a vacuum-assisted or forceps delivery. The studies are not perfectly clear in how long to wait to induce labor before this risk of infection goes up. This uncertainty is why there is some variation in doctors' practices and opinions, but most agree that, if you are GBS positive, induction will be recommended.

Q: I hear that oxytocin causes harder, more painful contractions. Is that true?

A: It is hard to know how true this is. Certainly, with oxytocin, we are encouraging your body to accelerate a process that naturally may take several hours or even days. It may or may not actually hurt more; it is hard to imagine how we could ever know for sure. If you are having an oxytocin induction of labor, try to ignore the oxytocin, focusing instead on your contractions and using all the coping strategies you were planning on using in labor anyway.

Q: Should I give myself an enema when I start labor?

A: No. Although enemas were standard practice many years ago, they are no longer recommended or required. Some women worry about pushing out stool as they deliver the baby, but you don't need to be concerned. Yes, it may happen, but who cares? Stool will not likely get on the baby, and if it somehow does, it will not increase the risk of infection to your baby or yourself. Don't worry about it.

Q: Do I need to shave?

A: No. It is neither necessary nor expected that you shave *anything* ahead of time (legs nor perineum). There seems to be a belief among some women that it is "polite" to their doctors to be clean-shaven … well, we should dispel that myth. Your doctors have seen every "hair" style and don't really care which one you are sporting. Nor will you be shaved in hospital. If your pubic hair extends up over the area where a Caesarean section incision might occur, then the hair just at that line may be clipped (not shaven). Shaving has been shown to increase surgical wound infections and is avoided.

Q: I hear about some women yelling during labor. Is that normal?

A: For some women, it is very normal, particularly if they do not have an epidural in place. Some women with an epidural even find themselves being pretty vocal at the time of delivery, too. Don't let it worry or scare you. The physical feelings and sensations can be very intense. You should not be worrying about repressing anything, even your voice, at this time.

What's next

While for most women, labor and delivery proceed spontaneously and smoothly, sometimes little things go wrong and, occasionally, some bigger things. That's why we're here — to assist you in giving birth to a healthy child and in staying healthy yourself.

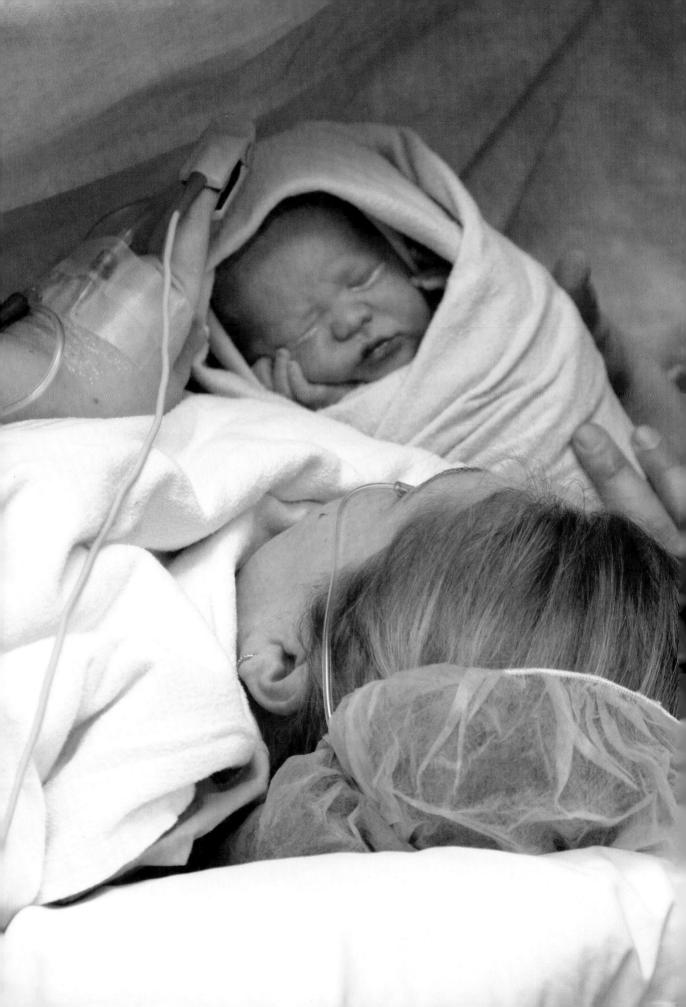

Part 11

Assisted Labor and Delivery

With a little help...

Almost a perfect design! A birth is always a miraculous event. The awe you will feel as your baby is born is an experience many health-care providers are lucky enough to witness every day in their professional lives. Most of the time, the birth proceeds easily, without any complications, but sometimes assistance is needed to solve problems that arise.

Interventions

The idea of intervention sounds a bit scary — vacuum extractors, forceps, and Caesarean section deliveries, in addition to labor induction procedures and medications. Try not to be intimidated by these interventions in your labor and delivery. At the end of the day, they may be needed to bring your baby into this world safely.

10 tips for coping with unexpected developments during labor and delivery

1. Keep an open mind. Situations change, and you need to be ready to adapt!

2. Be patient ... labor can be a long process. Sometimes not all the strength or willpower in the world can move things along.

3. Ask questions. Your health-care providers are always willing to spend time discussing your concerns.

4. Evaluate your options and weigh the risk of any procedure. It's your baby being born.

5. In an emergency, let your caregivers do their jobs without interference. They will explain what happened once the situation is stable.

6. Lean on your birth partner and delivery support team to make sure you have everything you need.

7. Don't be hard on yourself. Every birth is perfect.

8. Some things are not under your control, including complications in labor and delivery. Needing assistance is nothing to feel guilty about. It's not your "fault."

9. Have faith. Your baby will be born.

10. Laugh a little. Even if it hurts ...

Guide to ...

Kinds of assisted delivery

Assisted, or operative, vaginal delivery
A vacuum extractor or forceps are used to assist the doctor in delivering the baby vaginally.

Caesarean section

The baby is delivered through a surgical incision in the mother's abdomen. There are three circumstances that involve a Caesarean section:

- *Emergency Caesarean section:* The operation is performed on a woman in labor when an emergency arises (for example, signs of fetal distress or significant maternal bleeding) that makes a vaginal delivery too risky.

- *Urgent Caesarean section:* The operation is performed on a woman in labor when a vaginal delivery seems risky or unlikely (for example, a long labor with little cervical dilation).

- *Elective Caesarean section:* The operation is performed on a pregnant woman near term but not in labor. It is planned ahead of time. Common reasons include a previous Caesarean section or a breech presentation, or multiple babies beyond twins — and, in some cases, when the pregnant woman chooses to deliver by Caesarean section, rather than vaginally.

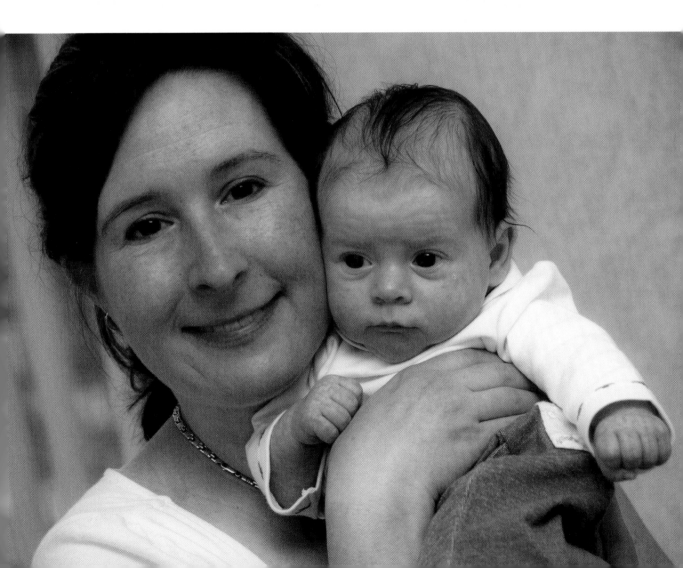

Poor progress in the first stage

During the first stage of labor, your progress can slow down if your cervix does not dilate at the expected rate of about 1 cm per hour. For example, your cervical dilation could stall at 5 cm for 3 hours, even though you are having contractions every 3 minutes.

In this case, there are three options for encouraging cervical dilation: wait a while longer, rupture the membranes, and/or augment contractions with oxytocin.

Wait

The first option is to wait longer to see if your cervix changes during the next 2 hours. It is possible that your cervix is just changing more slowly than the average. As long as you and your baby are otherwise well, waiting is a reasonable option.

Rupture the membranes

The next option is to rupture the membranes (if they are still unruptured), a procedure sometimes called an amniotomy. Rupturing the membranes releases prostaglandins that help stimulate uterine contractions. It also allows the head to apply more downward pressure on the cervix, without a pouch of amniotic fluid in the way. Rupturing the membranes has been shown to shorten labor by 1 to 2 hours and reduce the need for oxytocin by 20%.

Augment with oxytocin

The third option is to consider oxytocin augmentation of labor. This is usually done either after or in conjunction with rupturing the membranes. Oxytocin is a hormone your body makes during labor to stimulate uterine contractions. Giving you extra oxytocin will increase the strength and frequency of your contractions. This should help your cervix dilate a little more rapidly. Oxytocin is usually administered intravenously.

Guide to ...
Amniotomy procedure

The procedure for rupturing the amniotic membranes is no more painful than a vaginal exam to check cervical dilation. It will not hurt the baby. An amni-hook, an instrument that looks a little like a crochet hook, is used to rupture amniotic membranes.

- The hook is gently introduced into the vagina and guided through the cervix (with the hook along the doctor's finger) and then rotated until the very thin amniotic membranes are snagged in the hook. When the hook is pulled down, this causes a tear.

- Amniotic fluid pours out of the vagina at this stage. The color and quantity of fluid will be noted (normally, it is clear). From this point on in your labor, you will leak amniotic fluid continuously.

Oxytocin is given in very low doses initially, and if you and the fetus tolerate the oxytocin, the dose is slowly increased until your contractions are coming every 2 to 3 minutes. They will feel very strong. The fetal heart rate will be monitored continuously once you are receiving oxytocin. If there is any sign, such as a drop in heart rate, that the baby does not tolerate the increased strength and frequency of contractions, the oxytocin infusion will be stopped.

Arrest of labor

If oxytocin has been used in appropriate doses for 2 to 4 hours, and the cervix still hasn't dilated further, it is not likely that the cervix will be able to dilate enough to allow a vaginal delivery. This is called arrest of labor. At this point, your doctor will likely recommend a Caesarean section.

Causes of labor arrest

Problems of slow labor and labor arrest in both the first and second stage can be attributed to one of the three P's: power, passenger, or passage.

- "Power" refers to the frequency and strength of the uterine contractions. Sometimes, the contractions are not frequent enough to cause cervical dilation. Other times, the uterine muscle doesn't contract strongly enough to push the baby out. If the frequency and strength of the uterine contractions have been increased with oxytocin, and the cervix still doesn't dilate, there is nothing else that can be done to increase the strength of the contractions.

- "Passenger" refers to the baby and "passage" refers to the birth canal, or pelvis, of the mother. There are a few reasons why the passenger might not fit through the passage. The passenger is too big, or the passage too small. Or, perhaps, the passenger is not positioned in the best way to allow delivery. For example, if the baby is facing the mother's front, it is harder for the baby to fit through the maternal pelvic bones than if it faced her back. While the baby's position might be manipulated, there is nothing that can be done in the first stage of labor to modify a poor fit between the passenger and the passage.

Risk factors for arrest of labor in the first and second stage

- Advanced maternal age
- Complications in pregnancy
- Non-reassuring fetal heart rate
- Epidural
- Big baby
- Pelvic contraction (that is, a small pelvis)
- Baby facing the mother's front
- First pregnancy
- Short stature (less than 4 feet, 9 inches (150 cm) tall)
- Chorioamnionitis (infection in the fluid and membranes around the baby)
- Overdue pregnancy
- Maternal obesity

Second stage labor arrest

You have done very well, coped with labor, reached full dilation, perhaps even pushed for an hour or more … but … the baby … still … hasn't … come … out. The baby's heart rate is typically fine, but the head still isn't crowning. This very frustrating situation is called second stage arrest. It has the same potential causes and risk factors as first stage labor arrest.

Keep going

If the baby is coming down through the birth canal in an appropriate position, and if it feels as if your pelvis will accommodate the baby, the first option is to keep going. You are almost there! It is very hard to muster the final bit of energy you need to push that baby out the last few centimeters, but with an encouraging and supportive team helping you, it can be done. Close your eyes, rest deeply between contractions, and visualize your baby in your arms … Now: push hard!

Augment with oxytocin

Oxytocin will strengthen your contractions and make them come a little bit closer together, allowing you to push your baby out with a little more force. Sometimes, just a touch of oxytocin seems to make the difference.

Assessing progress

If the head descends closer and closer to your perineum with oxytocin and pushing, then you are making good progress. If not, it may be time to consider an assisted delivery.

Guide to…

Management of second stage arrest

At this point there are several options. Which one is best for you will depend, in part, on an assessment of your baby's position and station and the shape of your pelvis.

- *Position:* If the baby is facing your spine, then this is the optimal fit between your baby's head and your pelvis. If the baby is coming down the birth passage facing sideways or forward, we know that it is significantly harder, sometimes impossible, for the mother to push the baby out. Sometimes, oxytocin and continued pushing will encourage the head to turn. Sometimes, the head can be turned manually by your doctor or midwife. And sometimes, an assisted delivery with a rotation may be appropriate.

- *Station:* How deeply the baby's head has entered the pelvis and how close it is to the perineum indicates how soon the baby might be delivered. If the head is still very high in the pelvis, a vaginal delivery is less likely.

- *Pelvic shape:* The internal shape of the maternal pelvic bones will indicate if the baby can pass through them easily. Some mothers have a very narrow pelvis, and vaginal deliveries of "bigger" babies can be almost impossible.

Assisted delivery options

- If the head is low enough, your doctors can help you have a vaginal delivery with the assistance of either forceps or a vacuum extractor.

- If you are fully dilated, but the head is still high, a Caesarean section will be advised over a vacuum-assisted or forceps delivery. These kinds of vaginal deliveries are not safe when the head is high.

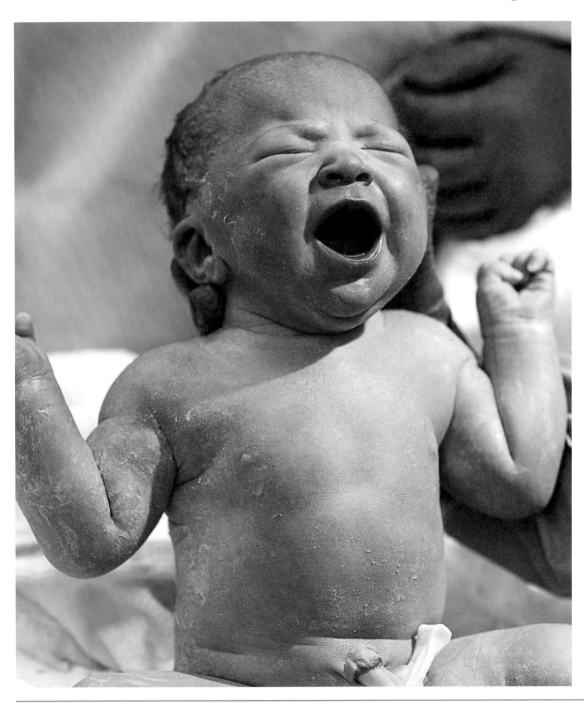

Non-reassuring fetal heart rate

The baby's heart rate will be monitored during the first and second stage of labor, either intermittently following contractions or continuously using a monitor belted to your belly. The purpose of monitoring the fetal heart rate is to ensure that the baby is coping with labor well. If the intermittent monitoring reveals a concern, then continuous monitoring should begin.

Fetal heart tracing

The monitoring will produce a graph, referred to as a fetal heart tracing. If the fetal heart rate has an abnormal pattern, it may be a sign that your baby is having trouble. Obviously, if the baby is not coping well, she should be delivered very soon, by Caesarean section if necessary, but if the tracing is normal, indicating that the baby is coping well, there is time to wait for your labor to progress naturally.

Fetal scalp sampling

Some patterns — such as a deep and prolonged drop in the fetal heart rate — can be interpreted as distress with a fair amount of certainty. Other patterns have a less precise interpretation, and although distress is suspected, the only way to know for sure is to do a fetal blood test, known as fetal scalp sampling. Fetal scalp sampling is a way to reduce your chances of having a Caesarean section. If the fetal scalp sample is normal, then it will probably be fine to continue labor. If fetal scalp sampling is not available (some hospitals do not have the ability to do this test), then a non-reassuring fetal heart rate tracing should lead to an expedited delivery.

Guide to ...
Scalp-sampling procedure

A fetal scalp blood sample involves taking a few drops of blood from the fetal scalp and testing the blood for its pH (or acidity) to determine how much oxygen the baby is getting. The test sounds scary but is safe and relatively painless.

- A small plastic cone is used to hold the walls of your vagina open (like a Pap test) and enables the examiner to see the baby's head.
- A pinprick is made in the scalp, and a tiny amount of blood (only a few microliters) is collected.
- The blood is analyzed right away, so your delivery team should have an answer within 5 minutes.
- If the test shows that the baby is coping well, labor can progress normally.
- If the baby is not coping well, immediate delivery is advised. The test is sometimes repeated periodically if the fetal heart rate does not improve.

Assisted vaginal delivery

About 6% of deliveries are assisted vaginal deliveries (sometimes called operative vaginal deliveries). A vacuum extractor or forceps are used to assist delivery of the baby. This can only be done when the cervix is fully dilated and the baby's head has descended low enough in the pelvis.

Evaluating the situation

For most parents, it is very scary to think of someone manipulating their baby's head with instruments in order to help delivery. Your doctor knows this situation is difficult for everyone — scary for you and your family, a bit riskier for the baby than a spontaneous delivery, and more challenging for the doctor.

Ultimately, if you are in the situation where the baby seems "stuck" or the fetal

Reasons for intervening in vaginal delivery

An assisted vaginal delivery is used in one of two circumstances:

1. The fetal heart rate is not reassuring and delivery must be expedited for the well-being of the baby; **or**

2. The mother is having difficulty delivering the baby past a certain point on her own and needs some assistance with the last part of the delivery. Most often, this happens because

   • the baby is positioned in an awkward way

   • the mother is exhausted and can no longer push effectively

   • the mother has a condition that makes a lot of pushing dangerous for her (some heart conditions, for example)

heart rate is not reassuring, you may need to ask yourself, "Would I rather have an assisted vaginal delivery or a Caesarean section?" Often, however, a Caesarean section at this stage is also a difficult procedure. With the head wedged deep in the pelvis, a Caesarean section is associated with a higher risk of complications than a Caesarean section performed before labor begins. Tough decisions may need to be made.

Vacuum-assisted delivery

In a vacuum-assisted delivery, a suction cup is applied to the baby's head. Suction is generated with the assistance of a pump that applies a downward force on the baby to encourage its delivery. A vacuum extractor is a very effective instrument to use when the baby does not need to be rotated and when the head is not very high. You must still push to help deliver the baby.

Vacuum-assisted delivery complications

Complications are unusual but do occur in about 5% of vacuum-assisted deliveries. Most problems are related, not surprisingly, to the scalp where the vacuum cup is applied. There can be abrasions (small cuts) on the scalp, as well as bruising underneath where the suction cup is applied (a condition called a cephalohematoma). The incidence of retinal hemorrhages is also higher in

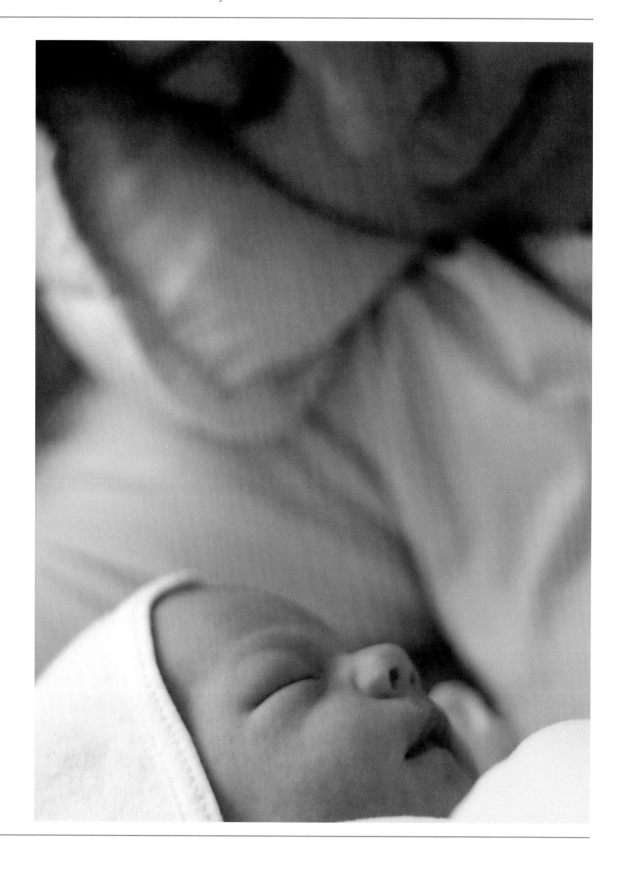

Guide to ...

Vacuum-assisted delivery

- Before a vacuum-assisted delivery, your doctor will make sure that your bladder is empty by using a small catheter to empty it.

- Your doctor will also ensure that you are as comfortable as possible, either with an epidural, with nitrous oxide, or with a local anesthetic injection.

- Your legs will probably be supported in a flexed position, either by stirrups, foot pedals, or a helper's hands.

- The vacuum cup will then be gently placed on the baby's head.

- When a contraction begins, the suction will be applied and you will be encouraged to push as hard as you possibly can while the doctor will gently pull in a downward direction on the handle of the vacuum extractor.

- It may take several pushes during two to three contractions until the baby delivers.

- Once the head is delivered, the vacuum cup will be removed and the remainder of the delivery will proceed as usual.

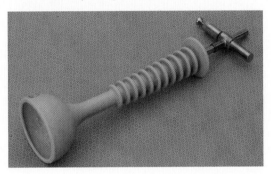

vacuum-assisted deliveries than in other types of deliveries. These complications generally resolve on their own with no serious or long-term consequences. Much rarer, although more serious, is bleeding within the baby's head.

If the head does not deliver with the assistance of the vacuum extractor, you will likely proceed to a Caesarean section.

Forceps delivery

Forceps are designed to be inserted into the vagina and placed around the baby's head, cradling the cheeks on either side. By gently pulling on the handle of the forceps, the baby is delivered. Forceps can also be used to coax a baby to turn into a more amenable position for delivery. If the baby is transverse or occiput posterior, turning the forceps can help the baby turn into an occiput anterior position, where the diameter of the head is a little smaller and a better fit for the maternal pelvis, easing delivery.

Forceps complications

You may see some red marks over the baby's cheeks. These forceps marks will disappear within about 24 hours. Nerve injuries to the baby's face and skull fractures are also more likely than in a spontaneous delivery, although still very rare. Long-term developmental outcomes have been studied, and there does not appear to be any increased risk of adverse outcome with forceps deliveries. For the mother, there is a greater chance of vaginal lacerations, episiotomy, and perineal pain after a forceps or vacuum-assisted delivery than following a spontaneous delivery.

If the head does not deliver with the assistance of forceps, you will likely proceed to a Caesarean section.

Guide to ...

Forceps-assisted delivery procedure

- Before a forceps delivery, your doctor will make sure that your bladder is empty by using a small catheter to drain it.

- Your doctor will also ensure that you are as comfortable as possible, either with an epidural, with nitrous oxide, or with a local anesthetic injection.

- Your legs will probably be supported in a flexed position by stirrups.

- The forceps will be gently introduced into your vagina and will slide into position around your baby's head, one side at a time, between contractions.

- Once both sides are in place, the doctor will carefully check the position of the forceps to make sure that they are positioned correctly in relation to the baby's skull bones. It is very important that they are placed in the right position.

- Once the correct position is confirmed, you will be encouraged to push very hard with your next contraction while your doctor pulls gently on the handles of the forceps. Ideally, your baby will deliver over the next one or two contractions.

- The forceps are gently removed, and then the remainder of the baby is delivered in the usual fashion.

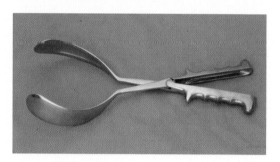

Application of Forceps

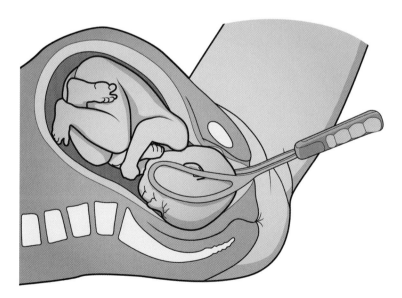

Shoulder dystocia

Shoulder dystocia is the technical name for "the shoulders get stuck." It is an obstetric emergency and can be quite scary as the delivery team responds quickly and in force! All of a sudden, lots of people will appear in your delivery room to help the delivering doctor and prepare for the baby's arrival.

Stuck

With a shoulder dystocia, the head delivers vaginally, but then one of the baby's shoulders gets stuck behind your pubic bone, preventing easy delivery of the rest of the baby. This condition affects between 1% and 2% of deliveries.

There are specific maneuvers that are done in order to free the "stuck" shoulder. Your entire delivery team will be well versed in these maneuvers and always ready to perform them if necessary. Listen carefully to their instructions.

Injury

Your baby will be carefully examined by a doctor following a shoulder dystocia to make sure that any injuries, if present, are identified early. The nerves between the neck and shoulder can be stretched inadvertently in an effort to deliver the shoulder, which sometimes leads to an injury called a brachial plexus injury. This will be suspected if the baby seems to have difficulty moving her arm. Most of these nerve injuries are temporary and resolve within a few days to months, although sometimes physical therapy is required. There is also the possibility of a fracture to the clavicle, which will usually heal quite well. Very rarely, there is a permanent injury.

Risk factors for shoulder dystocia

Shoulder dystocia is very hard to predict. Many babies who have shoulder dystocia have no risk factors, and most babies with risk factors do not have shoulder dystocia.

- Big babies with birth weight of more than 9 pounds (4 kg), which is often difficult to predict ahead of time
- Maternal diabetes, which leads to bigger babies with big chests and shoulders
- Vacuum-assisted or forceps delivery
- Previous baby with shoulder dystocia
- Maternal obesity and high weight gain in pregnancy

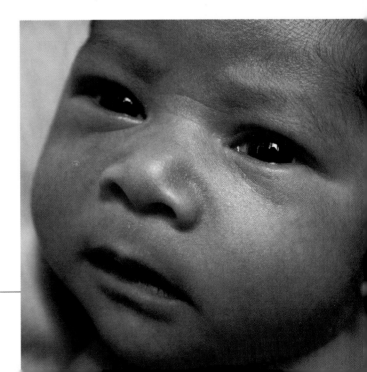

Vaginal tears

Vaginal tearing is common following a vaginal delivery in a first-time mother. Tearing is usually less, and sometimes absent, in subsequent deliveries. The amount of tearing is quite variable and depends on a number of factors, but the size of the baby seems to play a key role in how severe a tear will be. Forceps or vacuum-assisted deliveries are associated with more tearing than is a spontaneous delivery.

Tearing concerns

Many women fear vaginal tearing, perhaps more than any other result of labor and delivery. They are concerned about their pain, both immediately and postpartum, stitches, sexual function, and pelvic floor strength. For most women, the tearing is not very severe, and postpartum pain is not great. The stitches will heal quickly, in about 2 weeks.

For guidelines in caring for vaginal stitches, see Part 12, Caring for Your Baby and Yourself (page 414).

Vaginal lacerations grading

- *First degree:* superficial laceration involving only the skin or mucosa (the shiny skin-like tissue layer that lines the vagina)
- *Second degree:* laceration involving the muscles of the perineum
- *Third degree:* laceration involving the anal sphincter
- *Fourth degree:* laceration involving the anal sphincter and the rectum

Lacerations can also involve the labia and tissue near the clitoris and the urethra.

Did You Know?

Hematomas

Injuries to the tissues and muscles of the perineum and vagina can occur following any kind of delivery but are more common if a vacuum extractor or forceps have been used. Most lacerations are small, and the bleeding is well controlled by the judicious placement of sutures. Occasionally, bleeding can occur in the deeper tissues of the vaginal wall and sometimes the labia. If this happens, there is a possibility of developing a collection of blood, called a hematoma, in these areas.

A hematoma can collect a surprising amount of blood, leading to reduced blood counts. They are also usually quite painful because the pressure of the collected blood presses on nerves in the area. If the hematoma is getting bigger, it is important to stop the bleeding and it may be necessary to do this surgically, under general, local, or epidural anesthesia. If the hematoma is not getting any bigger, it is sometimes better to leave it alone. Painkillers can be given, with ice and pressure placed on the area to minimize further expansion.

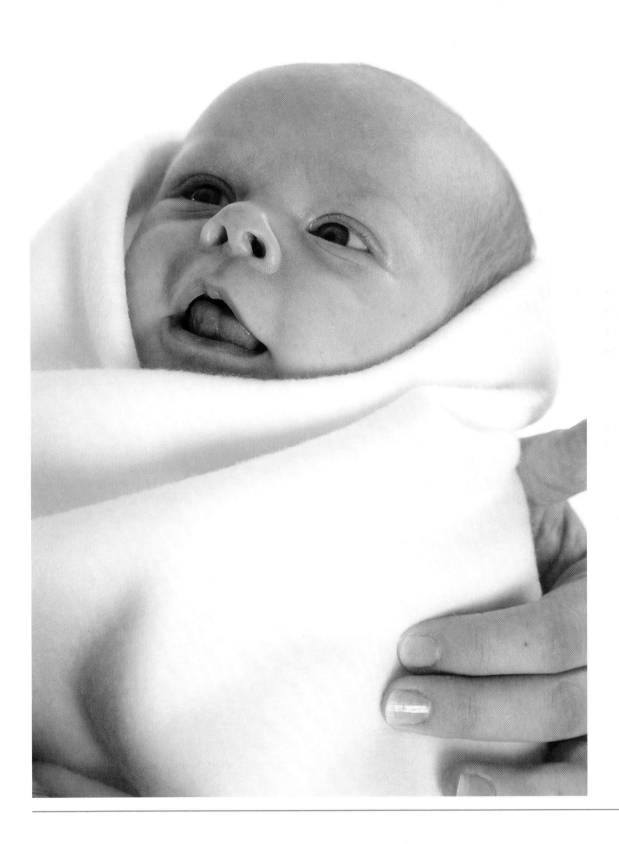

Caesarean section

No obstetric situation is perfectly predictable, so it is wise for you to be prepared for at least the possibility of Caesarean section. In general, a Caesarean section is done when the benefits to the mother or the baby outweigh the benefits of vaginal delivery. Caesarean sections are either unplanned and urgent because of circumstances arising while you're in labor, or planned and scheduled ahead of time because of maternal or fetal risks. More recently, elective Caesarean sections are sometimes done because the mother requests one.

Increasing incidence

Although we don't really know what the optimal Caesarean section rate should be, the World Health Organization suggests between 10% and 15%, balancing the risks and benefits of Caesarean section to both the mother and the baby. However, the percentage of deliveries by Caesarean section is higher in North America and increasing. In Canada, for example, about 25% of babies are now born by Caesarean section. Why is this so?

The increasing rate of Caesarean section has been attributed to the perception of risk during labor on the part of physician and patient, changes in clinical practice (fewer forceps deliveries, more inductions of labor, fewer vaginal births after Caesarean section), and medical-legal concerns. Other reasons include the increased average age of pregnant women; the increased number of multiple births following assistance with reproductive technologies, such as in vitro fertilization; and the increased levels of obesity in our society (including pregnant women).

Unscheduled Caesarean section

The most common reasons for a Caesarean section in this circumstance are a non-progressive labor or a non-reassuring fetal status. Once the decision to proceed with a Caesarean section has been made by you and your caregivers, the procedure will usually go rather quickly. National guidelines advise that a Caesarean

Did You Know?

Unnecessary Caesarean sections

Many women are concerned that they will have a Caesarean section unnecessarily. If this is concern of yours, discuss with your health-care provider specific things that you can do to reduce your chance of Caesarean section. For example:

- If your baby is breech, you can discuss an external cephalic version (ECV) procedure to try to turn the baby to a head-down position.

- If you have had a Caesarean section before, you may be a candidate for a vaginal birth after Caesarean section (VBAC).

- If a nurse or midwife is not available continuously, consider having a supportive friend join you or consider hiring a doula, which has been shown in some studies to lead to a modest reduction in Caesarean sections.

Guide to...

Reasons for Caesarean section

1. Labor does not progress. Either the cervix does not dilate enough or the head does not descend enough to allow a vaginal delivery. By the time a Caesarean section is advised, there is likely no other way to deliver the baby. About 30% of Caesarean sections happen for this reason.

2. The baby is not tolerating labor. This is suspected primarily if the fetal heart rate is not reassuring. By the time a Caesarean section is considered, the baby likely needs to be delivered quickly because she may not be getting enough oxygen inside the uterus. The baby will be healthier if delivered sooner rather than later, so Caesarean section is offered as a rapid way of delivering the baby. About 10% of Caesarean sections happen for this reason.

3. The baby is not in a lie that allows labor to proceed safely. The safest lie for a baby during a vaginal delivery is head down. If the baby is sideways (transverse) in the uterus, it is impossible to deliver the baby vaginally. If the baby is head up (breech), most doctors believe that the safest way to deliver the baby is by Caesarean section. About 10% of Caesarean sections occur because the baby is not in the head-down position.

4. A previous incision on the uterus, either because of a Caesarean section or because of other surgery, such as a myomectomy to remove fibroids. About 30% of Caesarean sections occur because of previous surgery.

5. The remaining 20% of Caesarean sections occur for a number of much more unusual conditions:

   - Abnormalities in the placenta, such as placenta previa

   - Maternal infection, such as herpes or HIV, that can be passed to the fetus during a vaginal delivery

   - Maternal illness, such as severe pre-eclampsia, where the mother cannot tolerate either a vaginal delivery or the time necessary to wait for a vaginal delivery

   - Fetal concerns, where the fetus is suspected of having a problem while still in the uterus that suggests a vaginal delivery might be more dangerous than a Caesarean section

   - Twins (particularly if the bottom twin is not head down), triplets... or more.

   - The mother requests a scheduled Caesarean section.

section for urgent reasons should be started within 30 minutes of the decision.

An unscheduled procedure is more difficult than a scheduled Caesarean section for a number of reasons. Mentally and emotionally, you may not be as prepared for a Caesarean delivery. Perhaps you had your heart set on a natural and spontaneous vaginal delivery. Perhaps you are afraid, both for yourself and the baby. You may already be exhausted after a long labor, having missed a night of sleep, and because of the pain you have been having in labor.

Guide to...

Choosing an elective primary Caesarean section over a vaginal delivery

While some doctors are willing to perform a primary elective Caesarean section, citing the patient's right to surgical intervention, others are not, citing the position papers issued by national medical associations. Despite these positions, there are strong pros and cons for this means of delivery.

Position papers

ACOG (American College of Obstetrics and Gynecology): "In the case of an elective Caesarean delivery, if the physician believes that Caesarean delivery promotes the overall health and welfare of the woman and her fetus more than does vaginal birth, then he or she is ethically justified in performing a Caesarean delivery. Similarly, if the physician believes that performing a Caesarean would be detrimental to the overall health and welfare of the woman and her fetus, he or she is ethically obliged to refrain from performing the surgery. In this case, a referral to another health-care provider would be appropriate if physician and patient cannot agree on a method of delivery."

SOGC: The Society of Obstetricians and Gynaecologists of Canada does *not* promote Caesarean sections on demand. "The Society has always promoted natural childbirth" and "believes that the decision to perform a Caesarean section during labor and delivery should be based on medical indications."

FIGO (International Federation of Obstetrics and Gynecology): "At present, because hard evidence of net benefit does not exist, performing Caesarean section for non-medical reasons is ethically not justified."

Pros of elective primary Caesarean section

1. Delivery day can be scheduled with some certainty, although the possibility of going into spontaneous labor prior to the scheduled day always exists.
2. No labor pain.
3. Lower chance of postpartum hemorrhage following a planned Caesarean section compared to a vaginal birth or an urgent Caesarean section following labor.
4. No perineal tearing.
5. Short-term reduction in the risk of urinary incontinence.
6. Fetal problems related to vaginal birth avoided; in particular, injuries related to the delivery of a large baby whose shoulders get stuck at delivery (shoulder dystocia).
7. Cases of stillbirth can be averted (because stillbirth at this gestational age is so rare, 1000 Caesarean sections would have to be done to avoid stillbirth).

Cons of primary elective Caesarean section

1. Risk of major illness, or morbidity, in the mother are much higher following a planned Caesarean section than a planned vaginal delivery. Conditions more common following Caesarean delivery include: blood clots in the legs or lungs, heart attacks, infections, significant bleeding, and significant bleeding leading to the need for hysterectomy. The risk of one of these events is low but is still three times higher than with a planned vaginal delivery. (There are 9 cases of major morbidity per 1000 planned vaginal deliveries.)

2. Longer recovery period following Caesarean section, with greater pain during the recovery period, although by 3 months any differences in pain between the two groups have disappeared.

3. Baby at higher risk of breathing problems than after a planned vaginal birth.

4. Risk to a future pregnancy. A Caesarean section leaves a scar in the uterus and in the surrounding tissues and skin. These issues may not be of concern if you are only planning to have one child.

   a. Scarring in the surrounding tissues and skin means that each subsequent Caesarean section is more difficult, and the risk of injury to other organs, such as the bowel and bladder, is increased.

   b. Scarring in the uterus is an area of weakness and is at risk of opening or rupturing in a subsequent pregnancy.

   c. Scarring in the uterus also predisposes a subsequent pregnancy to problems with placental growth:

   i. *Placenta previa:* The placenta grows too low, covering the cervix and sometimes leading to bleeding in a pregnancy.

   ii. *Placenta accreta and increta:* The placenta penetrates into the muscle of the uterus in an abnormal way, leading to a virtual inability to deliver the placenta following birth, sometimes making a hysterectomy the only solution.

5. Health-care costs associated with Caesarean section are higher than for vaginal delivery, both because of operating room costs and longer in-patient hospital stays.

Debatable points

Some popular issues involved in choosing between Caesarean section or vaginal delivery lack scientific substance:

1. *Sexual function:* Sexual function following vaginal delivery and Caesarean section seem to be about equivalent in studies done to date.

2. *Maternal mortality:* Maternal death is a very rare outcome in North America, and it does not seem to be more likely following a Caesarean section.

3. *Pelvic floor damage:* The muscles of the pelvic floor do sustain damage during pregnancy, which can sometimes lead to urinary incontinence and prolapse (or "dropping") of the uterus, but research studies to date have not been able to conclude definitively that Caesarean section will prevent damage to the pelvic floor. Because the medical evidence is poor in this area, it is not advisable to use this as a reason to justify a Caesarean section.

Summary

In sum, a vaginal delivery is associated with a net benefit over elective primary Caesarean section, at least as far as the medical community is aware at this time. This is why you may encounter some reluctance on the part of doctors to perform a Caesarean section without a medical reason.

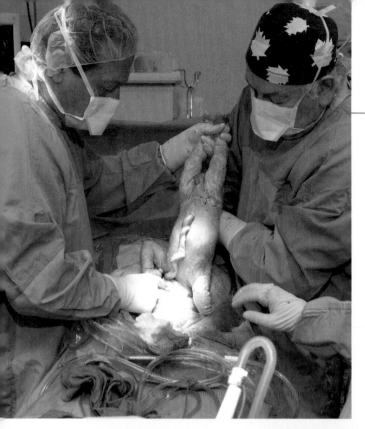

Guide to ...

Caesarean section procedure

A Caesarean section will take place in an operating room, with an anesthesiologist present, as well as at least one extra nurse and a surgical assistant, in addition to the obstetrician. Usually, your labor support partner is able to join you in the operating room.

1. Your anesthesiologist will make sure that you will be comfortable during the operation, usually by giving you a spinal anesthetic or by increasing the amount of medication in your epidural. Less frequently, a general anesthetic is given.

■ Breech birth. The legs and the body are delivered before the head in this Caesarean section.

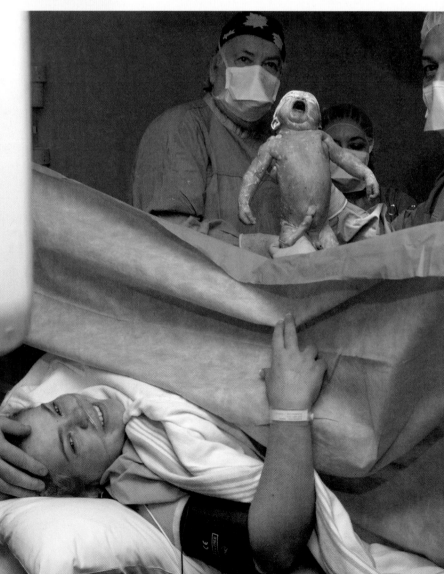

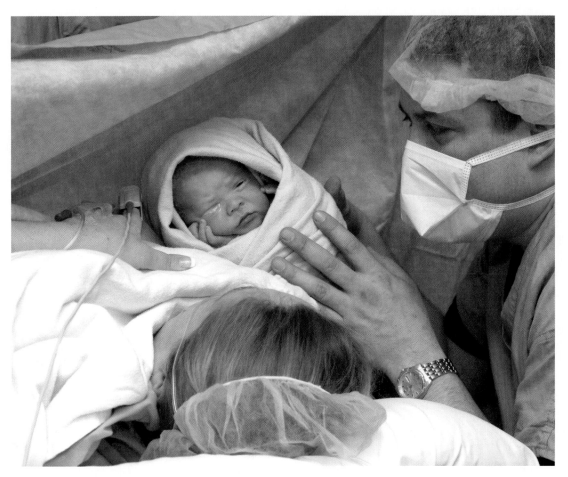

2. A catheter will be placed in your bladder.

3. Your abdomen will be cleansed with an antiseptic.

4. You will be covered in sterile drapes so that, from your chest down, only your belly shows.

5. Your obstetrician or surgeon will make an incision in the skin of your abdomen, usually very low down and side-to-side, just above your pubic hair line.

6. Your abdominal muscles will be gently separated in the midline (not cutting them) until finally your uterus is incised.

7. Your obstetrician or surgeon will reach into your uterus and lift your baby out.

8. Your baby is born. Congratulations!

9. Your baby's umbilical cord will be clamped and cut, and your child will be handed to the waiting nurse or respiratory therapist.

10. Your obstetrician will then deliver the placenta and close the uterus, while your baby will go to the baby warmer to be checked over and wrapped up.

11. As long as all is well, you and your birth partner can hold your baby and visit for a few minutes.

12. Your skin incision will be closed with staples or stitches and bandaged. You will be cleaned up before being transferred to the recovery room.

Scheduled Caesarean section

The most common reasons for a scheduled Caesarean section are previous uterine surgery (including previous Caesarean section) and breech presentation.

If you have planned a Caesarean section and go into labor or your membranes rupture, you should go straight to the hospital for an assessment. It may be necessary for the Caesarean to be performed sooner than you expected.

Timing

Most elective Caesarean sections will be scheduled at around 38 to 39 weeks. There

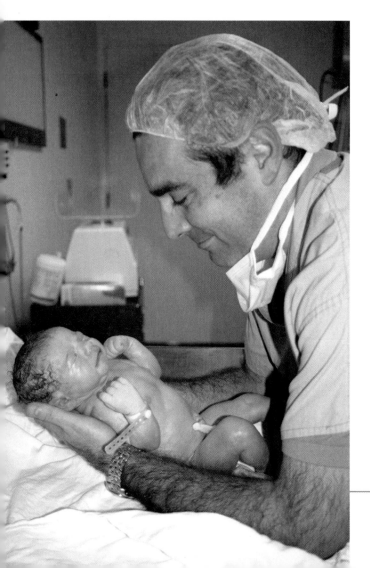

is a balance being struck here. The chance that you go into labor spontaneously needs to be reduced, but the Caesarean section should not be planned too much before 40 weeks because there is a risk that the baby's lungs will not be fully mature and she will have trouble breathing at birth, requiring an admission to the NICU and possibly use of a ventilator.

Elective primary Caesarean section

An elective primary Caesarean section is done at a woman's request in the absence of any medical reason that would necessitate this procedure. Recently, this delivery choice has become popular among celebrities who are "too posh to push." In Brazil, for example, the primary elective Caesarean section rate is as high as 80% in some portions of the affluent population. It has been reported that 33% of doctors would choose primary Caesarean section for themselves or their wives. This elective procedure remains controversial, however, because of potential operative and post-operative risks to the mother and baby.

Did You Know?

Infection risks

If your membranes were ruptured for a long time before your Caesarean section, your risk of endometritis (an infection of the uterus) may be as high as 20% to 25%, and your risk of a wound infection up to 15%, even with a dose of preventive antibiotics. If you have a Caesarean section with intact membranes and no labor, your risk of endometritis and wound infection is much lower, only 1% to 2%.

Risks of Caesarean section

Fetal risks are low for scheduled, elective, and even unscheduled operations. There are several significant maternal risks peripartum and some longer-term complications of Caesarean section, particularly as they relate to future pregnancies.

Fetal breathing problems

In vaginal deliveries, the stress of labor helps the baby produce steroids that help the baby get ready for breathing, and the process of squeezing through the birth canal helps push amniotic fluid out of the lungs. Following a Caesarean section, some babies have some water persisting in their lungs, which can give them a little bit of difficulty breathing well for a few days. This is called transient tachypnea of the newborn (TTN). (Tachypnea means fast breathing.) This condition can be the result of immature lungs at the time of Caesarean section, but it can be minimized if the Caesarean is booked at 39 weeks or later. TTN is about three times more likely after elective Caesarean delivery than after vaginal delivery. The chances of a baby having TTN following an elective Caesarean section is 35 in 1000 vs. 12 in 1000 following Caesarean section in labor, and 5 in 1000 following vaginal delivery.

Fetal trauma or injury

In all Caesarean sections, there is a very small risk of trauma or injury to the baby during delivery, usually limited to a small scrape or cut from the scalpel used in the operation. Injury is more common during an emergency Caesarean section, presumably because the operation is proceeding at a much faster than usual rate.

Causes of hemorrhage at Caesarean section

- Failure of the uterus to contract well is the most common cause of hemorrhaging. Usually, there is a good response to medications to control the bleeding. In rare cases, the bleeding cannot be stopped with medications. If that is the case, there are a number of special techniques your obstetrician will use to control the bleeding.

- Injury to a blood vessel is another cause. Careful surgical technique will allow identification and treatment of this problem.

- Placental abnormalities can also contribute to bleeding. Treatment will depend on the situation.

Endometritis

This infection of the lining of the uterus can occur following a vaginal delivery but is more common after a Caesarean section. It typically shows up a few days to a week post-Caesarean. Symptoms include fever and lower-abdominal pain, as well as a sudden increase in your vaginal bleeding or a foul-smelling vaginal discharge.

In order to reduce the chance that endometritis develops, you will be given a dose of antibiotics in the operating room. If you do develop endometritis, you will be treated with antibiotics, usually with oral medication as an outpatient, but, if it is severe, in-patient, intravenous antibiotics may be recommended. All antibiotics you will be treated with will be safe for breastfeeding.

Wound infections

You can develop an infection in your wound as well. If you have a wound infection, you may have any of the following symptoms: your incision and the skin around it may appear very red and feel hot to the touch, you may have a fever, you may have a lot of pain around the incision, and/or the incision may be leaking fluid. The incision may look as if it is gaping open in places.

If you have a wound infection, you need to see a doctor right away. The incision may need to be opened up to allow pus to drain out. If it is not severe, antibiotics alone may be enough.

Bleeding (hemorrhage)

Blood loss at delivery is generally more at a Caesarean section than at a vaginal delivery. The average blood loss at Caesarean section is thought to be about 1000 cc (1 liter) vs. 500 cc (500 mL) at a vaginal delivery, although the exact amounts are hard to determine accurately. Bleeding in excess of this is considered hemorrhage.

Injury to other organs

As in all surgeries, other organs are at risk of being inadvertently injured during a Caesarean section. The organ most at risk is the bladder, with an injury occurring on average in 1 in 400 Caesarean sections. The risk of injury to bowels or bladder also increases during an emergency Caesarean section. Usually there is just a small area of injury that is quite easily repaired.

Blood clots

The risk of developing a blood clot in your legs (known as deep venous thrombosis, or DVT) or lungs (pulmonary

Did You Know?

Blood transfusion

About 2% to 3% of women who have a Caesarean section end up needing a blood transfusion.

Most doctors recommend a transfusion only if hemoglobin is low and the patient is also symptomatic. Symptoms of low blood levels (anemia) include a racing heart (palpitations); a rapid heart beat; a low blood pressure; dizziness, especially when rising; and extreme fatigue.

If the situation is not acute, you will have ample time to discuss these risks with your doctor to ensure that you are comfortable with the decision to transfuse. In some cases, transfusion is a lifesaving measure.

embolus, or PE) in pregnancy and the postpartum period is anywhere from 0.2% to 2%, depending on your risk factors. A Caesarean section increases your risk of a blood clot three to five times over the risk following a vaginal delivery. The most important thing that you can do to reduce your risk of blood clots is to get up and move around the day after your operation. This will get your blood moving and help prevent blood clots.

Long-term maternal risks

Most long-term complications of Caesarean section are related to subsequent pregnancies:

1. The frequency of placenta previa is more common in women who have had a Caesarean section. The risk of abnormal placental development (placenta accreta and increta) is

higher in women who have had a Caesarean section.

2. In a subsequent pregnancy, mode of delivery must be considered carefully. While a vaginal delivery after Caesarean section (VBAC) is possible, there is a risk of the uterine scar opening up, which is called uterine rupture. The incidence of this is 1% to 2% if a VBAC is attempted.

3. If VBAC is either not attempted or unsuccessful, and a Caesarean section ensues again, this second and subsequent Caesarean sections will each be longer and often complicated by more scarring, which in turn increases the risks of bladder injury and bleeding.

4. Another complication of Caesarean section is numbness and/or pain around the incision site. This can sometimes occur because of unavoidable injury to nerves in the abdominal wall at the time of surgery; as the incision is made, these nerves are always cut. Sometimes, the nerves become entrapped as they heal, causing pain, burning, and numbness. Fortunately, this is unusual.

Post-operative recovery

Recovering from a Caesarean section can be challenging. It is hard to look after a newborn baby, and it is hard to recover from major surgery. Now you have to do both. This is the time to call in all your extra resources and support — all those people who told you to "just call if you need anything" should be called.

Bowel discomfort

Post-operative bowel function is not always normal. During an operation, your intestines are often moved around a little or touched. This causes them to stop their normal function of passing food, drink, and gas, which leaves you feeling bloated and a little nauseous. Once you are passing gas out your bottom, it is a sign that all is well. Sometimes, it can take a day or two for the gas to pass, and you may have gas pains until it does. Gas pains can hurt a lot, sometimes more than the incision itself. Get up and walk around — activity will help the gas move. You may find yourself fairly constipated in the beginning, perhaps in part due to any narcotic medication you may have received. Sometimes a rectal suppository can help.

Incision care

The incision will be covered with a dressing until the second post-operative day. Once the dressing is removed on day 2, the skin itself will have closed over.

Did You Know?

Keeping risks in perspective

All of these risks sound very alarming, and you may wonder why anyone would ever consent to a Caesarean section given these risks. Remember that these risks are always being weighed against the benefits of a Caesarean section in your situation. Although a risk of 15% of developing a wound infection or a 1% chance of developing a blood clot seem like big risks, if a Caesarean is ultimately deemed to be the safest way to deliver your baby, most women are prepared to take these risks.

Now you can leave the incision open to the air. You can also have a shower (you have never had a shower that feels as good as this one). Let the water run over your incision, don't use any soap directly on the incision, and pat it dry gently. If you have staples or stitches that need to be removed, they will usually be removed on the third day if you have a transverse (side-to-side) incision. If the incision goes up and down, then the staples or stitches will need to stay in for a week.

Pain management

Continue taking the pain medication as long as you need it. In the hospital, you will often be prescribed an anti-inflammatory medication as well as acetaminophen and narcotic painkillers. Once you go home, you may continue to need pain medication, usually only for a week or two. Continue with an anti-inflammatory medication and

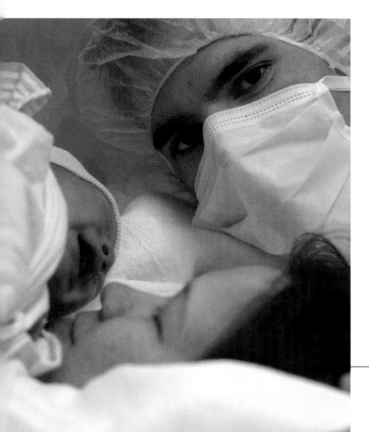

Guide to...

Hospital recovery after Caesarean section

You will recover quite soon after your operation and will likely be ready to go home with your newborn baby 3 days after the surgery.

- *Day of surgery:* Oral intake limited mostly to fluids. You will spend the time mostly in bed. Breastfeed (if you've chosen to).
- *Day 1:* Catheter in bladder and IV in arm will be removed. Get up and walk around a little. Increase your food intake with a light meal. Breastfeed (if you've chosen to).
- *Day 2:* Dressing will be removed and incision examined. Move around a lot more. Eat normally. Breastfeed (if you've chosen to).
- *Day 3:* Stitches or staples will be removed from incision. Breastfeed (if you've chosen to). Plan on going home.

acetaminophen for a few days and then start reducing the pain medication. In this way, you may be able to avoid severe pain and the need to take narcotic medications, which can make you and the baby sleepy, and you constipated.

Bleeding

You will have light vaginal bleeding after your Caesarean section, just as you would if you had had a vaginal delivery. It will last a couple of weeks. If the bleeding increases to the point where you are soaking two pads an hour for 2 to 3 hours in a row, contact your doctor immediately to rule out the risk of serious postpartum hemorrhage (PPH).

Vaginal birth after Caesarean section

It used to be said, "Once a Caesarean, always a Caesarean." We now know that this is not true and that vaginal birth after a Caesarean section (VBAC) is possible and beneficial in many cases. In general, the benefits of a VBAC are a faster recovery and lower maternal risk than with repeat surgery. Overall, the success rate of VBAC is approximately 75%.

VBAC risks

The risk of serious complications arising during the labor of a woman attempting a VBAC is between 0.8% and 1.6%. These risks include assisted delivery, uterine separation, infection, and blood transfusion. A separation of the Caesarean scar on the uterus is the most serious potential complication during labor. This is an unusual event, which happens in only 1 out of every 100 attempted VBACs. This may require you to have immediate

Guide to ...

Evaluating the possible success of a VBAC

Well in advance of your due date, even during your pre-pregnancy planning for a second child, discuss these issues with your doctor. Remembering as much as you can about the first delivery will help you and your caregiver formulate the best plan for you in a subsequent pregnancy.

- What is the ideal timing for a second delivery? The time between the two deliveries should be at least 2 years. If this time is shorter, it could increase the chance of the uterine scar opening up.

- How did your previous pregnancy progress? Was the Caesarean section scheduled or unscheduled? It is helpful to have a copy of your antenatal record and your doctor's operative note from the first Caesarean. This is especially true if you

are moving to a different doctor, hospital, city, or country.

- If your surgery was unscheduled, what was the reason? If the Caesarean section occurred because the baby's heart rate was non-reassuring, your pelvis is "untried" — that is, you don't really know if a baby will fit through your birth canal. Probably it will.

- If the Caesarean section was performed because the baby did not fit through your birth canal, what was the size of the first baby? Were you fully dilated at the time? Did you push? If so, for how long? The answers to these questions can help your health-care provider estimate the chances of a successful VBAC.

- If your delivery was scheduled, what was the reason? A Caesarean section performed before labor for a breech has the best chance for a successful VBAC in a subsequent pregnancy.

surgery. If the scar opens, there is a risk of bleeding and premature separation of the placenta. In some very rare circumstances, the oxygen flow to the baby can be affected.

Because of the concern of uterine rupture and its potentially serious consequences, it is advisable for women attempting VBAC to labor in the hospital and to be carefully monitored throughout labor.

Did You Know?

VBAC caution

The risk of uterine rupture increases if prostaglandins are used to induce labor. If an induction of labor is considered (perhaps because you are overdue), then it is safer to rupture your membranes and use a small amount of oxytocin. If your cervix is not ripe, some doctors will advise a repeat Caesarean section rather than an attempted VBAC.

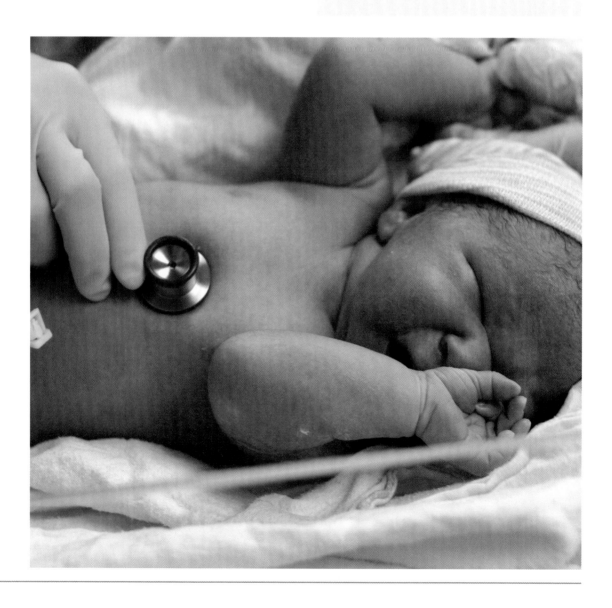

Postpartum hemorrhage

Excessive bleeding, or postpartum hemorrhage (PPH), affects approximately 1% to 5% of women giving birth. It can occur following either vaginal or Caesarean delivery. Postpartum hemorrhage is an obstetric emergency, but your delivery team is well-prepared to identify and treat the causes.

Lochia

For the first few days after delivery, the uterine discharge, or lochia, is mostly blood and red in color (lochia rubra). After 3 to 4 days, it becomes paler in color (lochia serosa), and by day 10, it usually has become white or yellowish (lochia alba). It takes about 4 to 6 weeks for the lochia to stop completely. You may notice a stopping and starting pattern, where you bleed for a few days, stop, and then bleed for another few days. This, too, is normal.

Excessive bleeding

The usual definition of excess bleeding is more than 2 cups (500 mL) of blood loss at a vaginal delivery or more than 1 quart (1 L) of blood loss at a Caesarean section. Excessive bleeding, or hemorrhage, can occur either immediately (early postpartum hemorrhage) or somewhat delayed (late postpartum hemorrhage). Late hemorrhage may develop anywhere from 1 day to 12 weeks after you are home from hospital. Excessive late bleeding is quite uncommon, happening to less than 1% of women.

Causes of excessive bleeding

1. *Uterine contractions:* The placenta attaches to the wall of the uterus and receives maternal blood from big open sinuses in the uterine muscle wall. After delivery of the placenta, the muscular tissue of the uterus is supposed to contract and close off these openings for blood flow, like a valve closing a pipe. If the uterus does not contract well or enough, blood can flow out of these openings in the uterine muscle, and, since the placenta is no longer there, the blood essentially spills out of the uterus into the vagina.

2. *Retained tissue:* There is some retained placenta, membranes, or blood clots in the uterus. In this case the uterus may have trouble contracting enough because the tissue or blood clot inside acts like a balloon holding the uterus open.

3. *Trauma:* There is some trauma to the tissues of the uterus, cervix, or vagina, such as a tear that has not yet been fixed or sutured, that is leading to continued bleeding.

4. *Coagulation abnormalities:* There is some reason why the body is unable to clot its blood properly, referred to as a coagulation abnormality. This can happen all on its own or with any one of the other causes.

Early PPH

Health-care providers can reduce the chance of postpartum hemorrhage by 40% by routinely giving oxytocin after delivery of the baby and placenta. If you are bleeding too much after delivery, other medications can be used to stimulate the uterus to contract more effectively. You will be simultaneously examined to look for bleeding tears and lacerations, as well as retained tissue in the uterus. A catheter will be placed in your bladder to make sure that a full bladder does not prevent the uterus from contracting fully. If necessary, you will receive a blood transfusion. Most bleeding settles down at this stage.

Occasionally, more drastic measures need to be taken, including procedures to block blood vessels to your uterus, either surgically or using a newer technique called

Postpartum Hemorrhage Fact Sheet

Reason for postpartum hemorrhage	Cause	Risk factors	Treatment
Uterus unable to contract	Uterus over-distended	Multiple pregnancy (twins, triplets, etc.) Macrosomia (big baby) Polyhydramnios (excess amniotic fluid)	Give medication to help uterus contract
	Uterine muscle relaxation	Fast labor Long labor High parity (many babies previously)	Give medication to help uterus contract
	Intra-amniotic infection (infection within the uterus)	Fever Prolonged time with ruptured membranes (waters broken)	Give medication to help uterus contract, as well as antibiotics
Retained products of conception	Abnormal placenta	Abnormal placenta may be seen on ultrasound	
	Retained products	Previous uterine surgery (placenta more sticky at scar, less likely to separate completely) High parity Incomplete placenta noted at time of delivery when inspected	Remove retained placental pieces. Usually the doctor can reach inside the uterus and do this immediately after delivery. Alternatively, a D&C to do this.
Trauma	Lacerations of the cervix, vagina, or perineum	Fast delivery Delivery with vacuum extractor or forceps	Identify and suture the lacerations

embolization. Very, very rarely, if the bleeding does not stop, the uterus is removed by hysterectomy in order to save your life.

Late PPH

Excessive bleeding after the first 24 hours following birth is usually caused by a small piece of retained placenta or an infection in the uterus. Your doctor or midwife will examine you for infections, test your blood, and order an ultrasound to make sure the uterus is empty of any retained placenta. Medications to help the uterus contract and to expel the excess tissue may be prescribed, along with antibiotics. Sometimes, a D&C (dilatation and curettage) will be done to remove the retained tissue. After any bleeding episode, iron supplements can help your body replace the hemoglobin lost during bleeding.

Reason for postpartum hemorrhage	Cause	Risk factors	Treatment
Trauma (continued)	Extensions or lacerations at Caesarean section	Deep engagement of head when Caesarean section performed. Malposition of baby's head at time Caesarean section performed	Identify and suture the lacerations
	Uterine rupture	Previous uterine surgery (including Caesarean section)	Identify and suture the lacerations
	Uterine inversion (turning inside out)	High parity. Placenta attached at top of uterus	Return the uterus to the right position
Coagulation abnormalities	Pre-existing health problems (e.g., hemophilia A, von Willebrand's disease)		Replace the missing blood components
	New problem acquired in pregnancy		Replace the missing blood components
	Anticoagulation with medications (e.g., heparin, low molecular weight heparin)		Replace the missing blood components

F.A.Q.

We answer many questions from pregnant women and their partners. Here are some of the most frequently asked questions. Be sure to ask your health-care providers any other questions that may arise. If they don't have the answers, they will refer you to a colleague who does.

Q: Is it true that some women have "childbearing hips" that make labor and delivery easier?

A: Unfortunately, it is impossible to tell if a woman truly has childbearing hips by looking at her from the outside! What really counts is the internal diameter of her pelvis. We have all seen women with ostensibly tiny hips easily deliver big babies, while larger women with a very narrow internal pelvis have trouble with smaller babies.

Q: What do I need to do to prepare for an elective Caesarean section?

A: On the day of your surgery, follow your doctor's instructions about fasting. Prior to any major surgery, it is important that you have an empty stomach. This makes the anesthesia and surgery much safer for you, significantly reducing the risk that any recently ingested food or drink that might be in your stomach comes back up your throat and into your lungs. This is called aspiration and is a serious complication that can lead to pneumonia, lung damage, and a need to stay on a ventilator in an intensive care unit.

Q: How long does a Caesarean section take?

A: Although the time can vary between different surgeons and different patients, on average a Caesarean section takes about 1 hour from start to finish, with only about half of that time being direct operating time.

Q: How long do I have to stay in the hospital after a Caesarean section?

A: You will probably be discharged from the hospital on the third post-operative day, unless you are having a problem. You can anticipate being a little slow on your feet, especially on stairs. It will be a week or two before you are up to taking short walks. You will need to arrange for someone to drive for you as well. You should not drive for at least a few weeks. In some parts of the world, auto insurance is invalid for 6 weeks after a Caesarean section. Do not lift anything heavier than your baby for several weeks. If you have a toddler at home, encourage the older child to climb into your lap for visits.

What's next

Your pregnancy is still not over! According to most authorities, pregnancy includes the 6 to 12 weeks following the birth of your baby, commonly known as the postpartum period.

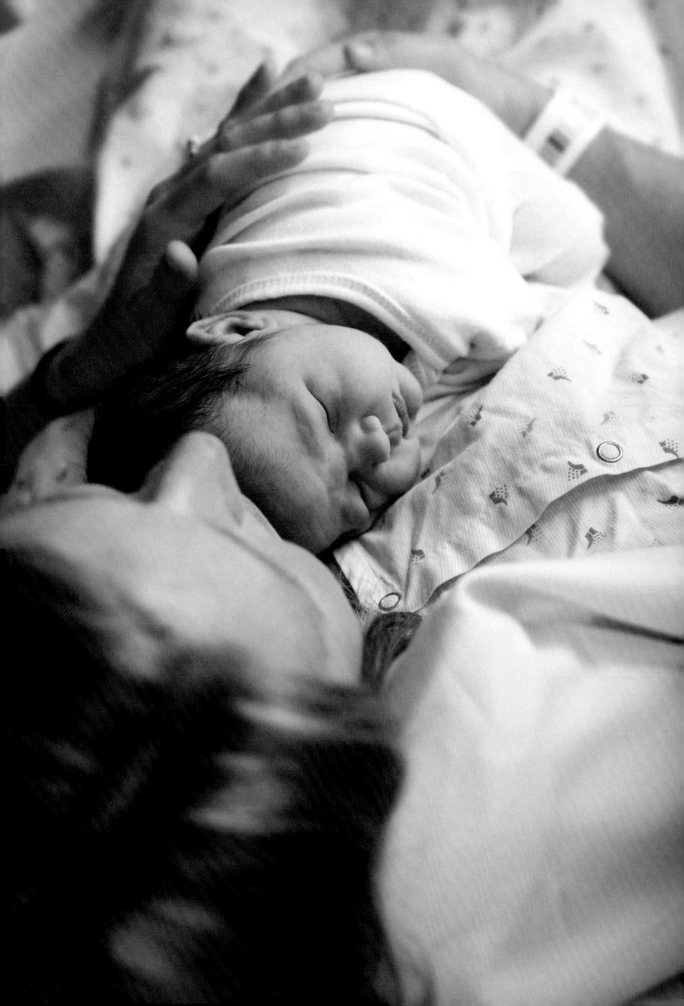

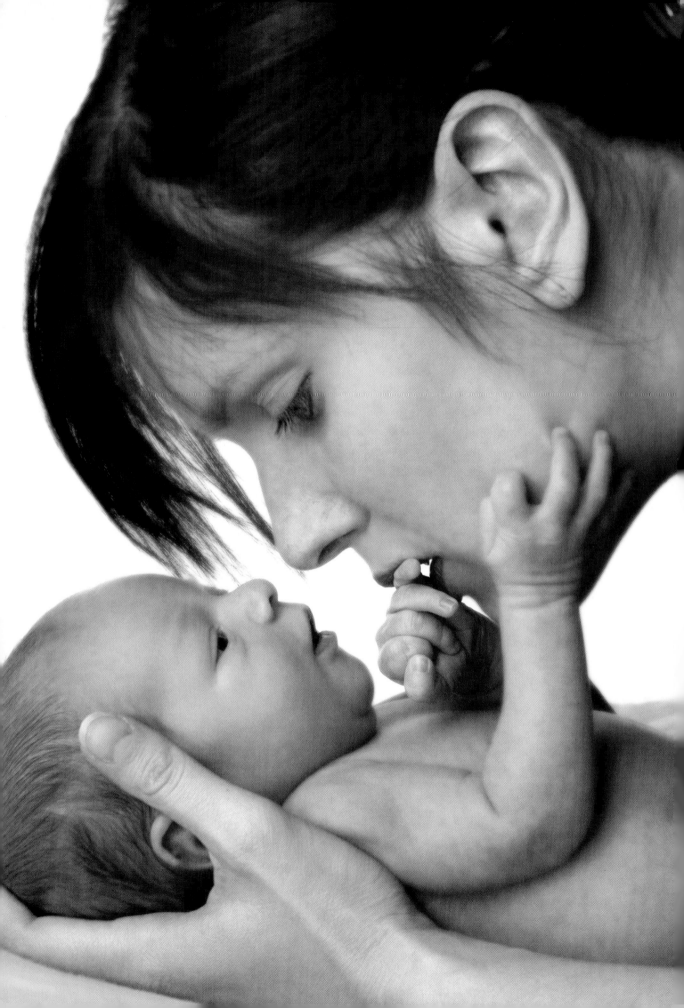

Part 12

Caring for Your Baby and Yourself

In the beginning

You did it! There's your baby in the hands of your doctor or midwife, and ready for your care. To start, your job is easy — just cuddle, nurse, and admire this marvelous child while your delivery team attends to some routine tasks. Later, you'll have some more work to do as the two of you get acquainted. The first 12 weeks after delivery are sometimes called the "fourth trimester" — your baby is as dependent on you for warmth, food, and waste management (diaper changes!) as he was in the womb, but it takes a lot more work now.

First minutes

It can be busy in the first few minutes after delivery as everyone welcomes your baby into the world and checks to be sure everything is going well. Your delivery team will ensure that your baby is adapting to extra-uterine life and breathing well — a big job for a newborn!

Warming your baby

Your baby is born at body temperature and slippery wet from the amniotic fluid. The first job is to get your baby dry so he doesn't get cold in the cooler air of the room. If your baby is doing well after an uncomplicated delivery, he is often placed right on your chest to be dried off with soft, warm towels.

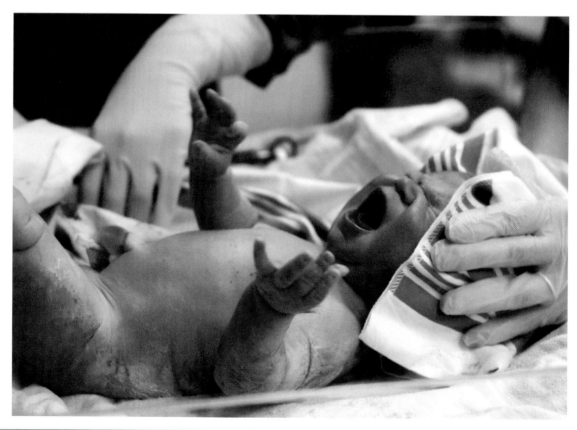

Did You Know?

Picture perfect

When you first lay eyes on your baby, she will be beautiful, of course, but not picture perfect. She may be covered in vernix caseosa (a white creamy coating that protected her skin as a fetus) and spotted with some blood left from the delivery process. If her birth was assisted, there may be some light bruising from the vacuum extractor or forceps. There may also be signs of caput and molding, two specialized terms used to describe normal effects of delivery:

- *Caput:* This refers to a soft tissue swelling on the top of the baby's head that results from pushing. There can be as much as 1/2 to 3/4 inch (1 to 2 cm) of caput. This is why some babies have heads that look a little "pointy" right after a delivery. But don't worry; the swelling disappears within 24 hours.

- *Molding:* This refers to a special feature of baby's skulls that allows them to pass through the narrow birth canal. The skull bones are able to shift a little bit, overlapping each other to allow the head to fit through the pelvis. Again, don't worry about this — the head will resume its normal shape after delivery.

Once your baby is dry, he can stay with you on your chest, covered in a blanket. Hold and cuddle your baby, skin to skin, if you wish. And if you have chosen to breastfeed, now is a good time to give it a try.

Your baby will not be bathed properly for several hours, because new babies are not very good at regulating their body temperature. So ignore the vernix and those little smears of dried amniotic fluid and blood on his body, and remember that, in this case, cleanliness takes a back seat to warmth!

In a few minutes, your newborn will need a little bit of attention from the nurses or midwives, who may take him away to the "baby warmer," a heated bed where it is easy to observe him. This bed can also act as a resuscitation unit if the baby needs help breathing. Your doctor or midwife may take this time to place a few stitches in your perineum if there was a tear. By the time you are all tidied up, your baby will be ready to come back to you.

First Hours

In the first hours, your baby will undergo a few routine checks and procedures to ensure his good health.

Weight

Your baby will be weighed and possibly measured for length, usually while in the delivery room.

Eye drops

Your baby will receive antibacterial eye drops to prevent serious eye infections that can be passed on from bacteria in your vagina. These eye drops are given within the first hour of life. They may make your baby's eyes look a little "goopy" for a little while, but that will go away soon.

Vitamin K

Your baby will also receive an injection of vitamin K, which helps blood form clots and prevents serious bleeding. Newborn babies are more prone to bleeding than adults, but a dose of vitamin K prevents a serious disease called hemorrhagic disease of the newborn. Vitamin K is given by injection into the thigh.

Umbilical cord

The umbilical cord will be trimmed to a short length (if it wasn't already cut short by the delivering doctor or midwife).

First diaper

Your baby is usually diapered early for obvious reasons. Many nurses ask the baby's father or your birth partner to prove their prowess in diapering at this time! Nurses may give you or your partner coaching support with other chores, such as holding, bathing, and dressing him.

Breastfeeding

If you are breastfeeding, you will be encouraged to start right away. For the first few hours, nurses will monitor your progress and lend a helping hand.

HOW TO...
Swaddle your baby

A well-swaddled baby will stay warm. Nurses and midwives are fantastic at swaddling babies, and you may wish to follow their directions:

1. Start with a square or rectangular blanket.
2. Fold in one corner a little and place the baby diagonally on the blanket, with the baby's head on the folded part.
3. Wrap one corner over the baby and tuck it tightly in behind her.
4. Fold the bottom corner up and over her feet and legs.
5. Then wrap the remaining corner across and behind the baby, stretching the blanket tightly.
6. Now the baby should look like a little baby burrito ... or spring roll ... or cabbage roll. Top her off with a little hat or bonnet.

Apgar score card

Sign	Score of 0	Score of 1	Score of 2	Total
Appearance (skin color)	blue all over	blue at extremities, body pink	body and extremities pink	
Pulse (heart rate)	absent	< 100 beats per minute	> 100 beats per minute	
Grimace (reflex irritability)	no response to stimulation	grimace/feeble cry when stimulated	sneeze/cough/ pulling away when stimulated	
Activity (muscle tone)	none	some flexion	active movement	
Respiration (breathing)	absent	weak or irregular	strong	
Score				/10

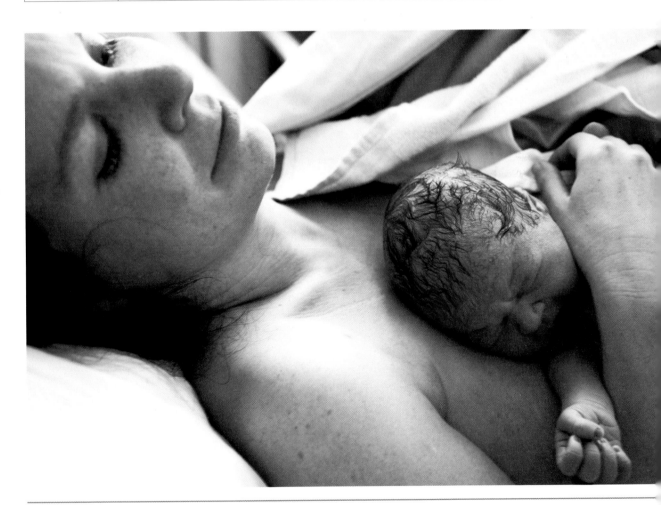

Newborn examination

Before going home from the hospital, your baby will be examined by your family doctor, your midwife, your pediatrician, or an on-call doctor. This first physical examination assures everyone that your baby is thriving. Use this opportunity to ask any questions you may have about caring for your baby for the next few days.

Newborn screening

Not all medical problems can be detected at birth or during the newborn examination. However, some of these rare conditions can be screened for with blood tests (pin prick in the heel) and treated successfully if diagnosed early. In some states in the United States and Canadian provinces, babies are screened for more than 25 conditions, while all states and most provinces screen for three important conditions. In most states and provinces, hearing is also tested.

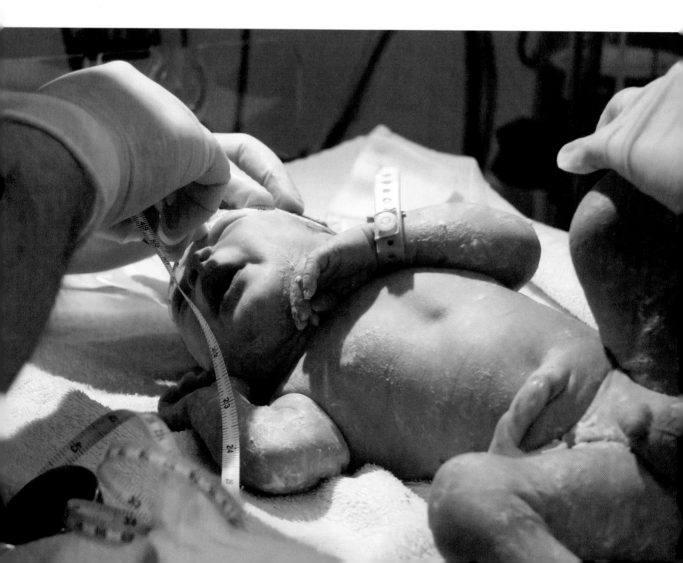

- Phenylketonuria (PKU): This metabolic disease can lead to developmental delay if not identified and treated early in life.
- **Congenital hypothyroidism:** This hormonal disorder can cause developmental problems, poor growth, and cretinism if not treated.

- Galactosemia: This blood sugar disorder can lead to blindness, developmental delay, and death if not treated.
- **Hearing disorders:** If hearing loss is diagnosed (using a small microphone in the baby's ear) before 6 months of age, this improves the chances of the baby's speech and language developing normally.

Guide to...

Special features of the newborn examination

This is a general examination from "head to toes" (or "toes to head" if she is squirming) with some concerns specific to newborn babies, including:

Growth charts

Your baby's weight, length, and head circumference will be measured and plotted on a growth chart that compares her to other newborn babies. This serves as a benchmark for charting her growth at subsequent medical check-ups.

Fontanelles and palate

The fontanelles, two soft spots in the skull (one on top of the head and one at the back of the head), will be examined to ensure there is adequate room for skull growth. Likewise, your baby's mouth will be examined to make sure that the palate, or roof of the mouth, is whole, enabling your baby to suck from the breast or bottle. The doctor will also check to see if there are any abnormal features to your child's face that may indicate a genetic abnormality.

Hips and testicles

Your baby's hips will be examined by rotating her legs to ensure that they are properly in their sockets. For a boy, the testicles will be palpated to check that they have descended from the abdomen (where they start off in fetal life) into the scrotum.

Spine and skin

Your baby's back will be checked for any tuft of hair or spinal dimple that may indicate spina bifida, a neural tube defect. Your baby's skin will be checked for jaundice (yellow discoloration), rashes, and any congenital defects or birthmarks. As early as the first day, newborns can develop several rashes, including milia and acne. Most resolve on their own.

Reflexes

Your baby has several unique reflexes that will be tested to check her neurological system. These include the palmar grasp reflex (your baby's fingers and toes will curl around your finger when placed on the palm of the hand) and rooting reflex (your baby's head will turn toward you with her mouth open, looking for food, as you stroke her cheek alongside her mouth).

Day-to-day care

Once your baby has settled in, there are a few routine skills you need to master besides changing diapers — swaddling your newborn, carrying him, bathing him, and dressing him, to name a few — but you also need to be vigilant in caring for the umbilical cord stump and circumcision, if you have a boy. You may also be called on to care for a few common newborn illnesses, such as colic and jaundice. Caring for your baby can be a bit overwhelming at first, but in due course you will be a professional.

Caring for a circumcision

During a circumcision, the baby's foreskin is pulled out beyond the end of the penis and trimmed off. Immediately after the procedure, the baby should be nursed or given his bottle, held, and cuddled as much as possible. His penis will look slightly red and swollen. During the healing period, it is important to monitor and care for the area of the circumcision.

Sometimes the doctor performing the circumcision places a device called a plastibell on the penis after the operation. It takes about a week to 10 days for the scab over the incision or the plastibell to fall off. After the scab or plastibell falls off, no further care is needed outside of normal good hygiene. If the plastibell does not fall off after 2 weeks, contact your health-care provider.

Caring for the umbilical cord stump

After birth, the umbilical cord is no longer needed, so it's clamped and snipped. This leaves behind a short stump of tissue that is attached to your baby's navel. The umbilical cord stump gradually dries and shrivels, changing color from yellowish green to brown to black, until it falls off, usually between 1 and 2 weeks after birth. Good basic care helps prevent infection and may also help the umbilical cord stump fall off and the navel to heal more quickly.

HOW TO...
Care for a circumcision

1. Place an ointment-coated gauze over the site, and change it every time you change the baby's diaper.
2. Clean the area with warm water three or four times a day. Soap is not necessary.
3. Contact your health-care provider if you notice any of the following conditions:
   - Delayed healing of the penis
   - Excessive and persistent bleeding from the penis
   - Excessive redness or swelling of the penis
   - Pus or foul, persistent odor
   - Any signs of illness, such as a fever, a decrease in appetite, or irritability

Signs of infection

You may notice a red, raw-looking spot right after the umbilical cord stump falls off. A small amount of fluid, sometimes tinged with blood, may ooze out of the navel area. This is normal. Rarely, the area can become infected. If your baby has an infection, prompt treatment can stop it from spreading. Call your health-care provider if you notice the following signs of infection:

- Pus around the base of the umbilical cord stump
- Red, tender skin around the base of the umbilical cord stump
- Foul-smelling discharge
- Baby cries when you touch the umbilical cord stump or the skin around it
- Fever
- Swelling and moistness on your baby's navel that lasts for more than 2 weeks after the umbilical cord stump has fallen off
- Bulging tissue around the navel after the umbilical cord stump has fallen off

HOW TO...

Care for the umbilical cord stump and navel

During the healing process, it's important to treat the navel area gently and to keep the umbilical cord stump and surrounding skin clean and dry.

Keep the area clean

1. Gently clean your baby's umbilical cord stump and the surrounding skin at least once a day or as needed during diaper changes or baths.
2. Soak a cotton swab in warm water and mild soap. Squeeze out the excess water, then gently wipe around the sides of the stump and the surrounding skin.
3. Wipe away any wet, sticky, or dirty substances.
4. Gently pat the area dry with a soft cloth.

5. After the umbilical cord stump falls off, continue cleaning around the navel at least once a day until the navel has completely healed.

Keep the area dry

1. Keep your baby's diaper folded below the umbilical cord stump to keep the stump exposed to air.
2. Bathe your baby carefully, preferably using sponge baths. In a regular bath, keep the umbilical cord stump above the water level until it falls off and heals.

Let the umbilical cord stump fall off naturally

1. Don't try to pull the cord stump off, even if it is hanging on by only a thread.

Multiples at home

Looking after multiples is quite an experience early on. Sometimes it seems like tag-team wrestling. One baby may be quiet and then the other starts up or needs changing. It takes a great deal of patience in the early going to survive the trials of looking after multiples. The first rule is, get help!

The saying that "it takes a village to raise a child" is even more true when it comes to multiples. This can be compounded if there is a toddler in the house already. Family is often your best resource for assistance. If you have the resources, you can consider hiring a nurse, doula, nanny, or student from a childhood education program. Somehow you will get through all of this, look back, and wonder how you did it.

Newborn health conditions

Babies have their fair share of minor health conditions, including several specific to their age, which may cause discomfort, but in most cases, they resolve themselves quite readily without further treatment. Still, these conditions can be disturbing to the parents and the baby. For more information on newborn health conditions, see *The Baby Care Book: A Complete Guide from Birth to 12 Months* (Toronto, ON: Robert Rose, 2007).

Colds

Healthy children can have six to eight colds in the first year of life, but, fortunately, they typically resolve on their own. In the meantime, maintain a healthy environment through hand washing, use a cool-mist humidifier (if the baby's nose is stuffed and the air is dry), and encourage feeding and hydration. If your baby has a high fever, difficulty breathing, poor feeding, or decreased urine output, seek medical attention.

Colic

Colic occurs in 10% to 15% of all newborn babies who are otherwise healthy. Colic can be a challenge, because your baby appears to be in inconsolable pain and you feel helpless. The only consolation is that the condition is temporary.

Colic is defined as persistent bouts of crying starting from 2 to 3 weeks after birth, with crying periods lasting for more than 3 hours a day and on more than 3 days a week. The abdomen is slightly distended and the legs drawn up. There is no known cause for colic, although many theories have been suggested, including milk protein intolerance, difficult temperament, over-feeding, an anxious mother or caregiver, or an immature gut.

Colic resolves on its own by 4 months of age. In the meantime, simethicone drops can help relieve gas, which, in turn, relieves symptoms of colic. Avoiding cow's milk protein in the formula or in the mother's diet can also be helpful.

Did You Know?

Tear duct blockage

Babies develop tear ducts in the first few weeks of life. Some babies have a blockage in these ducts that causes secretion, or discharge, in the corner of the eyes. The reason for this is not known. Treatment includes wiping away the discharge with a clean, wet washcloth or gauze. Usually, the problem resolves after the first 9 months. If it persists beyond the first year, the duct can be opened surgically. If you are considering gentle massage to open the tear ducts, discuss this procedure with your doctor.

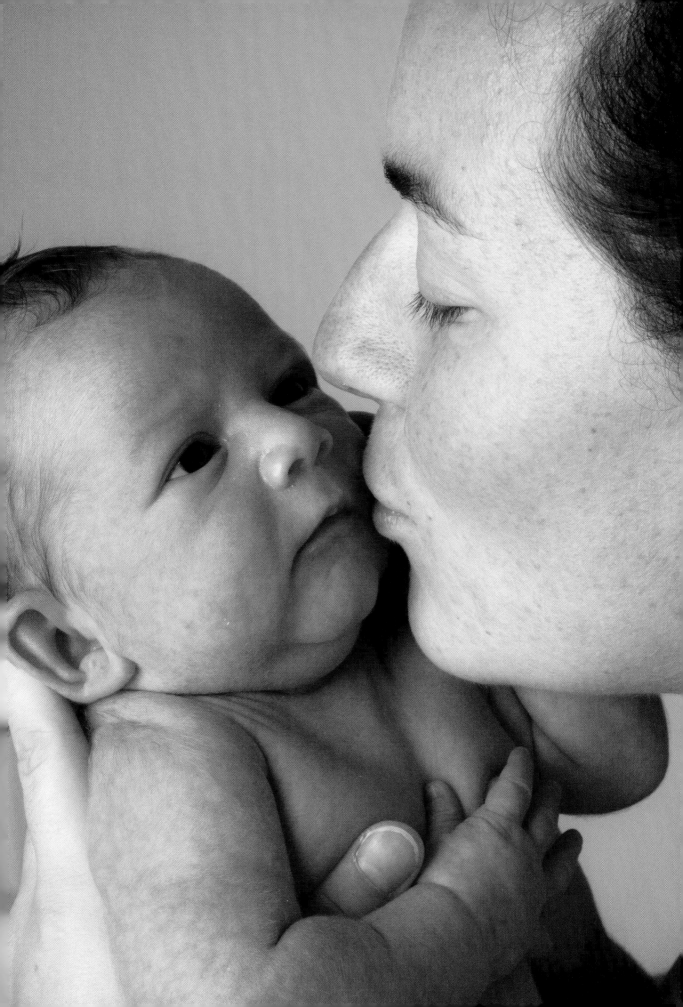

Did You Know?

Weight loss and gain

During the first few days, newborns can lose up to 10% of their birth weight through loss of fluids and waste (meconium). They also tend to be light eaters. Don't worry. Your baby will regain her birth weight by about 2 weeks of age and "put on" about 1 ounce (30 g) a day for the next 3 months. If she loses more than 10% of her birth weight or does not gain weight, your baby's doctor will discuss the next steps with you. This may be a sign that she is dehydrated or not getting enough to eat.

Constipation

Constipation in babies can be painful, but it is not all that common. It cannot be predicted by stooling patterns in newborns, which range in regularity from after each feeding to once a week. Babies eating supplemented formula usually have reduced frequency of bowel movements, but constipation is uncommon in breastfed babies. The usual treatment for constipation is reassurance and increasing fluid intake. If the baby does not pass any stool within the first 48 hours after birth, see your doctor. Laxatives or enemas should not be used without medical supervision.

Eczema

Eczema is a common skin rash in the newborn period and presents as a red, scaly, dry, and patchy eruption, most commonly found on the cheeks and trunk. The basic treatment is to stop the itch–scratch cycle by trimming the nails or putting cotton mittens on your baby's hands, moisturizing the area with petroleum jelly (or similar products), avoiding irritating fabrics or soaps, and, if necessary, applying corticosteroids prescribed by your doctor to reduce the inflammation.

Jaundice

Jaundice is a yellow discoloration of the skin and sclera (white part of the eyes), caused by increased bilirubin, a pigment produced by the breakdown of red blood cells. Bilirubin is normally metabolized by the liver, but some newborn babies have trouble doing so in the first few hours and days postpartum. Some breastfed babies develop a mild jaundice ("breast milk jaundice") that can last for a month or longer.

If your baby shows signs of jaundice, be sure to seek medical attention. If your baby is otherwise healthy, feeding well, and the bilirubin levels are not excessive, jaundice will resolve on its own. However, if jaundice persists and bilirubin levels become very high, the brain can be affected, leading to hearing loss, developmental delay, and behavior problems. Phototherapy using ultraviolet light is commonly used to break down the bilirubin pigment. This therapy will be recommended long before the levels become dangerously high.

Jaundice complications

These signs may indicate complications that require medical attention and monitoring of bilirubin levels:

- Jaundice appears within the first 24 hours after birth
- Your baby has difficulty in urinating or passing meconium (the baby's first stool)
- Your baby appears to have feeding difficulties, with signs of fever and infection

Feeding your newborn

By now you have likely decided either to breastfeed or formula-feed your baby. If you are breastfeeding, those childbirth classes on lactation, latching on, and expressing breast milk will come in handy. If formula-feeding, the nursing staff will show you how to mix up the appropriate infant formula in a bottle for you to serve your hungry newborn.

Breastfeeding

As with any new job or newly acquired skill, the first few days and weeks of breastfeeding can be the most challenging. Both moms and babies are learning this new skill together. The process often takes time and patience. Knowing what to expect in the first few days can help prepare you for these challenges.

How often

During the first month, newborns need to feed 8 to 12 times in a 24-hour period. It can be helpful to keep track of feeds. In the beginning, you may want to try nursing 10 to 15 minutes on each breast, and then vary the time as necessary.

Nocturnal feeding

It is not uncommon for newborns to sleep more during the day and feed more during the night. In fact, most newborns feed frequently and for long stretches during the nighttime hours. This is called cluster feeding. It's a good idea to get some rest during the day so you are better able to cope with the nighttime feedings. Don't worry about this pattern lasting forever. It won't. Over time, your baby will begin to sleep for longer stretches at night and increase his daytime feedings.

How much

Many new mothers worry that they won't be able to produce enough milk to nourish their baby; however, most women can produce enough milk for their baby, and even two or three babies! Only a very small number of women are physiologically unable to produce enough milk to nourish their babies.

Milk production is a process of demand and supply — the more milk that is demanded, the more the breasts supply. The most effective way to establish breastfeeding is to follow the baby's cues and practice early, frequent, untimed, and unrestricted feeding. This means you feed your baby whenever he is hungry, as often as he needs, for as long as he continues to feed, with no attempt to schedule or limit the baby's time at your breast. Once breastfeeding has been well established, your baby will settle into a more predictable pattern.

Did You Know?

Breastfeeding check-up

Breastfed infants should be seen by their doctor 48 to 72 hours after leaving the hospital. During this visit, the baby will be weighed and examined, and the mother's breastfeeding technique can be evaluated.

Guide to...

Starting up breastfeeding

1. Start breastfeeding as soon after birth as possible. Within the first hour is best. Research has shown that babies who breastfeed within the first hour of birth generally have more success with breastfeeding than babies who don't. Following this initial feeding, many babies will sleep for a 4- to 5-hour stretch as they recover from birth. It can be difficult to rouse baby for feeding during this time. Babies continue to be sleepy for the first 24 hours.

2. Plan on keeping your baby with you 24 hours a day so you can learn to recognize and respond to her feeding cues.

3. Plan on feeding your baby frequently in the first few days. She may be hungry often. Allow her to spend an unlimited time at your breast.

4. Gently rouse your baby every 2 to 3 hours and offer her the opportunity to breastfeed. If she seems too sleepy, unwrap her, taking off her clothes, and placing her skin to skin on your chest. This is all the encouragement most babies need to start looking for the breast and beginning to feed. Some babies will be more awake in the first 24 hours and should be fed as often as they demonstrate feeding cues.

5. Ensure your baby has a good latch on your breast. This will ensure you are both comfortable and successful — you in feeding, your baby in eating. An incorrect latch can result in significant breastfeeding problems. It's a good idea to ask for assistance from a trained lactation consultant or someone who has experience with breastfeeding.

6. Enlist the help of family and friends to assist with household chores and meal preparation. Keep visitors to a minimum. This gives you the time you need to focus on your new baby and for the two of you to begin to establish your breastfeeding relationship. Sleep whenever your baby sleeps. Having a new baby is exhausting — you need all the rest you can get to take care of your baby and recover from giving birth.

Once your milk supply is established, breastfeeding should be "on demand" (when your baby is hungry), which is typically every 1 to 3 hours. As newborns get older, they'll nurse less frequently, but they should not go more than about 4 hours without feeding.

In some situations, it may not possible to breastfeed, such as when a baby is sick or born prematurely. If you are in this situation, speak with your health-care provider about expressing and storing milk. Even if your baby cannot breastfeed, breast milk can be given via a feeding tube or bottle.

Expressing and storing breast milk

Expressing breast milk can be another way to provide your baby with breast milk benefits when you are separated. Expressed breast milk has the same nutritious and immunological properties as milk coming directly from the breast. Breast milk can be pumped and stored in the refrigerator for 72 hours. It can be frozen in a deep-freezer for up to 6 months. Frozen breast milk should be defrosted in the refrigerator (for 8 to 12 hours) or under warm running water. Do not defrost breast milk or warm it up with boiling water or in a microwave, because this will change the composition of the milk. After breast milk has been thawed, it should be used within 24 hours. Do not refreeze leftover thawed breast milk.

Breastfeeding multiples

With some perseverance, good instruction, and encouraging support, you should be successful in breastfeeding more than one baby. This is the time to call on a lactation consultant for advice.

As with singletons, the most effective way to establish breastfeeding is to follow cues from all your babies and practice early, frequent, untimed, and unrestricted feedings. And yes, in most cases, you will have enough breast milk for two or more. The true art of feeding multiples is orchestrating latching on to everyone's satisfaction.

If you are able to get both babies latched on at the same time, you will have more free time, but this can be difficult for everyone and sequential feeding may be the best option.

Despite good instruction, some mothers of multiples have a difficult time breastfeeding, which can lead to feelings of frustration, inadequacy, and depression. The babies can be frustrated, too, because they are not eating easily. If breastfeeding is still not working after getting help from a lactation consultant, go ahead with formula-feeding. You might even try a combination of breast and bottle, which gets your partner involved at the same time.

Did You Know?

First milk

For the first few days, your breasts produce a special kind of breast milk, called colostrum, that is small in volume but rich in antibodies. Around the third or fourth day, you will likely notice a dramatic increase in the volume of milk you are producing. Many women refer to this as their "milk coming in." You may notice that your breasts become quite hard, swollen, and painful to the touch during this period. It can be helpful to apply cold compresses to your breasts between feeds to help with the inflammation. Warm compresses or a warm shower just before a feed can help the milk flow more easily. You may also find you need to express a small amount of milk to soften the breast to help your baby latch on. Expressing milk will also help relieve the sensations of pressure and tenderness that accompany full breasts.

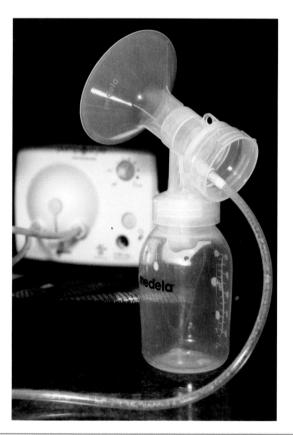

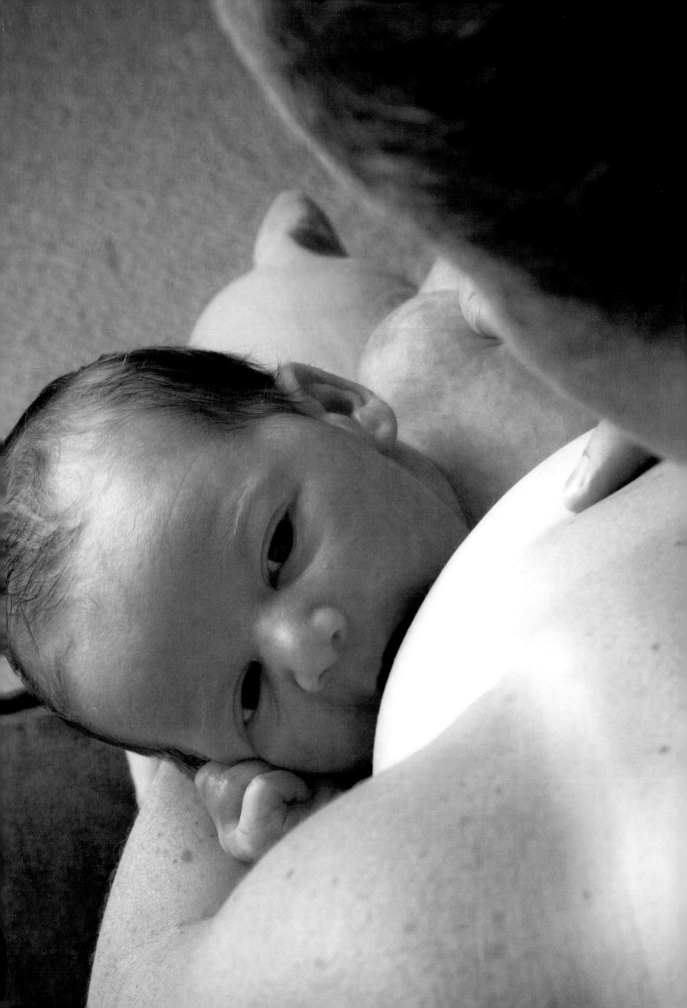

HOW TO...

Improve milk supply

If there is a problem with milk supply, initial interventions should be directed at increasing the demand on the breast, which will naturally increase the supply.

1. Ensure that baby is transferring milk effectively. Have your feeding technique reviewed and the baby's suck assessed by a lactation consultant or other professional knowledgeable about breastfeeding. Correct any identified problems.

2. Try using breast compressions while feeding to increase the amount of milk the baby is able to access during a feed.

3. Increase the frequency of feeds. The easiest way of ensuring an adequate milk supply is to feed your baby on cue, as often and for as long as she likes. Increasing the frequency of feeds increases milk supply by increasing the demand.

4. If factors exist that prevent you from increasing the amount of time the baby is spending at your breast, or if it has been determined that your baby is not removing milk from your breast efficiently, consider pumping your breasts. Adding pumping sessions between feeds or at the end of feeds will increase demand and consequently increase supply.

5. Take a nursing vacation. Remove all extraneous distractions and focus on you and your baby spending time together, doing nothing but eating and sleeping. A mini vacation of 2 to 3 days, with frequent feeding and lots of rest for you, can also work wonders for a low milk supply.

Galactagogues

When these measures aren't enough, you may want to consider the use of a galactagogue. Galactagogues are, by definition, substances that increase milk supply and generally fall into two categories, herbal preparations and prescription medications. Galactagogues should only be used in conjunction with other measures to increase breastfeeding frequency and milk transfer efficiency.

- **Herbal preparations:** Two of the most common herbs, used in many cultures, that seem to increase milk supply are fenugreek and blessed thistle. Be careful to get your herbs from a reliable source. No drug is considered 100% safe while breastfeeding, but the effects from fenugreek and blessed thistle on the baby are minimal, if any.

- **Prescription medications:** Domperidone (Motilium) is generally used to treat gastrointestinal disorders, but several studies have shown that use of this drug is effective in increasing milk production and that it is safe for both breastfeeding women and their babies.

Special nutrient needs

Women who are breastfeeding require additional calories, carbohydrates, iron, and fluids, even above pregnancy requirements. Many women continue their prenatal or multivitamin during lactation.

- **Calories:** During lactation, the DRI for energy is 500 calories more than pre-pregnancy intakes for the first 6 months of breastfeeding and an additional 400 calories after the first 6 months.

- **Carbohydrates**: Requirements are increased slightly to 7.5 ounces (210 g) per day.
- **Iron**: The DRI for iron during lactation is 9 mg per day.
- **Fluids**: Fluid requirements increase to 15 cups (about 4 L) per day during lactation, higher than during pregnancy.

Breastfeeding while pregnant

If you become pregnant while breastfeeding, you will need even more additional calories, protein, and fluid to support the growing fetus and maternal tissues. No set requirements have been established. In order to consume adequate amounts of energy, snacking on nutrient-rich foods between meals will likely be required.

Formula-feeding

If you are formula-feeding, be sure to choose a cow's milk formula that is iron-fortified to help prevent iron-deficiency anemia during the first 9 to12 months of life. Pasteurized whole cow's milk can be introduced at 9 months of age. Partly skimmed milks (2%, 1%, and skim) are not recommended for the first 2 years of your baby's life because the fat content of whole milk helps support his growth. Other formulas that are available for use, such as lactose-free, soy, non-iron-fortified, and specialty formulas, should be chosen only after consultation with a physician.

Newborn babies will take about 2 to 3 ounces (60 to 75 mL) of formula every 2 to 4 hours.

Introducing solid foods

Whether you are breastfeeding or formula-feeding, solid foods should not be introduced until the infant is 6 months of age. At that time, introduction of iron-fortified cereal is recommended, followed, in turn, by vegetables and fruit, milk products (such as cheese and yogurt), and meat and alternatives. Avoid honey and egg whites for the first year of life.

Did You Know?
Nicotine and alcohol
During breastfeeding, smoking and alcohol should be limited or avoided if possible. Nicotine metabolites remain in breast milk, and passive smoke (secondhand smoke) has also been detected in breast milk. Smoking more than 10 cigarettes a day can result in a reduction in breast milk production and cause poor weight gain and irritability in your infant. Alcohol appears in breast milk and can also interfere with milk supply. If you consume alcohol, wait at least 2 hours to breastfeed or "pump and dump" the milk. Surprisingly, caffeine does not pass into breast milk in large quantities.

Did You Know?
Essential fatty acid benefits
Essential fatty acids are passed to your infant through your milk, with the amount directly related to the amount you consume. Benefits from omega-3 fatty acids include ongoing development of the neural and visual systems. Be sure to include rich sources of omega-3 in your diet when breastfeeding. These include fatty fish, flaxseed and canola oils, and omega-3-fortified foods.

Breastfeeding challenges

Some lucky women are able to breastfeed easily and painlessly from their baby's first hours of life. For other women, breastfeeding is a challenge and a learned art, one that requires perseverance and dedication. If problems persist, see your doctor or midwife, who may refer you to a lactation consultant.

Managing common breastfeeding conditions

Condition	Signs and symptoms	Common treatment
Sore or cracked nipples Nipple pain can become so severe that you dread putting your baby to your breast	• Red, dry nipples • Visible cracks in nipples, bruising • Pain with breastfeeding, usually most severe when baby first starts to nurse • Nipple is "pinched" when baby comes off the breast	• Ensure that your baby is latching correctly — an incorrect latch is usually the cause of sore or cracked nipples. • After feeding, express a few drops of breast milk on your nipple and let it dry. • Make sure that your nipples always have a chance to dry after feeding. • Do not use breast pads that will not allow breast tissue to breathe. • Try lanolin ointment applied to nipples after each feed. • Do not apply creams or lotions that you need to remove prior to feeding. • When bathing, use only water (no soap) on breasts.
Leaking nipples Milk leaks out of nipple and onto bra/ clothing even when baby is not feeding or you are not with baby	• Breast milk comes out of nipples when you are not feeding	• None — this is a natural occurrence for some women. • To prevent leakage onto bra and clothing, use breast pads (cloth is best) to collect milk. • To prevent complications, such as dry, cracked nipples, use breast pads that are not lined with plastic.

continued on next page

Engorgement Breasts become too full with milk. Commonly occurs when milk first comes in or if feedings are missed	• Breasts extremely full and hard • Breasts may be painful to touch • Breasts are very warm • Areola are hard, difficult for baby to latch on	• Breastfeed more frequently. • Express breast milk frequently to relieve the pressure (preferably with a pump). • Apply warm compresses prior to feeding baby. • Apply cold compresses to breast between feeds for severe engorgement. • Massage breast, starting from your armpit and going down to your nipple, prior to feeding or expressing. • Consider pain medication as required (ibuprofen or acetaminophen). • Consider placing cold cabbage leaves inside the bra for 20 minutes or until the leaves soften — no evidence to support this treatment, but some swear by it.
Blocked duct One of the ducts that your milk flows through has become plugged	• One section of the breast is red, hard, and often painful • May feel a lump • Usually localized to one breast	• Feed frequently — suckling from baby will help to unblock duct. • Start the feed on the side that is blocked. • Try feeding your baby in different positions in an effort to unblock duct (for example, if you usually feed using a cradle method, switch to football hold) and try to position so the baby's jaw is on the side of the blocked duct. • Apply moist heat to affected area. • Massage the affected area. • Monitor this very closely — it can lead to mastitis if it is not treated.
Raynaud's phenomenon Vasospasm of the blood vessels — more common in other parts of the body (for example, the hands). Can be very painful	• Nipple turns white (vasospasm) after baby finishes feeding • After some time, color returns to nipples, but there may still be residual pain • When nipple is white, there may be a burning sensation, and when the blood/color return to the nipple, it may throb	• Fix latch first — pain is often secondary to a poor latch, and this pain increases exponentially when vasospasm occurs. • Apply a warm face cloth to the areola and nipple after breastfeeding and let it cool gradually. • In severe cases, you may require medication.

Mastitis Bacterial infection of the breast tissue (not a common problem)	• Pain or swelling in the breast similar to a blocked duct • Fever and other flu-like symptoms • Usually localized to one breast	• Try treatments as for blocked duct, but if persists for more than 24 hours, seek immediate medical attention and treatment with antibiotics. • Continue to breastfeed regularly. This infection does not affect the quality of the breast milk. Feeding may help treat the mastitis — abrupt stopping of breastfeeding will exacerbate the problem. • Start feeding on the affected side. • To prevent in the future, avoid pressure on the breast (from a poorly fitting bra, for example); try to feed baby regularly; and ensure that the baby has a good latch so that she is draining the breast effectively.
Yeast infection (*Candidiasis,* or thrush) May infect mother and baby and be passed back and forth May follow antibiotic use in mother or baby	• Mother may have pain while breastfeeding — lasts for entire feed and even after the feed in some instances • May have pain and very sensitive nipples while not breastfeeding — may be worse at night • Often described as a deep shooting pain or burning, which radiates deep into the breast • Baby may or may not have white patches (thrush) in her mouth or a persistent diaper rash	• Ensure that your baby is latching correctly — an incorrect latch will increase your pain. • Continue to breastfeed regularly, because this infection does not affect the quality of the breast milk. • Keep breasts dry and, if possible, expose them to the air as much as possible. • Do not use breast pads with plastic lining or wear a bra that traps in moisture around nipple. • Change your bra daily. • If the baby uses a bottle or pacifier, sterilize them daily. • Seek the services of a health-care provider. Topical treatments are generally used first, such as 1% gentian violet (for 4 to 7 days maximum) or topical antifungals (for example, clotrimazole). Treat the baby as well with gentian violet or a topical antifungal (for example, nystatin), because she may have oral thrush. Oral treatments can also be used (fluconazole for 2 weeks works well).

Adapted by permission from *The Baby Care Book: A Complete Guide from Birth to 12 Months Old* from The Hospital for Sick Children (Toronto, ON: Robert Rose, 2007).

Taking care of yourself

With so much attention justifiably being given to the care of your baby in the first few weeks, there's precious little time to care for yourself. Any labor and delivery is a stress on your body, even an easy delivery, and you need time to heal and recover. Resist the temptation to do too much. Persistent problems will be reviewed at your 6-week medical check-up, usually considered the end of the peripartum period. Take time to rest and heal so you can better enjoy the pleasures of being a mother.

Guide to...
Healing immediately after delivery

● Vaginal tears and episiotomy

Most stitches from a vaginal tear and episiotomy heal extremely well. After about 4 to 5 days, pain and swelling in the perineum should gradually decrease, and in about 2 weeks, the skin will be well healed, although possibly still a little tender. If you feel increasing pain or have a foul-smelling discharge, visit your health-care provider, who can examine your stitches to ensure they are not infected. You may need to take antibiotics, have sitz baths several times a day, and, on the very rare occasion, have more stitches put in. Infections in the perineum area are more common if third- or fourth-degree lacerations occur during delivery.

● Uterine contraction

Immediately after delivery, the uterus can still be felt in the lower abdomen, slightly below your belly button. It will slowly shrink. By 2 weeks, it is low enough to be in your pelvis, and by 4 to 6 weeks, your uterus will return to its normal size, shape, and position.

● Vaginal bleeding

Blooding, or lochia, gradually decreases in amount, and changes from bright red to pink and then yellow before stopping by 4 to 6 weeks. You should not be flooding through pads, changing pads more than once an hour, or passing large clots (small clots are normal immediately following delivery). Excessive bleeding following delivery can indicate a potential problem and needs to be brought to the attention of your doctor.

● Caesarean section incision

Generally, by the third day following surgery, the staples or skin sutures can be removed. It takes 6 to 8 weeks for full healing. You may notice numbness or a "pins and needles" sensation around the incision as the nerves heal at that site.

● Stretch marks

These will fade from red to silver but are permanent.

● Abdominal wall

The tone of your abdominal wall will be lax but will improve over several weeks. If you had a diastasis (separation) of the rectus muscles, this may persist.

Pain relief

Not only will you be exhausted from labor and sleep-deprived, but many women also have pain in the postpartum period. Typically, you will feel vaginal and perineal pain after vaginal delivery or abdominal and incisional pain after a Caesarean section.

Acute postpartum pain should be aggressively treated to allow you to carry out your daily activities comfortably and to prevent any long-term consequences related to chronic pain. Multimodal pain relief strategies are effective for postpartum pain.

- Caesarean delivery: If you have had a Cesarean section under general anesthesia, you may receive opioids via patient-controlled analgesia (pain pump). If you have had a Cesarean section under spinal or epidural anesthesia, a small dose of morphine will usually be included in the drug cocktail. The advantage of this is that when injected around the spinal cord, small doses of morphine have a prolonged effect, usually lasting for 18 to 24 hours. During this initial period, women usually do not require additional opioids, but start taking them on post-operative day 2.

- Vaginal delivery: If you have had a vaginal delivery and used an epidural for pain relief in labor, you may also receive morphine in your epidural. Again, this helps with vaginal and perineal pain for the first day after delivery. This is most commonly done for women who have suffered extensive vaginal tears. For more information on day-to-day pain relief strategies, see Part 7, Birth and Newborn Planning (page 259).

Breastfeeding safety

The biggest fear that most women have about pain relief after delivery is the effect of the drugs on breast milk and, in turn, the baby. However, common analgesics, such as acetaminophen and NSAIDs, are considered to be compatible with breastfeeding. While small amounts do end up in breast milk, these amounts are considered to be too small to have any effect on the newborn.

In general, opioids are safe, too.

Did You Know?
Codeine caution
Some women and babies have a gene that helps convert codeine to high levels of morphine very quickly, and, in these individuals, codeine can be dangerous. This gene is present in about 1% of Caucasians, but up to 30% of people from North Africa, Ethiopia, and Saudia Arabia. That said, it is exceedingly rare for codeine to be toxic to babies through breast milk. Still, be vigilant, and if your baby is sleepy or not rousing well for feeds, seek medical attention promptly. If you have any particular concerns, please discuss them with your obstetrician, midwife, or anesthesiologist.

Weight loss

Immediately following the delivery of your baby, you are going to feel lighter! Right away you lose between 11 and 13 pounds (5 and 6 kg) as you deliver the baby and the placenta. Then you usually lose another 4.5 to 6 pounds (2 to 3 kg) of excess fluid in your urine the first week.

Achieving a healthy weight

Further healthy weight loss will be much more gradual. Typically, if weight gain during pregnancy is within the target range, loss of pregnancy weight can be reasonably achieved by 1 year postpartum with balanced nutrition and regular exercise.

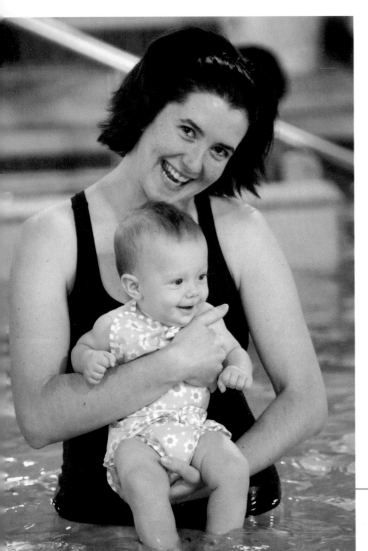

If your pre-pregnancy weight is not reached by 1 year postpartum, the risk of diabetes mellitus and heart disease is increased. Rapid weight loss (as a result of insufficient energy intake) can reduce your breast milk supply. Moderate weight loss of 1 pound (0.4 kg) per week is healthy and should not decrease your milk supply.

The metabolic demands of breastfeeding will help you lose some weight, but the last 10 pounds tend to persist. This may be a way of protecting the baby's milk supply.

Weight anxiety

Most women find it very frustrating that they cannot fit back into their favorite clothes months after giving birth, particularly when they see other new mothers looking trim. There are no standard patterns of weight loss, and every woman will lose her pregnancy weight at a different rate. Many factors are involved in the rate of weight loss, including rate of weight gain during pregnancy, dietary intake, physical activity level, and breastfeeding. Unreasonable weight loss expectations can be very disappointing and unhealthy for the postpartum woman.

Postpartum exercise

To achieve weight loss, you will likely need to exercise regularly, which will also help to restore muscle tone to your tummy. If you have had a normal delivery or even a Caesarean section, most standard activities can be resumed by the time you go home from hospital. You can walk, go up and down stairs, and take a shower. If you had a Caesarean delivery, you will be able to walk short distances, but you should use common sense. Avoid activities that increase discomfort in your incision, rest when your body tells you to, and avoid lifting heavy objects (or older children).

Walking it off

Walking is a great initial exercise. Begin with 15 to 20 minutes a day. By your 6-week check-up, if all is well, your doctor or midwife will likely advise you that you can start a regular exercise program regardless of how you gave birth. Don't forget that you will be more tired because of both the delivery and the care you are giving to your newborn baby. When re-establishing your exercise regime or starting one, you may find you need to work at both a lesser intensity and for a shorter time. Slowly increase both your aerobic and strength training, especially if you had a Caesarean section. Your level of discomfort should help guide you.

Breastfeeding before exercising

If you are breastfeeding, you may find your comfort is increased if you breastfeed your baby right before exercising. While exercise should not interfere with milk production or composition, lactic acid may increase in the breast milk temporarily if you are exercising at maximum intensity levels. While it is not clear if this lactic acid accumulation makes breast milk taste bad to your baby, if your infant does not feed well after you've been exercising, this is another reason to consider either feeding before exercise or postponing feeding until 1 hour after a tough exercise session.

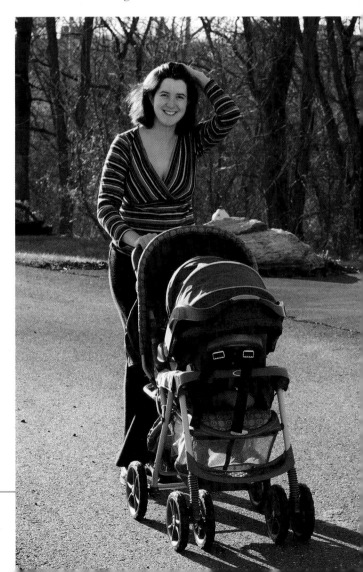

Sex after baby

While there is no definite time after delivery to resume sex, it's generally best not to have sex until at least 2 weeks after delivery to allow for any stitches to heal. Often, couples wait until after the 6-week check-up before starting, just to make sure the healing process is complete. While the bottle of champagne might be cooling in the refrigerator waiting for that go-ahead from your doctor, remember there is no right time for all women to resume sex.

Contraception

You have just delivered your baby a few weeks ago and, possibly, you are nursing around the clock. Why talk about contraception now? Be forewarned — it is possible to get pregnant only a few weeks after delivery, before your period returns, even while you are breastfeeding! You will ovulate again about 2 weeks *before* you see your first period. So unless you are ready to keep growing your family … think about contraception!

There are many methods of contraception you can use, depending on your medical history and current health, as well as the personal preferences of you and your partner. The only 100% foolproof way to avoid pregnancy is abstinence. While in the period following delivery this may seem like an excellent method, your libido will gradually return as the sleepless nights disappear, you physically heal, and you and your partner find time to be intimate again. Your health-care provider can help you find the right method for you.

Rule of thumb

A general rule of thumb is that if this is not the right time to get pregnant, then you should use something for birth control (even if you had trouble conceiving in the past). Fertility increases after pregnancy, so even if you required fertility treatments to conceive, you should consider yourself potentially fertile postpartum. Even breastfeeding women should use contraception. While women who are exclusively breastfeeding every 3 to 4 hours (including through the night) will have a delay of return of ovulation for up to 6 months after birth, you cannot rely on this 100% to prevent pregnancy.

Did You Know?

Lubrication

When you are breastfeeding, your body suppresses estrogen production. What that means for sex is that the vagina feels drier, with less lubrication even when you are aroused. You may need to use a lubricant. Water-based are best, readily available at your local pharmacy or most shops that sell condoms or sex toys. If you have had an episiotomy or tear, even though it is usually healed at 4 to 6 weeks, the area can still be tender for even up to a few more months. Try using the lubricant, but go slowly and gently and experiment with positions that are most comfortable and allow you more control. If the dryness is persistent and very bothersome, a vaginal estrogen cream can be prescribed to help.

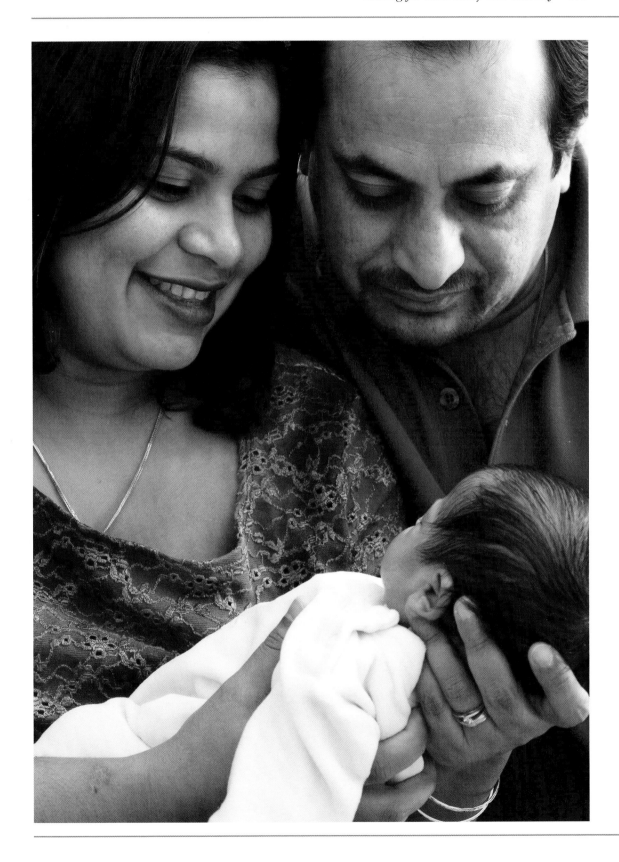

Postpartum infections

A fever of 38°C (101°F) or greater, especially if persistent over several readings, may indicate that you have an infection, most commonly in the urinary tract, genital tract or breasts. These infections are often related to your delivery or breastfeeding.

Postpartum infections

Infection	Signs and symptoms	Treatment
Bladder or urinary tract	• Pain when urinating • Urgent need to void • Blood in urine	• Urine culture • Antibiotics (safe for breastfeeding)
Kidney (pyelonephritis)	• Serious infection • Early symptoms similar to bladder infection • Tenderness over upper back and kidney • Spiking pattern of fever • Nausea and vomiting	• Intravenous antibiotics (for serious infection)
Uterine (endometritis)	• More common post–Caesarean section • Fever and chills • Abdominal pain • Uterine tenderness • Foul-smelling lochia • Possible increased vaginal bleeding	• Oral or intravenous antibiotic • 48–72 hour response
Caesarean section incision (wound infection)	• Occurs in 6% of cases • Red area around incision feels warmer than surrounding skin and spreads outward from incision into abdomen wall • Incision drains liquid, pus	• Antibiotics • Opening incision to drain pus (with local anesthetic) • Daily wound dressing (often by a visiting nurse)

Risk factors for postpartum infections

There are some factors in labor that may make an infection more likely:
• Prolonged rupture of membranes
• Prolonged labor
• Multiple cervical examinations
• Internal fetal monitoring

• Intrapartum chorioamnionitis (infection in labor)
• Preterm delivery
• Possibly, anemia and poor nutrition
• Some bacterial infections of the vagina

Weak bladder

Pregnancy and childbirth can weaken your pelvic floor muscles, causing urinary incontinence and leading to pelvic floor prolapse in some women. About 7% of women may notice this type of urinary incontinence after the birth of their first child. Many of the symptoms of pelvic floor weakness slowly get better after you deliver.

Risk factors

Risk factors that increase the chance of pelvic floor weakness include having a bigger baby, taking a long time to push your baby out once you are fully dilated, having a forceps delivery, and extensive tearing with delivery. Just being pregnant, even if you deliver by a Caesarean section, can lead to loss of strength in these muscles. Being overweight will worsen the symptoms.

Kegel exercises

To restore tone to these muscles, you should do pelvic floor exercises, known as Kegel exercises, 50 to 100 per day for 5 seconds at a time. You can do them pretty well anywhere — while breastfeeding, watching TV, or sitting on the bus. To learn how to do a Kegel exercise, try stopping your urine stream in the middle of urinating. Squeeze and hold these muscles. Now do the same action repetitively, holding for 5 seconds each time, when you are not urinating. Don't do this routinely as you urinate or you will run into more bladder problems.

Pelvic floor prolapse

If your bladder and bowel control symptoms are not getting better with time and Kegel exercises, speak to your health-care provider. Pelvic floor prolapse may require other treatments with supportive devices in the vagina (pessaries) or surgery. The choice and timing of treatment will depend on the severity, as well as whether you are planning to have other children. Since another child may negate the benefits of surgery, conservative non-surgical treatments will often be chosen until you have completed your family.

Symptoms of weak bladder

- Leaking (incontinence) of urine or even a lack of control of gas or stool from your rectum.
- Leaking happens when you cough, sneeze, or exercise — in other words, when you put increased pressure on your bladder.
- Leaking may be a small amount or, less often, a large amount requiring a pad.
- If leaking is constant or associated with pain while emptying your bladder, contact your doctor, because you may have a bladder infection, urinary retention, or an injury to your bladder or urethra from delivery (although this would be extremely rare).
- If you notice a bulge coming from the vagina, the bladder, uterus, and bowels may be pushing the vagina out due to pelvic floor muscle weakness. This condition is called pelvic floor prolapse.

Mood changes

In the first few days after delivery, following the stress of giving birth, women often feel let down or low. Fatigue from loss of sleep, anxiety about caring for your newborn, and the hormonal changes you are experiencing follow the stress of delivery, and it is not surprising that your mood might be affected. These mood changes can progress from the "blues" to chronic clinical depression. For more information on chronic mood disorders, see Part 13, Managing Medical and Environmental Risks (page 436).

Postpartum blues

At least half of women have some temporary "postpartum blues" in the first few days after delivery, and these can include feeling down, irritable, anxious, and teary, with rapid mood swings. If you are feeling the baby blues, make sure you take care of yourself as much as you can. Rest, eat, exercise, give yourself a mini break (even 15 minutes a day can be a boost), ask for help, or let those who offer

Did You Know?

Symptoms of postpartum depression

The symptoms of postpartum depression are similar to those of other types of depression. Symptoms can begin at any time within the first year after delivery, but the highest-risk period is the first month after birth. Here is a list of the symptoms of PPD. Read the list and see if any of the symptoms apply to you. If you have had some of these symptoms for more than 2 weeks, you may have PPD.

- My mood is very depressed most of the time.
- I am not enjoying anything.
- I do not want to care for my baby.
- I am having trouble bonding with my baby.
- My sleep is not my normal pattern: I have trouble sleeping even when my baby sleeps, or I sleep too much.
- I can't focus.
- My energy level is not what it was: My energy is either too low, or I feel agitated.
- My appetite isn't the same: I have no appetite, or I am overeating.
- I have trouble making decisions.
- My memory is terrible.
- I feel very nervous.
- I feel very guilty.
- I am very irritable and angry.
- I do not want to be around other people.
- I am crying a lot.
- I feel hopeless about the future.
- I am experiencing scary thoughts that do not go away.
- I have frequent thoughts about leaving or ending my life.

If you have thoughts about wanting to harm yourself or your baby, please seek help immediately, by calling 911 or going to your local emergency room.

help do so. Do not isolate yourself — go to a new-mothers' support group or talk to your partner, a friend, or a family member. With a little reassurance, this temporary mood change should resolve within 2 weeks.

However, if the blues last for a long time, start to interfere with your ability to care for your baby or yourself, or put stress on your relationship, this may be a more serious condition called postpartum depression.

Postpartum depression

Postpartum depression (PPD) is the most common complication of childbirth. It affects 15% to 20% of new mothers. While common, this condition often goes undetected and untreated. Many women are ashamed to say that they are suffering during what is supposed to be the happiest time of their lives, while others fear that they will be thought of as a "bad mother" if they are open about their feelings of despair. However, the good news is that postpartum depression is a very treatable illness that does have safe and effective strategies to help new mothers feel like themselves again and become the best mothers they can be.

Helping yourself

There are a few things that you can try at home to help yourself feel better. These include trying to get more sleep, eating well, going out at least once each day, doing light exercise, and asking other people to pitch in and help you and your family at this challenging time.

Getting professional help

Most women with PPD find that a combination of self-help activities and professional treatment is the best course of action. Most women who are pregnant or who have recently had a baby have ongoing contact with a family physician, obstetrician, or midwife. Telling these professionals that you are suffering is a great place to start. They may be able to help you or to point you in the right direction. There are psychiatrists who specialize in treating women who have PPD. Ask your doctor or midwife to refer you to one of these specialists. If they are not available in your area, seeing another psychiatrist will be helpful.

Treatment options

While PPD is a difficult illness to have, there are many proven ways to get well and to stay healthy so you can enjoy yourself and your new baby.

- **Talk therapy:** Talk therapy, or psychotherapy, is an excellent component of any treatment plan. In talk therapy, you will learn more about yourself and what is triggering your illness, as well as how to cope with your difficult thoughts, emotions, and relationships. Psychiatrists, psychologists, and other types of therapists can provide psychotherapy.

- **Medications:** Many women, particularly those who are suffering from more serious PPD, may require medications to feel better. Most antidepressants are safe to take while breastfeeding. Psychiatrists or family physicians can prescribe and monitor treatment with medication. For more information on safe medications for mood disorders, see Part 13, Managing Medical and Environmental Risks (page 436).

6-week check-up

Unless you have been instructed otherwise, you will see your doctor or midwife for a check-up 6 weeks after your delivery. This is a visit primarily for you — your baby has been getting regular check-ups already. If you are not sure your healing process is proceeding according to the typical timetable, or if a complication has arisen, call for an earlier appointment. If your health-care provider is also your baby's doctor, then aspects of your visit can be combined with a visit for your baby.

Labor and delivery review

At the 6-week check-up, your doctor or midwife will often start by reviewing with you your labor and your baby's birth, answering any questions you may have about how it went and any precautions that may be needed for future pregnancies, especially if there is a risk of recurrence of a complication.

Questions for discussion

- Are you still bleeding?
- Are you voiding (emptying) your bladder easily?
- Are you constipated?
- Do you have any problems with hemorrhoids?
- Do you have any pain from vaginal stitches (or from a Caesarean, if you had one)?
- Do you have any problems breastfeeding?
- Are you having sex again?
- How is your partner doing?
- How is your mood?
- Preterm delivery
- Possible anemia and poor nutrition
- Contraception

Routine tests

A few routine tests will be done, including a physical examination and a Pap test, and then you're out the door with a clean bill of health.

Physical examination

If you had stitches from either a tear or an episiotomy, your doctor or midwife will want to check to make sure these have healed. If there are any concerns about infection, vaginal and cervical swabs may be done to rule that out. Your uterus will be examined to ensure that it has contracted to a normal size.

Pap test

You may be in need of a Pap test if your last one was a year or more ago.

Diabetes test

If you had gestational diabetes mellitus, you will be booked for an oral glucose tolerance test at 3 months after delivery to ensure your glucose metabolism has returned to normal.

Au revoir

This 6-week visit marks the end of your pregnancy, looks forward to your ongoing good health and your baby's well-being — and opens a discussion of future pregnancies, if you are contemplating another one. Are you ready to do it all again?

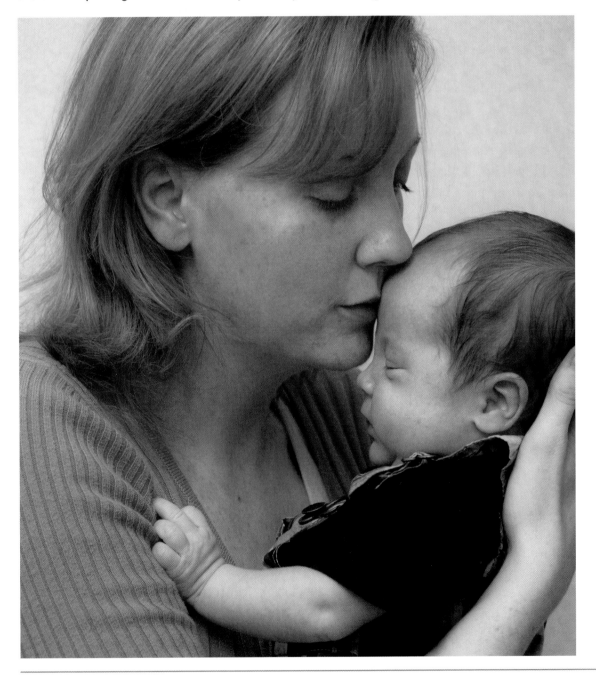

F.A.Q.

We answer many questions from pregnant women and their partners. Here are some of the most frequently asked questions. Be sure to ask your health-care providers any other questions that may arise. If they don't have the answers, they will refer you to a colleague who does.

Q: *What do I need to do to prepare myself to breastfeed?*

A: In the not-so-distant past, women were often told that all they needed to do was "toughen up" their nipples in preparation for breastfeeding. The descriptions of how to do this were enough to make even the most committed of women change their minds and reach for a bottle! Thankfully, research has shown that it is absolutely not necessary to prepare your nipples for breastfeeding. However, there are many other things you can do to prepare, including finding a support network ready to answer your questions and support you through your breastfeeding experience. La Leche League is an excellent support group. If you have any special concerns, you may find it helpful to meet with a lactation consultant to formulate a plan to maximize your success. Research has also shown that having a supportive partner is critical to breastfeeding successfully. Other important sources of support include mothers, sisters, and close friends.

Q: *How do I know if my baby is getting enough to eat?*

A: Most experts suggest you nurse or feed your baby whenever he seems hungry — a rigid feeding schedule is not necessary. Watch for signs that your baby is full (slow, uninterested sucking, turning away from the breast or bottle) and stop the feeding once these signs appear.

You can be assured that your baby is getting enough to eat if he seems satisfied, produces about four to six wet diapers a day, has regular bowel movements, sleeps well, is alert when awake, and is gaining weight. A baby who is fussing, crying, seems hungry, and does not appear satisfied after feeding may not be getting enough to eat. If you're concerned about it, speak with your health-care provider.

Q: *When can I try to get pregnant again?*

A: You can conceive again as soon as your body begins to ovulate, which varies depending on whether you are breastfeeding or not. Your return to fertility usually precedes your periods by about 2 weeks. If there were any complications during either your pregnancy or your delivery, this may affect your plans for the next pregnancy. Discuss your pregnancy experience with your health-care providers at your 6-week check-up. They can guide you on any additional precautions you should take either before you get pregnant or during your next pregnancy.

Q: Is it safe to have pregnancies close together?

A: There are some risks that may increase if the interval between pregnancies is too close together. Preterm delivery and babies that are small for their gestational age or have a low birth weight may occur if the time between the two pregnancies is shorter than 6 months. It is speculated that this is because your body needs some time to recover from the stress and nutritional burden of the previous pregnancy.

If you delivered by Caesarean section and are considering a vaginal birth for the next pregnancy, your health-care provider may suggest avoiding a short interval, which may be associated with a higher chance of uterine rupture with a VBAC (vaginal birth after Caesarean section). Many of us advise a year before conception in those who have had a Caesarean section, although there are few data to support this recommendation.

For women who are over the age of 35 or have a strong family history of early menopause, delaying too long before trying to get pregnant the next time may carry a risk of disappointment, because fertility does decrease with age.

What's next

From time to time in this book, we have referred you to Part 13 for more information on medical conditions and complications. Scan this section for information that may apply to your pregnancy.

Q: Why is my hair falling out?

A: Normally, hair cycles through growth and resting phases. During resting phases, hair is shed easily. During pregnancy, more of your hair is in a growing phase than a resting phase. In the postpartum period, this ratio switches and more of your hair is resting. You may notice increased hair loss that starts about 1 to 5 months after you deliver. Eventually, your normal hair growth patterns will return, but it may not be as thick.

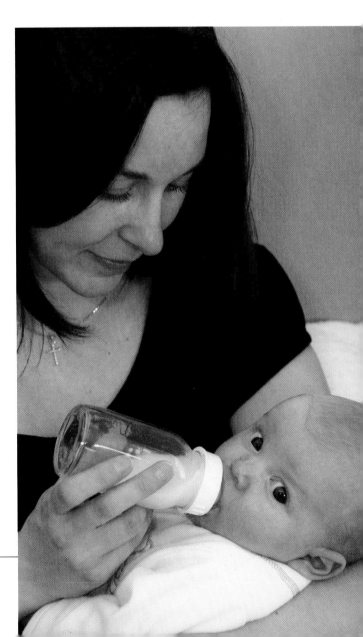

Part 13

Managing Medical and Environmental Risks

Risk management

Much of prenatal care is directed toward reducing the risk of serious complications. These risks include genetic diseases, chronic health conditions, exposure to substances harmful to the fetus, and pregnancy-induced conditions. The impact of these medical and environmental risks can be prevented or limited with careful management by you and your health-care providers.

Genetic diseases

To determine if you are carriers of a genetic disease, both partners should be screened before becoming pregnant or very early in your pregnancy. The best approach to managing these conditions is through prevention — genetic screening and counseling. If you and your partner test positive for being carriers of a genetic disease, you should seek counseling to discuss your options, ranging from accepting the odds of having a child with a genetic disease if you become pregnant to terminating a pregnancy in progress. For further discussion of your options, see Part 1, Planning Your Pregnancy (page 43).

Treatment plans

If your child is born with a genetic disease, you may not see any signs or symptoms until after birth, anytime from 3 months to 35 years (in the case of Huntington's chorea), at which time a treatment plan will be designed for current circumstances.

Common genetic diseases: onset and outcome		
Disease	**Onset**	**Outcome**
Cystic fibrosis	Infancy to adolescence	Excessive mucus production in lungs leading to respiratory disease
Hemophilia	Infancy	Blood coagulation disorder leading to excessive bleeding and bruising
Huntington's chorea	Adulthood (35–44 years of age)	Progressive neurodegenerative effect on personality and cognition with "chorea" (jerky movements)
Muscular dystrophy	Childhood (2–6 years of age)	Progressive muscular disease eventually affecting heart muscles and lungs
Sickle cell disease	Infancy	Anemia leading to lung disease, "sickle" pain episodes, and possibly stroke
Tay–Sachs disease	Infant (6 months) Juvenile (5–15) Adult (20s and 30s)	Progressive blindness, deafness, paralysis, and possible death
Thalassemia	Infancy	Anemia requiring frequent blood transfusions and leading to slow growth and enlarged spleen

Cystic fibrosis

Cystic fibrosis (CF) is caused by a mutation in a recessive gene, which leads to excessive mucus production in the lungs. Most of the time, the abnormal gene is inherited, although sometimes gene mutations can arise spontaneously in a developing embryo.

- *Screening*: Abnormal genes and gene mutations can be detected with a simple blood test.
- *Genetic counseling*: CF is an autosomal (not gender-related) recessive disease with two abnormal copies of this gene, one each from the mother and the father. Most common among Northern European populations.

Hemophilia and muscular dystrophy

Hemophilia (a blood coagulation disease) and muscular dystrophy (a muscular degeneration disease) are the classic examples of X-linked genetic diseases.

- *Screening*: Abnormal genes and gene mutations can be detected with a simple blood test.
- *Genetic counseling*: In X-linked genetic disease, the abnormal gene is carried on the X chromosome. Women have two X chromosomes; men have one X and one Y chromosome. While an abnormal recessive gene on one X chromosome will only make a female a carrier of a disease (since her other X is normal), a male will develop the disease because he does not have another X to balance the mutation.

Huntington's chorea

An autosomal dominant genetic disease, Huntington's chorea causes neurological deterioration in middle age, including chorea, or jerky movements.

- *Screening*: Physical examination usually reveals typical symptoms. Abnormal genes can be detected with a blood test.
- *Genetic counseling*: In autosomal dominant genetic diseases, dominant genes can cause disease if only one copy of the gene is abnormal. A parent with this disease has one abnormal gene and one normal gene. There is a 50/50 chance that each child will inherit the abnormal gene and have the disease.

Sickle cell disease

This disease changes the shape of the red blood cells from a perfect round doughnut shape into a crescent, or "sickle" shape, so that the red blood cells get stuck in tiny blood vessels, cutting off the blood supply to nearby tissues and causing pain. The abnormal red blood cells break down and cause anemia.

- *Screening*: Abnormal genes and gene mutations can be detected with a simple blood test.
- *Genetic counseling*: Sickle cell anemia is an autosomal recessive condition. In order for sickle cell anemia to occur, a sickle cell gene must be inherited from both the mother and the father. Inheriting one sickle gene is called sickle cell trait, a carrier state. Most common in families of African and African American descent.

Tay-Sachs disease

Tay-Sachs is a devastating neurological disease, in which a child faces progressive blindness, deafness, and paralysis. Death can ensue in early childhood.

- *Screening*: Abnormal genes and gene mutations can be detected with a simple blood test.
- *Genetic counseling*: Tay-Sachs is an autosomal recessive disease with mutations in both copies of the gene, most common in individuals of Ashkenazi Jewish, French Canadian, and Cajun descent.

Thalassemia

This group of blood disorders affects the hemoglobin molecule that carries oxygen in red blood, causing anemia. There are two main types of thalassemia: alpha and beta. Alpha thalassemia can have varying levels of severity. In the most severe form, fetal or newborn death results. Children with beta thalassemia may appear well at birth, but during the first year of life, they become pale and growth slows down.

- *Screening:* A simple blood test will reveal the alpha or beta thalassemia trait in parents. Testing can be done in utero to see if the baby has alpha or beta thalassemia.
- *Genetic counseling:* If only one parent is a carrier of a gene mutation associated with thalassemia and the other is not, the child may be a carrier but will not develop the disease. Most common in individuals of Mediterranean, Asian, and African descent.

Chronic health conditions

If you have a chronic condition pre-existing your pregnancy, you will certainly know the symptoms and will likely have a care plan in place. During pregnancy, these symptoms may flare and your management plan may need to be revised, especially any use of medications that could be harmful to the fetus. Some conditions present a higher risk than others to the fetus and to you. You will need to consult with your doctor before following any management plan, especially if medications are involved.

Asthma

Between 3% and 8% of pregnant women have chronic asthma, making it one of the most common medical conditions encountered in obstetric practice. As was the case before you were pregnant, it is important to have good lung function and prevent acute asthma attacks. Think about it this way — if you are having trouble breathing and getting enough oxygen, then so is the fetus. As always, the most important thing for a healthy baby is a healthy mother.

If your asthma gets worse, or you have any acute asthma attacks, they are most likely to occur in the second trimester. Very few women have an asthma attack during labor.

Managing asthma in pregnancy

- Ensure that your environment is as free of asthma triggers as possible.
- Don't smoke, or allow people around you to smoke.
- Avoid things you might be allergic to, such as pets and perfume.
- Avoid dust.
- Use protective covers on your pillows and mattress to avoid dust mites.
- Get a flu shot if you will be pregnant in winter months.
- If you have asthma, cooperate with your doctor in testing your lung function and monitoring your medications on a regular basis. Most of the commonly used asthma medications are safe for the fetus.

Asthma medications safe in pregnancy

- **Bronchodilators:** These medications relieve your acute sensation of wheezing or shortness of breath by relaxing your airways. A common example is Ventolin. Ideally, you will not need your bronchodilator very often if your asthma is well controlled, but if you do, you can feel comfortable that these medications are safe in pregnancy.
- **Corticosteroids:** Oral corticosteroids, such as prednisone, are generally considered safe to use in pregnancy, as are inhaled corticosteroids, used to reduce inflammation in the lungs. Common examples of inhaled corticosteroids include Pulmicort, Beclovent, and Flovent. Oral steroids, such as prednisone, are sometimes necessary if you have an acute exacerbation. Their use in the first trimester does increase the risk of cleft lip and palate. While there may be some risks associated with the use of oral steroids, in general, these risks are heavily outweighed by the benefit they confer.

Diabetes mellitus

If you have diabetes mellitus Type 1 or Type 2 before you become pregnant, you are probably an expert in monitoring and controlling your blood sugar levels. When you are pregnant, the job gets harder because of the action of placental hormones and the nutritional needs of the fetus.

Before the use of insulin, 50% of babies born to women with diabetes died late in pregnancy. With the excellent blood sugar control now achievable with insulin therapy, the numbers of babies who die before delivery has significantly decreased and is almost as low as in non-diabetic women.

Diabetes medications safe in pregnancy

- **Oral hypoglycemic agents:** Metformin and glyburide are being used increasingly during the first trimester, but are generally not considered good medications for use in diabetes during the second and third trimesters.

- **Insulin:** Insulin tends to achieve better control of the pregnant mother's blood sugars. In some cases, the pregnant woman may be switched from metformin or glyburide to insulin, which is safe in pregnancy. Women who are already on insulin may need to adjust their insulin doses, depending upon their diet and other circumstances, including whether they are suffering from nausea and vomiting.

Managing chronic diabetes mellitus in pregnancy

If you have Type 1 or Type 2 diabetes, you will need to be very active in managing your diabetes and your pregnancy, with guidance from your doctors, in order to minimize the risk of complications for you and your baby. Fortunately, with careful management, most women with diabetes are able to emerge from their pregnancy with a healthy baby — and as a healthy mother.

- **Blood sugar control:** If you have diabetes and are planning a pregnancy, the most important task is excellent control of blood sugar levels. If you use medications to control your diabetes, it is a good idea to switch to insulin before you become pregnant in order to ensure that your blood sugar control is stable before conception.

- **Complications control:** Your health needs to be evaluated carefully. Specifically, you need to be examined for indications of diabetes complications, including eye damage, nerve damage, hypertension, and heart disease. If you have any of these complications, the impact of pregnancy on the complications and their risk of progression in pregnancy need to be carefully considered.

- **Fetal monitoring:** The fetus will be closely monitored for growth and well-being.

Most of the birth defects associated with diabetes — typically involving the heart and the spinal canal — happen in the first 5 to 8 weeks of fetal development. Evidence suggests that careful control of blood sugar before conception and during the early weeks of pregnancy can greatly reduce, though not totally eliminate, the risk of these birth defects. Taking prenatal vitamins with folic acid before conception will also help.

For information on the management of pregnancy-induced gestational diabetes mellitus, see Part 6, Second Trimester Progress (page 226).

Higher-risk chronic conditions		
Chronic condition	Effect of condition on pregnancy	Effect of pregnancy on condition
Asthma	Small increases in risk of preterm labor, pre-eclampsia, and low birth weight	Conforms to the rule of thirds: One-third of women experience increased symptoms, one-third experience some improvement, and one-third experience no change in symptoms
Diabetes mellitus	Increased risk of caudal regression, spina bifida, miscarriage, pre-eclampsia, polyhydramnios, macrosomia, preterm birth, stillbirth, post-partum depression	Increased insulin requirements
Epilepsy	No effect from condition, but some anti-seizure medications increase risk of spina bifida and other neural tube defects and may have longer-term effects on a child's cognitive and neurologic function	No effect from pregnancy, but fatigue may contribute to seizures
Heart disease	If you were born with a congenital heart problem, your baby is at increased risk of also having a heart problem Preterm birth more common	Chronic heart disease can be made worse by pregnancy due to 50% increase in blood volume, making the heart work harder
Hypertension	Increased risk of placental abruption (placenta breaks off), preterm birth, fetal growth restriction, pre-eclampsia, and gestational diabetes	High risk of gestational hypertension and pre-eclampsia, with possible risk of developing diabetes
Mood disorders	Increased risk of preterm birth and complications	Increased severity of symptoms and higher risk of postpartum depression
Obesity	Increased risk of miscarriage, neural tube defects, gestational hypertension, gestational diabetes mellitus, preterm birth, high birth weight, delivery complications	Increased weight Can worsen complications of obesity (diabetes, hypertension)
Thyroid disorders: Hyperthyroidism	Increased risk of miscarriage, preterm birth, low birth weight, stillbirth	No effect on natural course of condition
Thyroid disorders: Hypothyroidism	Decreased fertility and increased risk of miscarriage and brain damage	No effect on natural course of condition

Epilepsy

Epilepsy is the most common neurologic disorder in pregnancy. All anti-epileptic drugs cross the placenta and some may harm the fetus. They will need to be replaced with safer choices. In general, most women with epilepsy do well in pregnancy, and so do their babies. Good medication planning, folic acid supplementation, and prenatal screening are important elements of good care.

Managing epilepsy in pregnancy

- If you are planning a pregnancy, discuss this with your neurologist so that it can be determined if you need to be on medications, and if so, which drugs pose the least risk to a fetus.

- If you are pregnant, medications need to be reviewed but not stopped. It's important not to precipitate a seizure.

- Because of the increased risk of birth defects, women on anti-seizure medication should take more folic acid than the general population of expectant mothers — 4 to 5 mg daily — for a few months prior to conception or as soon as you are aware of the pregnancy.

- Because there is some evidence that the mother's seizures may be harmful to the fetus, epilepsy management in pregnancy should aim to minimize the risk of seizures.

Epilepsy medications safe in pregnancy

- **Unsafe:** Drugs commonly used for seizures, including phenytoin, carbamazepine, phenobarbital, and valproic acid, have known effects on the fetus and should not be used in pregnancy.

- **Caution:** If these medications need to be used during pregnancy, they must be used with caution under the supervision of a physician. Newer anti-epileptic drugs, such as gabapentin and lamotrigine, cannot yet be recommended in pregnancy because there is not enough information on their fetal effects.

Heart disease

Chronic heart disease can be made worse by pregnancy. For example, if a woman had rheumatic fever as a child, she may have some narrowing of one or more of her heart valves. When she is not pregnant, she does not have heart problems, but in pregnancy, her blood volume increases by approximately 50%, making the heart work harder, particularly in the second trimester. This woman may develop signs of heart failure, making her pregnancy high-risk.

In other women, the rhythm of their heart is not steady, which again can be made worse by the increased blood flow in the heart during pregnancy. In this case, medication may be required to slow the heart down. In all cases, heart disease in a pregnant woman should be managed with the assistance of a cardiologist.

Managing heart disease in pregnancy

- If you were born with a congenital heart disease, your baby is at increased risk of also having a heart problem. It is important to share this information with your health-care providers (even if your problem is now fixed) so they can do a special ultrasound of the fetal heart (fetal echocardiography) before delivery.

- If you have acquired a heart disease (for example, valve disease due to rheumatic fever), this will not increase the risk of your fetus developing a heart problem.

- Treatment of your condition depends on the nature of your condition and its severity. You may be able to continue with your normal life, or, to minimize the overall risk to you and your fetus, you may need to stop working, rest in bed, or even be hospitalized for a time prior to labor.

- There may also be a greater need for help with child care after the birth.

- As always, adhering to a healthy lifestyle is a positive step. So watch your weight, get enough rest, eat properly, and avoid alcohol and tobacco.

- Exercise may or may not be advisable, depending on your situation. Consult your doctor for advice on exercise.

Cardiac medications safe in pregnancy

- Consult your health-care provider. There are many medications safe for use in treating cardiovascular conditions, and most are specific to the condition and the patient.

Chronic hypertension

Hypertension is similar to diabetes in that it can be a pre-existing condition (chronic hypertension) or can develop during pregnancy. If it develops during pregnancy, it is called pregnancy-induced hypertension (PIH) or gestational hypertension. Both chronic and gestational hypertension may progress to pre-eclampsia. If untreated, pre-eclampsia can cause dangerous seizures and even death. Hypertension can also lead to coronary disease, heart failure, stroke, and kidney failure. For more information on gestational hypertension and pre-eclampsia, see Part 8, Third Trimester Progress (page 291).

Higher risk

A pregnancy complicated by chronic hypertension is considered to be at higher risk for the mother and the fetus. Although most patients with mild hypertension do quite well and have healthy infants, high blood pressure can lead to placental complications and slowed fetal growth. These fetal risks are more frequent and more severe if hypertension is severely elevated as opposed to mildly elevated.

Managing chronic hypertension

- If you have chronic high blood pressure, seek medical counseling prior to becoming pregnant. Your blood pressure should be brought under control, and your medications changed to those that are safe to take during pregnancy.

- Severe chronic hypertension is treated with medications to reduce your blood pressure. It is less clear that mild hypertension should be treated with medications. You will need to discuss this with your doctor.

- If you are diagnosed with chronic hypertension while pregnant, your health-care provider will probably arrange for a few blood and urine tests to assess your kidney function, screen for diabetes, and monitor for pre-eclampsia.

- If you have not already done so, adopt a healthy lifestyle as soon as possible, including eating healthy foods, controlling your weight, exercising, and avoiding alcohol and tobacco.

Measuring hypertension

- Chronic hypertension is defined as blood pressure greater than or equal to 140/90 systolic/diastolic either before pregnancy begins or before the 20th week of pregnancy.

- Mild hypertension is defined as systolic BP in the range of 140 to 159 and diastolic BP in the range of 90 to 99 mmHg.

- Severe hypertension is defined as BP greater than 160/100 mmHg.

Fetal and maternal risks in chronic hypertension

Complication	Risk of complication developing from:	
	Mild chronic hypertension	Severe chronic hypertension
Placental abruption (placenta breaks off suddenly)	0.7% to 1.5%	5% to 10%
Preterm birth (at less than 37 weeks)	12% to 34%	62% to 70%
Fetal growth restriction	8% to 16%	31% to 40%

Hypertension medications safe in pregnancy

- Some women are on antihypertensive medications before pregnancy to control their blood pressure. Most of these medications are safe; however, some are associated with fetal abnormalities.

- If you are already taking a class of drugs called ACE inhibitors, you will need to switch to a safer drug, such as methyldopa, labetalol, or nifedipine, but be sure to consult with your doctor before making any changes.

Mood disorders

Pregnancy is assumed to be one of the happiest times in a woman's life, but 15% of women will develop a depressive or anxiety illness during pregnancy, and 50% of these cases go unrecognized and untreated. Depressed or anxious women may feel too ashamed or embarrassed to admit that they are having emotional struggles during this presumably happy period. In addition, physicians and other health-care providers may be too focused on the physical nature of the pregnancy and avoid direct questioning of the woman's mental health status. These women are left feeling significantly distressed and unable to cope.

Safe drugs for depression and psychosis

Major depression and schizophrenia are common during the reproductive years and often treated with medications. Some are safe, while fetal exposure to others is associated with fetal abnormalities, neonatal withdrawal, and long-term effects on the child. These issues need to be balanced with the risks to the mother of withdrawing the necessary medication.

Considered safe

- **Tricyclic antidepressants:** This class of antidepressants includes amytriptylline and nortriptylline. They are widely used to treat depression, anxiety, obsessive-compulsive disorders, migraines, and other problems. None of these drugs have been associated with congenital abnormalities when used in pregnancy.

- **Selective serotonin reuptake inhibitors (SSRIs):** These commonly used medications for depression and anxiety include fluoxetine (Prozac) and newer agents, such as fluvoxamine, paroxetine, and sertraline. Fluoxetine has been studied extensively and shown not to increase the risk of fetal abnormalities. Much less is known about the use of the newer agents during pregnancy, but none of the data suggest any negative effects. These agents have been generally considered safe for use during pregnancy.

- **Anti-psychotic medications:** Some anti-psychotic medications, such as chlorpromazine and haloperidol, may slightly increase the risk of fetal anomalies, but other types of anti-psychotic medications, such as olanzepine and risperidone, do not seem to increase the risk of anomalies, although the numbers studied are small.

Considered not safe

- **Monoamine oxidase inhibitors (MAOIs):** This is another class of medications used to treat depression. These groups of medications have not been studied enough to draw conclusions about their safety in pregnancy. Exposure should be avoided during pregnancy.

- **Mood stabilizers:** This class of drugs includes lithium, valproic acid, and carbamazepine, which have been identified as being associated with fetal abnormalities. They are not recommended for use during pregnancy, although for some women, their use is virtually unavoidable.

With caution

- **Anti-anxiety medications:** Valium and ativan have been associated with a slight increased risk of cleft lip after exposure during early pregnancy, but not a substantial risk, and may be used in pregnancy, but with caution.

Managing mood disorders in pregnancy

- Treatment for mood or anxiety disorders is required when the symptoms significantly interfere with daily functioning. Once a mood or anxiety disorder is diagnosed in pregnancy, it can be treated in a variety of ways.
- Every management plan should involve educating the mother and family about the symptoms, risk factors, and outcomes of the illness.
- Getting enough restful sleep is extremely important, as is added support from friends, family, and the community.
- Talk therapy is often helpful, with or without the addition of medication.
- If the symptoms become severe, some women will need to be referred to a mental health specialist (such as a perinatal psychiatrist).

Symptoms of clinical depression

The quality and severity of depression and anxiety in pregnancy differ from woman to woman. Typically, a pregnant woman with a mood or anxiety disorder will have five or more of the following symptoms:

- Depressed and/or irritable mood much of the time
- Bouts of crying
- Sleep disturbed by excessive worry
- Loss of appetite
- Anxiety or panic attacks
- Inability to take pleasure in anything
- Fatigue, apathy, loss of energy
- Loss of self-esteem or self-confidence
- Poor concentration
- Avoidance of social activities
- Frightening fantasies
- Excessive guilt
- Obsessive thoughts or behaviors
- Negative feelings about motherhood
- Regretful feelings about the pregnancy
- Suicidal thoughts or attempts

Masked symptoms

Differentiating normal mood changes in pregnancy from a clinical mood or anxiety disorder can be difficult. For example, insomnia, a hallmark of depression or anxiety, is a common experience, because many pregnant women have difficulty sleeping, especially in the third trimester, when they are physically uncomfortable.

In contrast, women with depression or anxiety cannot sleep because they cannot shut off their worries. Negative thoughts often interfere with the ability to fall asleep or stay asleep. In addition, physical symptoms, such as decreased appetite and lack of energy, may be seen as a normal part of pregnancy, especially if the woman is experiencing nausea or other medical problems. When the medical condition improves, she should start feeling better emotionally. If there is continued fatigue, lack of pleasure in activities, and social avoidance, she may be suffering from an underlying mental health disorder.

Obesity

In North America, obesity during pregnancy is becoming increasingly common. There are significant health risks related to being obese, and these are aggravated by pregnancy. If you are obese, you should attempt to lose some weight before becoming pregnant. Losing even as little as 5% to 10% of your body weight prior to pregnancy can help reduce the risk of serious complications.

Body mass index

To determine if you are overweight or obese, consult your health-care providers, who will help you calculate your body mass index (BMI), which is based on your weight and height. A BMI of 29.9 or more is considered obese. For more information on calculating your BMI, see Part 3, Eating Well for a Healthy Pregnancy (page 108).

Obesity risks in pregnancy

Before conception
- Reduced fertility and an increased risk of miscarriage

Once pregnant
- Increased risk of fetal congenital anomalies, particularly neural tube defects (spina bifida)
- Blood clots in your legs (deep vein thrombosis, or DVT)
- Gestational hypertension (high blood pressure in pregnancy)
- Pre-eclampsia (associated with the development of dangerously high blood pressure)
- Gestational diabetes

At birth
- Preterm birth
- High birth weight for gestational age
- Increased risk of labor problems, such as shoulder dystocia (obstructed delivery) or need for Caesarean section
- Increased surgical risk in obese women undergoing a Caesarean section

Managing your weight in pregnancy

- Before starting any diet or exercise program to lose weight before pregnancy and to manage your weight during pregnancy, consult with your doctor.
- For more information on healthy weight management, see Part 3: Eating Well for a Healthy Pregnancy (page 106) and Part 5: Exercising Safely in Pregnancy (page 166).

Thyroid conditions

Normal functioning of your thyroid gland is important throughout your life but has special importance in pregnancy for the mother and the fetus. If your thyroid is not functioning normally, you may have problems with your periods, you may have trouble conceiving, and you are more likely to miscarry if you do conceive. Postpartum, some women develop thyroid problems even if they have never had any before. Thyroid hormone is also essential to a developing fetus.

Hypothyroidism and hyperthyroidism

There are two types of thyroid disease: an underactive thyroid (hypothyroidism) and an overactive thyroid (hyperthyroidism). There is some evidence that the children of women with hypothyroidism have impaired neuropsychological development, even if the hypothyroidism is only subclinical (meaning hormone levels are low but not low enough for you to have obvious symptoms).

The most common cause of hyperthyroidism is Grave's disease, an autoimmune disease in which antibodies produced by your own body attack the thyroid, leading to excess release of thyroid hormone, although there can be other causes. An overactive thyroid gland produces too much thyroid hormone, which can have significant effects upon both how you feel and your pregnancy. If untreated, hyperthyroidism increases the risk of pregnancy loss, preterm delivery, low birth weight, and pre-eclampsia.

Screening

Because thyroid disorders are so common in women in general, some doctors use blood tests to screen for thyroid disease during pregnancy, so it is possible that you may be diagnosed for a thyroid condition even if you feel fine.

Managing thyroid conditions in pregnancy

Hyperthyroidism

- If you are diagnosed with hyperthyroidism, you will need to be treated by an endocrinologist.
- You will most likely be prescribed medications to control the amount of thyroid hormone produced.
- You may also need medication to lower your heart rate if you are having significant palpitations.
- In addition, your baby will need to be monitored for signs of thyroid disease after delivery, because some of the antibodies that act on your thyroid gland can cross the placenta and affect the baby's thyroid gland, too.

Hypothyroidism

- You should have your thyroid hormone blood levels measured frequently: at around 6 weeks gestational age, 4 weeks after any dose changes, and at least every trimester.
- If you are hypothyroid before you get pregnant, you are probably taking thyroid hormone pills (L-thyroxine). This medication is safe in pregnancy and breastfeeding, so you should continue taking it.
- About 75% or more of women with hypothyroidism in pregnancy will need to increase their dose of thyroid hormone in pregnancy, sometimes as early as the second month of their first trimester. Some doctors will advise you to increase your dose by 30% by taking an extra tablet 2 days a week, and then measuring your response to this a month later.
- After you deliver, you can probably return to your pre-pregnancy dose, but make sure you have your blood levels checked before making any changes.

Viral and bacterial infections

An infection occurs when your body is invaded by a bacteria, virus, fungus, or parasite. Some infections, such as the common cold, the flu, or stomach flu, will make you miserable for a short while but have no long-lasting impact upon your health or your baby. Normal precautions such as hand washing, flu shots, and taking care with local food and water will protect you.

Other infections, such as hepatitis B or HIV, may have few initial symptoms but be long-lasting and have life-threatening implications for both you and your baby. Unfortunately, pregnancy does not make you immune to the many bugs lurking in the environment, and you will come into contact with some of them. With some preparations and precautions, you can reduce, even avoid, your exposure to infections.

Fetal vs. maternal risk

When you have an infection during pregnancy, you must consider the impact of the infection on both you and the fetus. Sometimes, you will be just fine, maybe even barely notice the infection, but the microorganism can cause serious harm to the fetus, as in the case of toxoplasmosis (from a parasite picked up from cats). Sometimes health-care providers screen for a particular infection because identification and treatment will significantly reduce fetal risk. For example, medical treatment of HIV-infected mothers can significantly reduce the risk that the baby develops HIV. Some infections, such as influenza and varicella, pose more serious risks to women when they are pregnant.

Hepatitis C

Hepatitis C is a chronic infection transmitted by exposure to contaminated blood. In North America, transmission typically occurs through intravenous drug use and sharing of contaminated needles, as well as through contaminated blood transfusions, although blood used for transfusions is now tested for hepatitis C. It can also be sexually transmitted. In other parts of the world, transmission has also been reported to occur when medical equipment is not properly sterilized.

Maternal risk

Although most women with this infection do well in pregnancy — one study suggested that pregnancy may even slow the progression of liver disease — many people infected with hepatitis C will develop liver disease decades later.

Fetal risk

Hepatitis C is passed on to the baby in about 5% of affected pregnancies. Liver injury tends to be very mild in the first 20 years following infection for these children.

If you have hepatitis C and are breastfeeding, there is no risk of transmission of the infection to the baby through your breast milk. Caesarean section is not advised as a means to prevent infection, because it has not been shown to reduce transmission rates.

Managing exposure to hepatitis C in pregnancy

- Avoid intravenous drug use and sharing of contaminated needles.
- Avoid having casual unprotected sex. Use a condom.

Influenza

Although we commonly refer to the symptoms of fever, cough, and runny nose as "the flu," most of these infections are actually probably just a cold. Influenza tends to be more serious and last longer than a cold caused by a milder virus. The muscle aches and fever can be much more profound than with a cold.

Managing influenza in pregnancy

- Help prevent the flu by being vaccinated each year.
- Get plenty of rest and fluids.
- If your condition seems to deteriorate, particularly if you are having increasing trouble breathing, seek emergency care.

Maternal risk only

The risk of complications from influenza is higher than in the case of a cold, especially in pregnant women. In flu epidemics in the early and mid-20th century, pregnant women were among those who suffered the most from influenza, with high rates of mortality. Pregnant women are at higher risk of such complications as hospitalization and pneumonia. Fortunately, influenza does not seem to have any fetal effects. Your unborn baby is well protected inside of you.

Flu vaccine benefits

Flu viruses mutate rapidly, and, every year, an influenza vaccine is developed to combat the viruses in circulation. This vaccine is not only safe in pregnancy, it is highly advised. Using the vaccine will reduce the chance that you develop influenza, although it is unable to prevent it 100%. If you do develop influenza, and you have had the vaccine, the infection may be less severe.

You can protect your newborn from influenza, which could be very serious, by getting the flu shot and by encouraging other people who will be around the baby to be vaccinated. This will create a protective immunity in the people close to the baby.

Parvovirus

Also known as slapped cheek or fifth disease, parvovirus causes a non-specific flu-like illness, which you might just consider to be a cold. Sometimes, it causes no symptoms at all, but 25% of people infected with parvovirus will develop a rash or joint inflammation. The rash is much more common in children than in adults. The rash looks as if the person affected has red cheeks, hence the name "slapped cheek," and sometimes progresses to a lacy-looking rash on the trunk and limbs. Like so many infections, the infection is at its most contagious the week before the rash appears.

Managing parvovirus exposure

If you find out there is a parvovirus outbreak in your home, local school, or workplace, take the following steps to reduce your chances of becoming infected.

- Have your blood drawn to test your immune status.
- If you are not immune, decide whether or not to keep your other children or yourself away from the infected environment.
- If your child has the virus, reduce exposure by practicing good hygiene. This virus is carried on droplets, like the common cold, so wash your hands frequently, encourage the rest of the household to wash their hands frequently, and do not share food, cups, or dishes. Ask someone else in the household to take over care of the infected child.

Fetal risks

Although parvovirus does not cause any congenital defects in babies who have been exposed, it increases the risk of miscarriage and anemia.

- Miscarriage: Studies have shown that up to 15% of women infected with parvovirus before 20 weeks of pregnancy will miscarry. After 20 weeks, the risk of fetal loss is much lower, less than 3%.

- Anemia and hydrops: In about 1% of infected fetuses, the virus can attack developing blood cells, causing these cells to die, leading the baby to develop anemia. The fetus can then develop a condition called hydrops, which is associated with swelling of many different tissues in the fetus, and, sometimes, fetal death. Fortunately, the incidence of fetal death has been significantly reduced in recent years. If parvovirus is suspected, your doctor will arrange for you to have frequent ultrasound tests to detect hydrops. If hydrops is detected, it is now possible to give the fetus a blood transfusion while you are pregnant.

Exposure risk

Children are the most common source of parvovirus, so pregnant women who have small children at home or who care for small children in their work are at the highest risk of exposure. If someone in your household is infected, there is about a 50% chance that a non-immune person will become infected herself. If a child in a teacher's classroom is infected, there is a 20% to 30% chance the teacher will become infected. The chance of a mother passing the infection on to her fetus is 20% to 30%.

There is nothing that can be done to treat the infection; it will resolve on its own. Nor is there any vaccine for the virus. Once you have had parvovirus, you are immune. Most people are infected as children. Immunity can be detected with a blood test. About 60% to 70% of pregnant women are found to be immune to parvovirus.

Rubella

If you have rubella (German measles) during pregnancy, there is a very good chance of passing the infection on to your fetus. If the infection occurs before 16 weeks, there is a chance the fetus will develop congenital anomalies in hearing, vision, and the heart. After 16 weeks, these anomalies are unlikely to occur, but there may be slow intrauterine growth and neurological problems. Fortunately, because most of the population is immunized, outbreaks of rubella are rare and even the non-immune woman will be safe.

If you contract rubella, you can expect to have a mild, flu-like illness that progresses to a red rash. There is usually no treatment required other than acetaminophen. Take care to avoid contact with pregnant women.

Managing rubella exposure

- If you are planning a pregnancy, make getting immunized against rubella a high priority. Most women in the United States and Canada are immunized against rubella as children, but occasionally, the immunity wears off. Your health-care providers will test your rubella immunity early in your pregnancy, and if your vaccine seems to have worn off, you will be offered a booster shot, but not until after the birth of your baby.
- Women arriving in the country after childhood or children who have been adopted internationally should have their immunization status checked and upgraded as necessary.
- Because the rubella vaccine is a live, attenuated vaccine (meaning it is a live virus, but one that has been altered so as not to induce illness, just immunity), it should not be given to pregnant women. If your pregnancy is confirmed shortly after getting a rubella vaccine, do not worry. Congenital rubella syndrome has never been reported after a vaccination.
- All women who are not immune in pregnancy should be vaccinated post-partum.

Bacterial vaginosis

Although uncomfortable, this bacterial infection poses limited risk to the fetus. Bacterial vaginosis (BV) is associated with an abnormal vaginal discharge, often with a fishy smell, that may be worse after sex, but BV can be present and you can have no symptoms. Although having new or multiple sexual partners is a risk factor for the condition, it is not generally believed to be sexually transmitted. The infection itself represents an overgrowth of bacteria that are normally present in the vagina at much lower levels, although why this happens is not well understood. If you are concerned that you have BV, a vaginal examination and assessment of the discharge will be able to diagnose it.

Managing bacterial vaginosis

- In general, if you have no symptoms, there is no need to treat BV, because eventually the bacterial balance in your vagina will normalize.
- If you have symptoms, antibiotic treatment is available.
- Because a connection has been made between preterm birth and bacterial vaginosis, you may be screened and treated for BV in pregnancy, especially if you have had a previous premature delivery.

Varicella

While planning your pregnancy, check to be sure you are immune to the varicella virus, commonly known as chicken pox, to protect yourself and your child. While many of us have this image of chicken pox as a fairly benign childhood disease characterized by an itchy red rash, it can be more serious in adults, and even more so in pregnant women. The fetus may also be infected.

Maternal risk

Potentially serious complications of chicken pox for pregnant women include lung, liver, and brain infections. A pregnant woman who develops complications of chicken pox, particularly pneumonia, is more likely to be very seriously ill than her non-pregnant counterpart.

Fetal and newborn risk

Congenital varicella syndrome is associated with maternal chicken pox infection in the first and second trimester and involves scarring of the skin, abnormal limb development, developmental delay, and eye problems in the child. Fortunately, this syndrome occurs in less than 1% of pregnancies affected by chicken pox. A further risk occurs when mothers develop chicken pox in the few days prior to delivery and up to 2 to 3 days after delivery. The newborn baby has a high chance of acquiring chickenpox and becoming seriously ill.

Managing exposure to varicella

- If you are not immune, plan to get vaccinated at least 1 month before you begin your pregnancy.

- If you are exposed to someone who develops chicken pox shortly after you become pregnant and you are not immune, you should be very concerned about your risk and the baby's risk of infection.

- Because the vaccine to protect against chicken pox is not safe for pregnant women, your doctor may prescribe varicella antibodies (known as VariZIG), which can help prevent you from getting the infection.

- Act quickly if you think you have been exposed and you lack immunity, because the VariZIG must be given within 96 hours of exposure in order to be effective.

- If you develop chicken pox, an antiviral mediation called acyclovir may be prescribed in an effort to reduce the severity of the disease.

- If you are in the first or second trimester, it is generally advised to have fairly frequent ultrasound monitoring of your pregnancy to determine whether the fetus has developed congenital varicella syndrome. The incidence of this syndrome is low, and your health-care providers can recommend a course of action if it should develop.

Yeast infections

During pregnancy, increased estrogen levels seem to make women more prone to developing a vulvar or vaginal yeast infection. The most common symptom is vulvar itching, soreness, and irritation. Sometimes there is some pain when you urinate. Sometimes there is a vaginal discharge associated with yeast infections, and although it can often be thick, white and clumpy, it can also have other appearances. If you have any doubt about your symptoms, see your health-care provider, who can examine you and perform a simple vaginal swab to confirm the diagnosis. Rest assured that although vaginal yeast infections are a nuisance, they will not harm your baby.

Managing yeast infections

It can be difficult to eliminate these infections completely in pregnancy, so the focus is usually on symptom control. The treatments advised in pregnancy are all intravaginal.

- Use a 7-day intravaginal treatment. The 1-day and 3-day treatments are often not long enough.

- Commonly used medications considered to be safe in pregnancy for intravaginal use include miconazole, clotrimazole, and terconazole. In most jurisdictions, these medications are available over the counter, without a prescription.

- If you are fairly confident that your symptoms are related to yeast, go ahead and treat yourself, but be sure to let your health-care providers know at your next visit.

- If you are unsure for any reason, see your health-care providers for an examination.

Sexually transmitted diseases

Some infections are transmitted sexually, not only from partner to partner, but also from the infected mother to the fetus, with serious outcomes for your baby. If you do not have a sexually transmitted disease (STD) prior to pregnancy, continue to protect yourself and avoid high-risk behaviors, such as unprotected sex. (Use a latex condom.) If you have an STD, be aware that some of these infections can be transmitted to the fetus, with serious consequences. If you suspect or know that you have an STD, talk to your health-care providers immediately to arrange for screening and suitable treatment.

Reportable infections

In many jurisdictions, STDs are "reportable infections," which means that the lab must notify your local public health department about your infection. You or your health-care providers may be contacted by a public health nurse to ensure that you have been treated and your sexual partners are tested and treated. If you do not wish to contact your sexual partners, someone from public health will often do so for you without revealing the source of their information. This seems intrusive but is done to protect the general population.

Chlamydia

This STD is becoming more and more common in the population, particularly among younger women, with serious outcomes for the mother and baby.

Maternal risk

Chlamydia infects the cervix. If symptoms are present, you may have an abnormal vaginal discharge, painful urination, abdominal

Managing chlamydia in pregnancy

- **Screening:** In both men and women, chlamydia is often asymptomatic, so it is important to be screened to see whether or not you have the infection. Chlamydia can be detected with a swab taken from the cervix, often at the time of your Pap smear at your first prenatal visit to your doctor.

- **Antibiotics:** If you are found to have chlamydia, it will be treated with antibiotics that are safe in pregnancy. Your partner also needs to be tested and treated if necessary.

- **Test of cure:** Don't have intercourse until both of you have been treated, because otherwise you can pass the infection back and forth. You should also have a "test of cure," that is, a repeat swab to ensure that the treatment was successful.

- **Condom:** Transmission of chlamydia can be prevented by using a latex condom during sex, so use one every time, even if you are already pregnant.

pain, or pain with sex. You may also have abnormal vaginal bleeding. Some people develop an inflammation in their eyes called conjunctivitis. If chlamydia is untreated, it can progress from being a simple cervical infection to a much more serious infection involving your fallopian tubes, ovaries, and pelvis, called pelvic inflammatory disease (PID), which is a major cause of blocked tubes and infertility, as well as ectopic pregnancy. Pelvic inflammatory disease in pregnancy can also be associated with preterm labor and delivery

Baby risk

If you have chlamydia at the time of delivery, there is up to a 50% chance that you will pass the infection on to your baby. A baby who develops chlamydia can be quite sick. Up to 20% of these babies will develop pneumonia, and up to 20% will develop conjunctivitis.

Genital warts

The human papilloma virus (HPV) causes genital warts. There are many different types of HPV viruses — you may have heard about some types that are associated with abnormal Pap smears and even with cervical cancer — but the types associated with genital warts do not cause cancer. The warts appear as pink or skin-colored bumps, often with a raised and rough surface, around your vaginal opening or on your labia. They can also appear around your anus. The warts can appear weeks to months or even more than a year after you were exposed to the virus. Unfortunately, condoms do not protect you very well from getting genital warts from your partner or from giving them to your partner, because they tend to grow in places the condom doesn't cover.

Mother and baby risk

In pregnancy, genital warts can multiply, grow bigger, and become more sensitive. If this happens, don't worry, because the warts usually regress again after pregnancy.

There is a very small risk of passing the HPV virus on to your baby at the time of vaginal delivery, but most of the time, even if the HPV virus is passed on, the baby is not affected. Occasionally, the child can develop

Managing genital warts in pregnancy

- Warts can be treated with the application of various substances to the wart, but only one of these chemicals is safe in pregnancy — trichloroacetic acid (TCA). Alternatives include using liquid nitrogen (or cryotherapy) on the wart, or removing the lesion with a laser or with surgery.

- We do not know if performing a Caesarean section will reduce the chances of passing HPV on to a baby, so Caesarean section is not advised. However, if the warts are so large that they seem to be blocking the vaginal outlet, or if there is a concern that there will be a lot of bleeding from the warts at vaginal delivery, a Caesarean birth might be recommended.

Managing gonorrhea in pregnancy

- If you suspect you have gonorrhea, get tested with a cervical swab.

- If positive, you will be treated with antibiotics that are safe in pregnancy, if necessary.

- Make sure that your sexual partners are tested and treated, and that you have a test of cure to ensure that you have eliminated the infection before you have intercourse again.

- Like chlamydia, the transmission of gonorrhea can be prevented by using a latex condom during sex, every time, even if you are already pregnant.

warts as well, generally in the anal-genital region and sometimes on the vocal cords. Occasionally, children exposed to HPV in this way will develop breathing problems if the lesions spread in the lungs (recurrent respiratory papillomatosis).

Gonorrhea

Like chlamydia, gonorrhea is a reportable infection, and like chlamydia, gonorrhea is becoming increasingly common in our population, especially in younger women.

Mother and baby risk

If you have gonorrhea, you may have an abnormal vaginal discharge, painful urination, or pelvic pain. You may also have a sore throat, conjunctivitis, or more serious problems, such as inflammation of your joints, heart, skin, or brain tissues. If you pass gonorrhea on to your baby during your pregnancy, your newborn baby could develop a very serious eye infection or even a widespread infection, affecting almost every body system.

Hepatitis B

In North America, hepatitis B is usually a sexually transmitted disease, although it can also be passed on via contaminated blood, typically in IV drug users who share needles.

Managing hepatitis B in pregnancy

- Because you can carry hepatitis B without knowing it, all pregnant women should be screened for this infection.
- If the mother is hepatitis B negative, but other people living in the baby's family are hepatitis B positive, vaccination is recommended for the mother and her newborn baby.
- Theoretically, hepatitis B can be passed to the fetus at any time during the pregnancy, but most cases of transmission occur around the time of birth. To prevent transmission, all babies born to mothers with hepatitis B should receive immunoglobulin with special antibodies against hepatitis B and a vaccination at birth. This prevents 95% of hepatitis B infections in newborns.
- Provided that the baby has been vaccinated, it is safe to breastfeed.

In other parts of the world where hepatitis B infection is more common, hepatitis B is more likely to be transmitted through household contact with an infected person. For example, small breaks in the skin can lead to infection if someone in the household is infectious. Contact with the personal articles of an infected person, such as a razor or toothbrush, can also lead to transmission. Hepatitis B is also commonly transmitted from mother to child at birth.

Chronic carriers

This infection can persist in a lifelong, or chronic, state for many people. Chronic carriers of hepatitis B may have no symptoms, but are still able to transmit the infection to others, including the fetus or newborn. Some of these people will go on to develop liver disease later in life.

Fortunately, pregnancy seems to have no impact on the progression of hepatitis B in the mother, and hepatitis B has no impact on the pregnancy apart from the concern about neonatal infection.

Herpes

Genital herpes is a common viral infection in the population as a whole. The most obvious symptoms are blisters and sores in the genital region. The first infection is generally the worst, but, unfortunately, it can recur. Some people have recurrences monthly, while some people have them much less frequently. Outbreaks can continue to occur in pregnancy and, for some women, are more frequent in pregnancy. If you have your first herpes outbreak near term, there is a slight chance of passing the virus to the fetus through the bloodstream before labor, as well as passing it on during a vaginal delivery.

Baby risk

The chance of passing the virus to the baby at term depends upon whether or not the outbreak is a first outbreak or a recurrence. At a first outbreak, the chance of passing the infection on to the baby is 30% to 40%, but only 1% to 2% at the time of recurrences.

Babies infected with herpes can have different patterns of infection. About a third of babies will have herpes limited to their skin, eyes, and mouth. About a third will have herpes limited to their central nervous system. And about a third will have disseminated herpes affecting many organ systems.

Managing herpes in pregnancy

- Medication is available to prevent an outbreak during pregnancy. Acyclovir is considered safe, while valacyclovir and famcyclovir are probably safe, but there are less long-term data to support their use. You can also take acyclovir every day from about 36 weeks on to reduce the risk that you will have an active sore at the time of delivery.
- Most cases of transmission to the fetus happen at the time of delivery when the baby passes over a lesion in the vagina or on the vulva. If you have an active lesion at the time of delivery, your doctor will probably recommend a Caesarean section.

Human immunodeficiency virus

Human immunodeficiency virus, commonly known as HIV, is transmitted by exposure to body fluids contaminated with HIV, particularly semen and blood. Most women in North America infected with HIV have been infected through sexual contact. Infection with HIV cannot be cured, but it can be controlled with medications that slow the progress of the disease. Some people infected with HIV will develop AIDS, or acquired immunodeficiency syndrome, in which the immune system is unable to fight off infections and certain types of cancers. HIV in pregnancy is complicated, and infected women should be cared for medically by an obstetrician and a specialist in HIV.

Syphilis

This dangerous STD is, unfortunately, becoming more prevalent in some places. Usually, it causes a sore or an ulcer in the genital region, but not always. It is often followed months later by a rash, fever, and flu-like symptoms. Eventually, symptoms resolve on their own, even without treatment, but decades later, if syphilis is never detected

Managing syphilis in pregnancy

- Screening: Because of the severity of fetal infection, screening for syphilis is one of the routine blood tests in pregnancy.
- Penicillin: Syphilis is quite easily treated with penicillin. If you are allergic to penicillin, you will need to see an allergist to test for a true allergy and possibly for a desensitization program, because there are no other effective treatments.

or treated, people can end up with neurologic disease, including dementia, and heart disease.

Fetal risk

The fetal impact of syphilis can also be severe, causing premature delivery, congenital anomalies, low birth weight, and even fetal death. Babies who survive can be born with syphilis infections. Most potential cases of syphilis in newborn babies can be prevented if the infection is diagnosed and treated; for example, at least 80% of babies born to mothers with untreated syphilis will be affected, versus only 1% to 2% of babies born to mothers treated properly in pregnancy.

Managing HIV infection in pregnancy

- Screening: Because the initial infection with HIV often passes without many symptoms, women may be infected with HIV and not be aware of it when they become pregnant. The disease can be passed on to the fetus or newborn at delivery. For this reason, it is now advised that all pregnant women be screened for HIV infection early in pregnancy. That way, mothers with HIV can be diagnosed and treated, significantly reducing the chances that their babies will be born infected.
- Medications: Anti-HIV medications in pregnancy and at birth can reduce the risk that the baby of an HIV-infected mother develops HIV from 15% to 25% to under 2%. This treatment can literally save a baby's life. Some women know that they are HIV positive and

either become pregnant or wish to become pregnant. Because the current medications are so effective at reducing transmission to the baby, these women can now plan and undergo a pregnancy without worrying too much that they are passing on HIV to their baby.

- Breastfeeding concerns: Breastfeeding is generally not advised in women who are HIV positive because there is a chance of passing the infection through breast milk. In some parts of the world, such as Africa, where there is a great concern about clean water, HIV positive women do breastfeed their babies, but in North America, where you usually don't have to worry about cholera and other bacteria in the water supply, the baby is safer drinking formula.

Trichomonas

This STD typically causes an abnormal vaginal discharge, associated with burning and discomfort, as well as pain when urinating and sometimes pain with sex. If untreated, it can progress to a more serious infection affecting your uterus and fallopian tubes. In pregnancy, the principal concern is an association with premature rupture of the membranes. Trichomonas can be treated with antibiotics; your sexual partner should be treated as well.

Medications

Most over-the-counter (OTC) and prescription medications are safe in pregnancy, but some are known to be harmful to the fetus, especially when taken in the early weeks while the essential organs and body parts are developing. Your doctor will be able to prescribe safe substitutes in many cases. However, botanical medicines, or herbs, cannot be reliably classified as safe or unsafe because of limited scientific research. These medications are best avoided in pregnancy until their safety is proven.

Common drugs unsafe in pregnancy
Acne drugs

Sometimes, severe acne is treated orally with Accutane, or isotretinoin. Accutane can cause severe birth defects in exposed fetuses and should not be taken without very good contraceptive measures being used at the same time. You should not get pregnant for at least 1 month after stopping Accutane. Face creams or solutions that contain retinoids, such as tazarotene (Tazorac) and adapalene (Differin), should be not be used during pregnancy. Lotions that do not contain retinoids, such as benzoyl peroxide, are safe. Sometimes antibiotics are used in the treatment of acne; if this seems warranted, oral erythromycin is safe, as is oral or topical clindamycin.

Psoriasis drugs

Psoriasis is a skin condition that can vary greatly in severity. Mild cases can continue to be managed with topical corticosteroid creams. More severe cases are often managed with the use of retinoids, such as tazarotene, but this drug should not be used during pregnancy. Other systemic treatments include methotrexate, but, again, do not use treatments containing this agent during pregnancy.

A number of other immunosuppressive and immune modulator drugs may be advised; you should have a discussion with your dermatologist about the safety of these drugs in pregnancy before using them at this time. For many of these drugs, there are very few data about their safety in pregnancy.

Common drugs safe in pregnancy

Despite the long list of drugs and herbs to avoid in pregnancy, most over-the-counter and prescription medications pose no threat to the well-being of the mother and the fetus. These safe medications are often an integral part of your medical care and your baby's care. In looking for safe medications for various common conditions, see the partial list provided here, as well as *The Complete Guide to Everyday Risks in Pregnancy and Breastfeeding* from the Hospital for Sick Children (Toronto, ON: Robert Rose, 2004).

Pain killers

Acetaminophen is safe for headache, back pain, and other pain conditions in pregnancy. If stronger medications are needed, narcotics, such as codeine and morphine, are safe to use in pregnancy.

Antihistamines

Most antihistamines are safe in pregnancy and can be used for cold symptoms, as well as for hay fever and environmental allergies. Such medications include Benadryl and Atarax, both of which are safe to use in pregnancy.

Decongestants

The most commonly used oral decongestants include pseudoephedrine and phenylephedrine. These are felt to be safe in pregnancy. Topical nasal decongestant sprays, such as Otrivin, are also safe for use in pregnancy.

Cough suppressants

The most common cough suppressants are codeine and dextromethorphan, both of which are safe to use in pregnancy.

Antibiotics

Antibiotics are widely used in pregnancy to treat a variety of bacterial infections, including upper respiratory infections and urinary tract infections. Although almost all antibiotics cross the placenta, most are felt to be safe in pregnancy, except for ciprofloxacin, chloramphenicol, and tetracycline, which have been associated with congenital anomalies. Your health-care provider can prescribe a safe alternative.

Antifungals

Pregnant women can be particularly susceptible to vulvo-vaginal fungal infections, or yeast infections, after treatment with an antibiotic. Yeast infections can be easily and safely treated with a topical vaginal yeast preparation. Many of these preparations are available over the counter and contain common antifungal treatments, such as clotrimazole, miconazole, or nystatin. These agents are safe to use in the vagina during pregnancy, if taken as directed. Some of these agents, such as terazol, are given by prescription.

Anti-inflammatories

A number of creams and suppositories are available to help with the discomfort associated with hemorrhoids, all of which are safe during pregnancy. These agents include Anusol, Anugesic, and Proctosydl. Some products have additional hydrocortisone,

Unsafe drugs in pregnancy	
Antibiotics	Ciprofloxacin Chloramphenicol Tetracycline
Anticoagulants	Warfarin
Antifungal drugs	Griseofulvin Ketoconazole Itraconazole Triazoles Fluconazole, Terbinafine
Anti-inflammatory drugs	NSAIDs (3rd trimester) Colchicine
Antiparasitic drugs	Mebendazole
Cardiovascular drugs	Angiotensin-converting enzyme ACE inhibitors Angiotensin II inhibitors – Losartan
Chemotherapy drugs	Busulphan Cyclophosphamide Methotrexate
Endocrinological drugs	Radioactive iodine Sex hormones Octreotide
Thalidomide	
Vitamin A analogues	Etretinate Isotretinoin
Others	Misoprostol Mefloquine Statins Biphosphonates

an anti-inflammatory that helps with the inflammation of hemorrhoids. These are safe in pregnancy, but avoid NSAIDs (third trimester) and colchicine. Prednisone is also considered safe, especially after the first trimester.

Common cold remedies

There is no medication that will make a cold better. Most over-the-counter cold remedies have not been shown to have much benefit for managing symptoms or shortening their duration. In general, if you can manage your symptoms without medications, it is better to do so while pregnant. However, if you do wish to take a medication for your symptoms, choose carefully. Cough medicines containing iodine should be avoided because the iodine can impair the development of the thyroid gland in the fetus and thyroid functioning in the newborn.

Rash remedies

Certain conditions in pregnancy can cause itching of the skin. In addition to a good skin moisturizer, such as an Aveeno oatmeal bath, Benadryl or other antihistamines are safe for use in pregnancy. Serious rashes in pregnancy can be treated with topical hydrocortisone creams and by oral antihistamines to relieve the itchiness. If you develop a rash or itching in pregnancy, be sure to discuss this with your health-care provider.

Drug-free alternatives for common ailments

During pregnancy, most women should try to avoid as many non-essential medicines as possible. Here is a list of drug-free remedies for the treatment of common ailments:

Headaches or backaches

A head or neck massage can help relieve headache, while gentle stretching to relieve tight muscles can ease backache. Soaking in a warm bath can also work wonders.

Constipation

Drink more fluids and add more fiber (whole wheat bread, vegetables, fruit) to your diet. Bulking agents, such as bran, are safe. Put a few spoonfuls on your morning cereal.

Hay fever and allergies

Try to reduce your exposure to the allergens that trigger your reaction.

Coughs and colds

Try steam inhalations — they can help liquefy mucus, making it easier to cough up. Honey or glycerol cough lozenges coat the throat and are a safe cough-reducing option. Irrigation of your nasal and sinus passages can be undertaken with OTC saline solutions in order to minimize the risk of a sinus infection.

Complementary and alternative remedies

Complementary and alternative medications include vitamin and mineral supplements, herbal remedies (including teas), and botanical medicines. They are often called natural medicines, but this does not always mean they are safe, especially in pregnancy.

Vitamins and minerals

Use of prenatal multivitamins, often with supplemental iron, calcium, and folic acid, is commonly advocated by many health-care providers. These vitamins and minerals are not only considered generally safe, but, in the case of folic acid, protective against congenital abnormalities. Supplementation of iron in women who are iron deficient (anemic) can be helpful in improving their iron stores in preparation for blood loss at delivery. Calcium is also beneficial in women during pregnancy and breastfeeding.

Vitamin A caution

Vitamin A is the only vitamin that, when consumed at levels of more than 10,000 IU daily, can cause congenital abnormalities. If you are taking vitamin A, do not to exceed 5000 IU each day in supplement form.

Botanical and herbal medicines

Botanical or herbal remedies include traditional Western and traditional Chinese herbal medicine, as well as Indian (ayurvedic) and Native American herbal medicines. These products do not require a prescription. However, there is not enough scientific information about the safety of various herbal products to recommend their use during pregnancy and breastfeeding. The safety and effectiveness of even common herbal products containing echinacea, ginseng, evening primrose oil, and St. John's wort has not yet been established in clinical studies.

Did You Know?

Safety concerns

What we do know is that some herbal remedies contain chemicals that are as potent as prescription drugs — and that some can be dangerous to both you and your growing baby. Some herbal medications (such as dong quai and blue cohosh) are believed to cause uterine contractions. Sometimes, it might be desirable to cause uterine contractions with one of these medications (for example, if you are overdue), but using these uncontrolled and unregulated medications in an unsupervised setting is a dangerous way to go about an induction of labor.

Other herbal remedies can change the way prescription drugs work, interacting with them and causing serious side effects. Herbal medications are not regulated and controlled the way pharmaceutical products are, so different preparations of the same herb may contain varying amounts of the active chemicals. Because of these safety concerns, we advise pregnant women to avoid herbal remedies.

Environmental exposures in pregnancy

Pregnant women and their families usually want to learn what they can do to help minimize risks. A good place to start is by becoming aware of the elements of our environment that can potentially cause harm to a developing fetus, collectively known as teratogens, and then to avoid these risks or minimize exposure.

Teratogens tend to have variable effects upon developing fetuses, ranging from no effect to causing serious problems. This variability can be explained by different genetic susceptibilities, the timing of exposure (usually, first trimester is worst), the dose of the agent, and the length of exposure. For more information on environmental risks, see *The Complete Guide to Everyday Risks in Pregnancy & Breastfeeding* from the Motherisk Program at the Hospital for Sick Children (Toronto, ON: Robert Rose, 2004).

Lifestyle risks

Many women are accustomed to drinking alcohol, some women smoke, and a few use recreational drugs and drugs of abuse. These habits place the fetus at varying degrees of risk before you become pregnant. Try to break any lifestyle habits that put the fetus at increased risk of developing abnormalities.

Alcohol

There is no known safe level of alcohol consumption in pregnancy. National health agencies in the United States and Canada advise abstinence from alcohol during pregnancy, including early pregnancy (when you might not even know you are pregnant). Alcohol in your bloodstream passes through the placenta into the much smaller fetus in equivalent concentrations.

Recreational drugs and drugs of abuse

There is very little data about the impact of recreational drugs, such as marijuana, cocaine, methamphetamine, and heroin, on your fertility and your ability to conceive. However, we do know that these drugs can harm the fetus and the newborn baby. All women, especially pregnant women, should avoid these drugs.

Drug	Maternal, fetal, newborn, and long-term risks
Marijuana	Low birth weight Long-term cognitive problems, inattention, hyperactivity, depression, and substance abuse problems
Methamphetamine	Higher risk of poor growth Intuitively, a drug that is known to damage brain cells in adults is likely to cause fetal brain injury
Cocaine	Associated with increased incidence of heart attack, stroke, seizures, and sudden death for the mother Increased risk of miscarriage, premature delivery, placental abruption, high blood pressure, low birth weight, and fetal death Long-term problems, including lower IQ
Heroin	Associated with increased incidence of premature delivery, pre-eclampsia, antepartum bleeding, poor fetal growth, and poor fetal heart rate patterns Newborns may suffer from withdrawal symptoms, have behavioral and cognitive problems, and be at an increased risk of SIDS
Methadone	Used successfully to treat heroin addiction and, more recently, to treat chronic pain Preferable to use methadone under medical supervision than to use heroin, especially in pregnancy Methadone can be used while breastfeeding

Consumption of alcohol during pregnancy can result in a condition called fetal alcohol spectrum disorder (FASD). Affecting up to 1% of children, FASD is one of the most common causes of developmental delay in children. It can have a devastating, lifelong impact, leading to low birth weight, poor growth, abnormal facial features, and impaired cognitive development, as well as behavioral problems. The consumption of as little as 1 ounce (30 mL) of alcohol each day or one binge drinking session can result in FASD. In women who consume more than 2 ounces (60 mL) of alcohol daily in the first trimester, 30% to 40% of their children will have FASD.

Cigarette smoke

Quitting smoking is probably the single most important thing you can do to improve your health and that of your baby. Encourage everyone else in your family (especially if they will have contact with the baby) to stop smoking as well. If your partner still smokes, try quitting together. Ask your doctor for assistance with quitting smoking. There are special medications and programs available to help you.

Smoking can contribute to infertility. If you do get pregnant, smoking affects the ability of your placenta to grow and implant properly and can impede the delivery of oxygen to your baby. Smoking can lead to poor fetal growth, premature delivery, and placental abruption (premature separation of the placenta). Pregnant women who smoke are at increased risk of having a stillborn baby. In addition, an increased risk of sudden infant death syndrome (SIDS) has been linked to babies whose mothers smoke in pregnancy and continue to smoke or who live in an environment where smoking is allowed. There is also an increased risk of the child developing other problems, such as asthma, recurrent ear infections, colic, and allergies.

Hot tubs and saunas

Hot tubs and saunas may be relaxing, but anything that heats up your body (including steam baths) can theoretically heat up a developing embryo or fetus. Increased body heat can be a result of having a fever because you are sick, or artificially increasing your body temperature by using a hot tub or sauna. While frequent hot tub or sauna use is not forbidden during pregnancy, it's wise to limit your exposure. High body temperature in the first trimester has been associated with double the risk of miscarriage, a two- to three-fold increase in the risk of neural tube defects, and a drop in blood pressure that could reduce the oxygen and nutrition getting to the fetus. Miscarriage risk is slightly lower for sauna use.

While a hot bath will cool down, hot tubs and saunas are kept at a constant high temperature, making it more likely that risk is increased by use of a hot tub or sauna.

Precautions

To be on the safe side, avoid hot tubs and saunas in the first trimester, and later on in your pregnancy, avoid them because they may cause your blood pressure to drop and make you feel faint.

If you do use a hot tub or sauna:
- Don't let your body temperature get higher than 102.2°F (39°C) for more than 10 minutes.
- Sit with your arms and upper torso above the water in a hot tub to keep your body temperature down.
- Check the water temperature with a thermometer.
- Pay attention to the warning signs of overheating, such as dizziness, faintness, chills, or nausea.
- If you begin to feel unwell, leave the tub or sauna and seek medical attention immediately.

Food-borne bacteria and parasites

Food-borne illnesses caused by bacteria, such as salmonella, E. coli, and listeria, should be avoided during pregnancy. While these bacteria can make you ill, listeria, in particular, can be passed to the fetus and may cause significant illness. For more information on preventing food-borne illness, see Chapter 3, Eating Well for a Healthy Pregnancy (page 125).

Toxoplasmosis

This disease occurs following infection by a parasite called *Toxoplasma gondii*. The parasite exists in a few different forms. One form, the oocyst, is shed in cat feces. Other forms can exist in the meat of animals we eat, especially lamb and pork, but also in beef and chicken. It can also be carried in the soil and be found on the surfaces of unwashed vegetables.

Most women who are infected with toxoplasma are asymptomatic or have only a mild flu-like illness. Despite this, transmission to the fetus can occur with serious consequences, although the severity of the effect on the fetus is significantly reduced as the pregnancy nears term. If you get a toxoplasma infection in pregnancy, antibiotic treatment may reduce the risk of transmission to the fetus.

Managing exposure to *Toxoplasma gondii*

If you are immune to toxoplasma (which can be determined with a blood test), then you don't need to worry; you cannot be reinfected. If you are not immune, you should follow a few precautions to prevent infection:

- Don't change the kitty litter — let someone else do it. If you must do it, wear gloves and wash your hands carefully after handling the feces. (Petting and handling your cat cannot pass on the infection. House cats that eat cooked food are not at risk of developing or passing on toxoplasma.)
- Wash vegetables carefully.
- Make sure your meat is cooked to at least 100°F (70°C) or has been frozen for at least one day (freezing to −18°C, or 0°F, kills the parasite).
- Avoid cured or brined meats — curing and brining do not kill the parasite.
- Avoid raw eggs, unpasteurized milk, and unfiltered water.
- Wear gloves when gardening.
- Wash your hands carefully after handling unwashed vegetables, raw meat, and kitty litter and after gardening.
- Clean your hands and utensils in a dilute bleach solution (1 tsp/15 mL bleach in 3 cups/750 mL water) after handling raw poultry and meat.

Managing mercury exposure

There are many different guidelines concerning the quantity of high-mercury-containing fish that can be safely consumed during pregnancy. The United States Food and Drug Administration (USFDA) has strict guidelines. For example, the USFDA recommends that pregnant and breastfeeding women limit their consumption of canned albacore, or white, tuna to one 6-ounce (170 g) can a month, and that they avoid entirely fish with known high levels of mercury (fresh or frozen tuna, swordfish, orange roughy, shark, marlin, tilefish, and king mackerel). Health Canada's guidelines are more liberal and suggest that it is safe to have a small amount of fish with higher mercury levels — but not more than once a month.

Food contaminants and additives

Some healthy foods can be contaminated by toxic substances in the environment they grow or live in, especially certain species of fish.

Mercury in fish

Most fish is a healthy food choice during pregnancy. For expectant mothers, it is an excellent source of protein, high in omega-3 fatty acids, and low in saturated fat. However, some fish contain unsafe levels of mercury, a teratogen that can cross the placenta.

In high concentrations, mercury may contribute to cerebral palsy, poor physical and mental development, and blindness or deafness in the infant. This degree of mercury contamination is very unusual in North American populations, so don't panic if you have been eating lots of fish. Be aware, however, if there are concerns about mercury contamination in the water in your community.

High-mercury-containing fish
Health Canada recommends that all pregnant and breastfeeding women limit their consumption of the following high-mercury-containing fish to one meal of no more than 1 cup (150 g) a month:

- King mackerel
- Marlin
- Orange roughy
- Shark
- Swordfish
- Tilefish
- Tuna, fresh or frozen

Health Canada also recommends that pregnant and breastfeeding women limit their consumption of canned albacore, or white, tuna to 2 cups (300 g) per week, which is equivalent to 4 servings where 1 serving = $\frac{1}{2}$ cup (75 g).

Low-mercury-containing fish
Health Canada recommends that consumption of the following fish and seafood be limited

to no more than two meals a week, each containing no more than 1 cup (150 g), to obtain health benefits from fish and seafood:

- Char
- Cod
- Herring
- Mackerel
- Mussels
- Pollock
- Salmon
- Sardines
- Scallops
- Shrimp
- Sole
- Tuna, light canned (skipjack or yellowfin)

Polychlorinated biphenyls

Polychlorinated biphenyls (PCBs) are toxic environmental pollutants found in very low levels in food, in the soil, and in the air. PCBs concentrate in animals, with the highest levels found in humans. People who eat game and sports fish are at greatest risk. In the past, there has been concern about PCBs in salmon, but more recent data suggest that PCB levels in both farmed and wild salmon are well within safe limits.

Check with your regional authorities about the safety of the game and fish you are eating, and minimize your exposure to PCBs by discarding the inner organs, removing all visible fat, and preparing the food to eat by grilling, broiling, baking, or boiling — not frying, which preserves the fat where PCBs are concentrated.

Caffeine

Motherisk conducted an analysis of scientific studies of the effect of caffeine in pregnancy and concluded that 150 mg of caffeine did not trigger any adverse effects, but if more than 150 mg caffeine was consumed daily in the first trimester, there was a higher incidence of miscarriage and low birth weight.

Besides the caffeine in a cup of coffee, tea, or can of pop, some amount of caffeine is naturally found in many foods. There are also hidden sources of caffeine in some foods and herbs. Guarana is an example of an herb that contains caffeine. High-energy drinks or sports drinks may contain this herb or caffeine itself. Be sure to read the label before consuming sport drinks or high-performance beverages.

Herbal teas

Some herbal teas are made from plants that may have medicinal effects upon pregnancy, but information about herbal teas changes often, so if they are currently a part of your diet, ask your health-care provider for the most up-to-date information. The two most commonly consumed teas in pregnancy are ginger tea, which can be safely used to calm morning sickness and nausea, and raspberry leaf tea, which is advocated by some people for use late in the third trimester to shorten labor. This claim has not been proven objectively, nor has the safety of raspberry leaf tea been proven.

Safe herbal teas

Health Canada says that it is safe to consume 2 to 3 cups (500 to 750 mL) of the following herbal teas daily:

- Blackberry
- Citrus peel
- Ginger
- Lemon balm
- Linden flower (this tea is not safe if you have a heart problem)
- Orange peel
- Rose hip

Unsafe herbal teas

It is not safe to consume any amount of the following teas during pregnancy, because they can cause uterine contractions:

- Chamomile
- Dong quai
- Sassafras

Managing Medical and Environmental Risks

Artificial sweeteners

Artificial sweeteners (non-nutritive sweeteners) are substances that sweeten foods and beverages without adding calories or increasing blood sugars. In general, moderate use of artificial sweeteners is considered safe in pregnancy, but some sweeteners can cross the placenta and should be avoided.

Sweetener safety

- Aspartame is safe in pregnancy as a table-top sweetener and as a food additive.
- Health Canada recommends against using cyclamate (Sugar Twin, Weight Watchers, and Sucaryl) and saccharin (Sweet'N Low and Hermesetas) as tabletop sweeteners during pregnancy.
- Cyclamate is not allowed as a food in the United States.

Caffeine content in common foods and drinks

Recommended intake: no more than 150 mg per day

Food or drink	Serving	Caffeine
Coffee, Starbucks, grande	16 fl. oz (500 mL)	330 mg
Coffee, Starbucks, latte	16 fl. oz (500 mL)	150 mg
Coffee, plain, brewed	8 fl. oz (250 mL)	95 mg
Coffee, instant	8 fl. oz (250 mL)	93 mg
Coffee, espresso	1 fl. oz (30 mL)	64 mg
Coffee, decaffeinated, instant	8 fl. oz (250 mL)	2 mg
Coffee, decaffeinated, brewed	8 fl. oz (250 mL)	2 mg
Black tea, brewed	8 fl. oz (250 mL)	47 mg
Black tea, decaffeinated	8 fl. oz (250 mL)	2 mg
Green tea, brewed	8 fl. oz (250 mL)	30–50 mg
Snapple iced tea	16 fl. oz (500 mL)	18 mg
Nestea	12 fl. oz (355 mL)	17 mg
Coca-Cola Classic	12 fl. oz (355 mL)	3 mg
Diet Coke	12 fl. oz (355 mL)	47 mg
Pepsi	12 fl. oz (355 mL)	38 mg
Diet Pepsi	12 fl. oz (355 mL)	36 mg
Mountain Dew, Diet	12 fl. oz (355 mL)	54 mg
Dr. Pepper, Diet Dr. Pepper	12 fl. oz (355 mL)	42 mg
Sprite, Sprite Zero	12 fl. oz (250 mL)	0 mg
7 Up	12 fl. oz (250 mL)	0 mg
Häagen-Dazs Coffee Ice Cream	½ cup (125 mL)	30 mg
Hershey's chocolate bar	1.55 oz (16 g)	9 mg

Chemical pollutants

Pollution — of all kinds — is one of the greatest risks to public health, contaminating the air we breathe and the water we drink. What are the risks of pollution to the fetus? How concerned should you be? And what can you do about it? To start, know the enemy.

Household risks

Tobacco, air fresheners, cosmetics, pesticides, household cleaners, and molds are among the potential indoor dangers, along with organic compounds found in new carpet and paints. You might even want to avoid standing in front of your microwave oven when it's on, or to have it checked for leaks. Although with most hazardous substances used in the home, a pregnant woman would have to be exposed to a large amount for a long time in order for them to harm her baby, it's easier to stay safe and avoid potential problems.

Carbon monoxide

Carbon monoxide is a colorless and odorless gas emitted from wood-burning, oil-burning, and gas-burning furnaces, stoves, and fireplaces. If this gas is not properly exhausted from the home, the home's inhabitants can suffer serious illness and death. If the carbon monoxide levels are so high that a pregnant woman loses consciousness, the fetus can suffer brain damage, leading to developmental delay, and intrauterine or postnatal death.

Be sure to check your heating and cooking systems for carbon monoxide leaks and install a carbon monoxide detector and alarm system in your home. If you think you have been exposed to carbon monoxide, go to an emergency room right away. But remember, if the levels haven't made you or other family members symptomatic, any significant effects upon the baby are unlikely.

Organic solvents

Many household cleaners contain solvents. Solvents are chemicals that dissolve other substances and include such common products as degreasers, paint thinners, and varnish

Managing solvent exposure

- Pregnant women who work with solvents — even women who do arts and crafts at home — should minimize their exposure by making sure their work space is well ventilated and by wearing appropriate protective clothing, including gloves and a face mask. Never eat or drink in the work area.

- Although some household cleansers contain solvents, there are many safe alternatives. Pregnant women should read labels carefully and avoid products (such as some oven cleaners) with labels stating that they are toxic. You might also try substituting safe, natural products. For example, baking soda can be used as a powdered cleanser on most surfaces, and a solution of vinegar and water can effectively clean many surfaces.

removers. Lacquers, silk-screening inks, and paints also contain these chemicals.

Outdoor air pollution

Many studies have shown that babies whose mothers are exposed to high levels of air pollution are more likely to be born prematurely or with a low birth weight. Precautions are advisable, although millions of women who live in big cities with higher-than-average levels of air pollution have healthy babies.

Managing air pollutant risks

- Monitor local air quality conditions, and when the air is poor, limit the time you spend outdoors, including driving.

- Avoid smoke-filled rooms — and, obviously, don't smoke yourself.

- Keep the air conditioning on in your car when you're in congested traffic.

- Reduce the amount of time you spend in areas where there is a high volume of vehicular traffic.

Trihalomethane

In municipal water supplies, chlorine is added to drinking water to kill disease-causing microbes, but, paradoxically, when chlorine combines with other materials in water, it forms potentially harmful byproducts called trihalomethanes. In recent years, there have been concerns about possible pregnancy risks from these byproducts.

Managing water safety

- Drinking tap water is probably safer than drinking bottled water, which is not subjected to such rigorous quality control and testing. It is also an environmentally friendly choice.
- Drinking water from wells also can become contaminated with pesticides, lead, arsenic, and other heavy metals, as well as bacteria-laden runoff from farmer's fields.
- If you suspect that your water supply is polluted, have it tested and drink bottled water until you receive the results.

Lead

Specific heavy metals and minerals can pass across the placenta when ingested, inhaled, or even touched. They are toxic to the fetus and newborn. Exposure to high levels of lead during pregnancy has been shown to contribute to miscarriage, preterm delivery, low birth weight, and developmental delays in infants.

Lead was used for many years in gasoline, paint, and other commercial and home products. Other possible sources of lead in the home include lead crystal glassware and some ceramic dishes, arts and crafts materials (oil paints and ceramic glazes), old painted toys, and cosmetics containing surma or kohl. You might also be exposed to lead in drinking water if your home has lead pipes, lead solder on copper pipes, or brass faucets.

The amounts have decreased greatly since the 1970s, when non-leaded gasoline and paints were introduced in the market and legislated in some jurisdictions.

Managing lead contamination

- **Lead-based paint:** If you live in an older home, you may be exposed to lead in deteriorating lead-based paint. If lead-based paint needs to be removed from your home, make sure you stay away until the project is done. Leave the job to the experts, who use proper precautions.
- **Lead pipes:** If your home has lead pipes, lead solder on copper pipes, or brass faucets, you might consider replacing these with non-leaded products. If not replaced, water from the cold water pipe, which contains less lead than hot water, should be used for cooking and drinking during pregnancy, and for preparing baby formula. Running the water for 15 to 30 seconds before drinking or using it for cooking helps reduce lead levels. Contact your health department or water supplier to find out how to get pipes tested for lead.

Mercury

Besides the risk of mercury contamination from eating certain species of fish, elemental (pure) mercury is used in thermometers, dental fillings, and some batteries. It's recommended that dentists avoid using dental amalgam (a silver-colored material that contains mercury) to fill cavities in teeth of pregnant women, although there is no evidence that it will harm their babies. Talk it over with your dentist.

Arsenic

Arsenic is another metal suspected of posing pregnancy risks, although the small amounts normally found in the environment are unlikely to harm a fetus. Arsenic enters the environment through natural sources (forest fires and weathering of rock) and manmade sources (mining and electronics manufacturing).

Women who may be exposed to higher levels of arsenic include those who work at or live near metal smelters, hazardous waste sites, and incinerators, or live in agricultural areas where arsenic fertilizers were/are used on crops.

If you live in an area that may have high arsenic levels, you'll want to protect yourself from exposure by limiting your contact with soil.

Managing pesticide exposure in pregnancy

- Remove food, dishes, and utensils from the area before the pesticide is applied.
- Close all windows and turn off air conditioning when pesticides are used outdoors so fumes aren't drawn into the house.
- Have someone else apply the chemicals while you leave the area for the amount of time indicated on the package instructions.
- Afterwards, have someone open the windows and wash off all surfaces on which food is prepared.
- Wear rubber gloves when gardening to prevent skin contact with pesticides.
- Try using less toxic products — there are more on the market than ever before.
- Use safe insect repellants. DEET (diethyltoluamide) is among the most effective at keeping insects, such as mosquitoes and ticks, from biting. Preventing insect bites is important during pregnancy because mosquito- and tick-borne infections, such as West Nile virus and Lyme disease, may be harmful in pregnancy. There is no evidence that DEET is harmful in pregnancy to the mother or the fetus.

If you use well water, have it tested for arsenic to determine whether it is safe to drink, or drink bottled water.

Until 2003, arsenic was included as part of a preservative for pressure-treated lumber used to build decks and outdoor play sets. It's recommended that you apply a sealant to these structures at least once a year to reduce exposure to arsenic.

Pesticides

There is little proof that exposure to pest-control products at levels commonly used at home pose a risk to the fetus. However, all insecticides are to some extent toxic, and some studies suggest that high levels of exposure to pesticides may contribute to miscarriage, premature delivery, and birth defects. Therefore, pregnant women should avoid pesticides whenever possible.

Occupational hazards

One study has shown that women factory workers, laboratory technicians, artists, graphic designers, and printing industry workers who were exposed to solvents on the job during their first trimester of pregnancy are more likely than unexposed women to have a baby with a major birth defect, such as spina bifida, clubfoot, heart defects, and deafness. Other studies have found that women workers in semiconductor plants exposed to high levels of solvents called glycol ethers were almost three times more likely to miscarry than unexposed women. Glycol ethers also are used in jobs that involve photography, dyes, and silk-screen printing.

Managing chemical hazards at work

In general, you can reduce the risk of working with or around chemicals by taking the following precautions:

- Discuss any exposures in your workplace with your health-care provider to determine whether additional on-the-job protections or an alternative assignment is advisable. This is especially important for women who work in high-risk industries, such as agriculture and refining.
- Be sure your workplace has good airflow.
- Wear gloves, special clothing, and respirators.
- Store chemicals in sealed containers.
- Do not eat near chemicals.
- Wash your hands after contact with chemicals and before eating or drinking.
- If chemicals are spilled on your clothing or skin, change immediately and follow the directions for cleaning off the chemical.
- Change out of your work clothing and wash your hands well before leaving your workplace.
- Do not store or wash work clothes with street clothes; if possible, wash work clothes at work.
- Leave work clothes and accessories at work.
- Most workplaces have preventive measures in place to help reduce exposures to chemicals and radiation in some occupations.

Pregnancy-induced conditions

Certain medical conditions are induced by pregnancy. The most common are summarized in this chart, listed in alphabetical order with page numbers that lead to more detailed information available in previous chapters.

Condition	Key Signs and Symptoms	Management
Anemia (page 230)	• Excessive fatigue • Shortness of breath • Pale skin, conjunctiva	• Increase intake of iron-rich foods • Take iron supplements
Back pain (page 207)	• Pain, often in lower back • May be worse with exertion	• Gentle exercise • Rest as necessary • Acetaminophen as needed
Blocked duct (page 412)	• Pain in breast • Lumpy breast	• Massage quadrant of breast affected, especially while nursing • Hot compresses to breast prior to nursing
Breast engorgement (page 412)	• Full breasts, firm to touch • Tenderness	• Nurse baby • Cold cabbage leaves
Carpal tunnel syndrome (page 208)	• Pain and tingling in fingertips/hands • Worse in mornings	• Wrist splints, at minimum at night, maybe more often
Cholestasis (page 210)	• Itchy skin, usually in absence of rash	• Fetal monitoring • Antihistamines for itch • Urso to reduce bile acids
Common Cold (page 448)	• Runny nose • Cough • Fever	• Rest • Fluids • Acetaminophen as necessary
Constipation (page 136)	• Difficulty passing stool	• Increase fiber intake • Increase fluid intake • Consider stool softeners
Ectopic pregnancy (page 158)	• Pain in lower abdomen • Dizziness • Unusual bleeding • Often asymptomatic	• Immediate medical attention required • Surgery (possibly) • Methotrexate (possibly)

Eczema (page 404)	• Itchy skin • Dry, scaly skin	• Eliminate irritants • Avoid over-drying of skin • Corticosteroid cream
Fatigue (page 138)	• Reduced energy • Tired • Sleepiness	• Rest • Increase intake of iron
Gestational diabetes mellitus (page 226)	• Usually no symptoms	• Dietary modifications • Exercise • Insulin (possibly)
Gestational hypertension (page 291)	• Usually no symptoms	• Rest • Monitoring • Medication (possibly)
Gingivitis (page 137)	• Bleeding gums	• Soft toothbrush • See dentist
Group B streptococcus (page 289)	• Usually no symptoms	• If GBS is found in urine, treat with antibiotics • Antibiotics when in labor
Headaches (page 139)	• Usual headache pain	• Acetaminophen • If no response to acetaminophen, seek medical opinion
Heartburn (page 136)	• Pain behind breastbone • Worse after eating • Worse when lying down	• Smaller meals • Sleep propped up • Antacids (Maalox, Gaviscon) • H-2 receptor blockers (ranitidine or Zantac)
Hemorrhoids (page 304)	• Pain in rectum, worse with bowel movement • Occasionally, blood in stool	• Stool softeners • Sitz baths • Hemorrhoid cream • Steroid suppositories
Incompetent cervix (page 222)	• Vaginal bleeding • Increased vaginal discharge • Pressure in pelvis	• Bedrest • Cervical cerclage
Intrauterine growth restriction (page 282)	• Poor fetal growth measured by serial ultrasounds	• Careful fetal monitoring • Reduced activity • Possibly, early delivery
Leg cramps (page 278)	• Sudden, intense pain in calf • Muscle contraction • Often at night	• Stretch calf muscle • Increase fluid intake

Mastitis (page 413)	• Fever • Pain in breast • Portion of breast is hot, red, tender	• Continue nursing • Acetaminophen • Antibiotics
Miscarriage (threatened) in first trimester (page 156)	• Vaginal bleeding • Cramping	• If bleeding heavy (> 2 pads/hr for 2 hrs in a row), seek urgent medical opinion • If not heavy, ultrasound in next 1 to 2 days to establish diagnosis
Miscarriage (definite) in first trimester (page 156)	• Heavy vaginal bleeding • Cramping • Tissue passed vaginally (possibly)	• If bleeding very heavy (> 2 pads/hr for 2 hrs in a row), seek urgent medical attention • Otherwise, seek medical advice next day • May need RhIg if blood type is Rh−
Molar pregnancy (page 159)	• Abnormal vaginal bleeding • Nausea & vomiting (possibly)	• Ultrasound • D&C
Mood changes (page 139)	• Depressed mood • Anxiety	• Seek medical opinion • Psychotherapy (possibly) • Medication (possibly)
Nausea and vomiting (page 134)	• Nausea • Vomiting • Inability to tolerate food/drink	• Small, frequent meals • Avoid triggers • Diclectin • Gravol • Other medications may be required
Nipples leaking (page 411)	• Milk leaking when not nursing	• Nurse often • Wear breast pads
Nipples sore (page 411)	• Painful nipples • Bruised/bleeding nipples • Worse with baby latching	• See a lactation consultant • Latch needs to be corrected • Put a few drops of breast milk on nipples and allow it to dry
Pelvic floor prolapse (page 421)	• Postpartum drop of uterus to level of vaginal opening • Pressure sensation	• Pessary surgery
Placenta previa (page 298)	• Painless vaginal bleeding	• Ultrasound to confirm diagnosis • Urgent medical care if bleeding • Avoid putting anything in vagina • Bedrest (possibly) • Caesarean section
Postpartum depression (page 422)	• Depressed mood • Inability to enjoy life/baby • Fear of self-harm or harming baby	• Seek medical care • Seek support • Psychotherapy (possibly) • Antidepressants

Pre-eclampsia (page 293)	• Headache • Visual changes (floaters, spots) • Pain under ribs on right side • Swelling	• Seek medical care urgently • Immediate delivery may be required
Pubic symphysis separation (page 296)	• Pain over pubic bone • Difficulty walking (sometimes)	• Acetaminophen • Physiotherapy
PUPPP, prurigo, and pruritic folliculitis (pages 211 and 212)	• Itchy rash with red spots • Starts on abdomen and spreads	• Cooling skin cream • Antihistamines • Corticosteroid cream
Urinary incontinence (weak bladder) (page 421)	• Leaking urine • Usually worse with cough/laugh/sneeze	• Kegel exercises
Urinary tract infection	• More frequent urination • Painful urination • Cloudy urine • Often no symptoms	• Antibiotics • Drink lots of fluids
Varicose veins (page 208)	• Prominent veins in legs • Achy and sore (sometimes) • Worse with prolonged standing (sometimes)	• Elevate legs • Wear support hose
Yeast infection (page 443)	• White, itchy vaginal discharge	• Antifungal vaginal suppositories

F.A.Q.

We answer many questions from pregnant women and their partners. Here are some of the most frequently asked questions. Be sure to ask your health-care providers any other questions that may arise. If they don't have the answers, they will refer you to a colleague who does.

Q: I had a few drinks in my first trimester before I knew I was pregnant. What can I do?

A: Although we believe that it is safest if no alcohol is consumed at any time during pregnancy, we know that at least 50% of pregnancies are unplanned and that this is a common situation. Many women are racked with guilt about this, but there's nothing to be done but to stop drinking from this point forward and stop worrying — the odds are that everything should be fine. It is highly unlikely that a few drinks early in pregnancy will have any significant effect or cause fetal alcohol spectrum disorder (FASD). If, however, you are a heavy drinker or an alcoholic, see your health-care provider immediately.

Q: I don't understand why I can eat some kinds of tuna without worrying about mercury but not others.

A: Not all tuna is the same… Mercury accumulates as it travels up the food chain. There is less mercury in small fish, but as big and bigger fish eat the smaller fish, mercury levels become concentrated in the bigger and older fish. The tuna that you eat fresh or frozen tends to be from a bigger and older fish than the tuna that gets canned, so it has higher levels of mercury and thus should be consumed less often (not more than once a month). Likewise, not all canned tuna is the same… Albacore, or white, tuna has a higher level of mercury than other kinds of tuna labeled "light tuna" (yellowfin, skipjack, and tongol). So even though canned albacore tuna has acceptably low levels of mercury in it, if you eat a tuna fish sandwich every day made with this tuna, you will be getting too much mercury. A sandwich or two a week will keep your mercury consumption levels in a low, safe range.

Q: Are deli meats safe to eat in pregnancy?

A: For some of us, it is hard to imagine lunch without a sandwich filled with sliced ham or turkey. Although low, there is a risk of contamination with listeria. It is advised by the USFDA and Health Canada that deli meats and hot dogs be heated until steaming hot prior to consumption by pregnant women. Dried meats, such as salami and pepperoni, are safer because listeria is less likely to grow in the dry environment.

Q: How much caffeine is safe to consume in pregnancy, if any at all?

A: Two reputable groups have addressed this question. Health Canada advises consumption be limited to no more than 350 mg of caffeine a day, while Motherisk is more conservative in their recommendation of 150 mg of caffeine daily, which is 1 to 2 cups (250 to 500 mL) of regular coffee. If in doubt, ask your favorite coffee shop how much caffeine is in their blends.

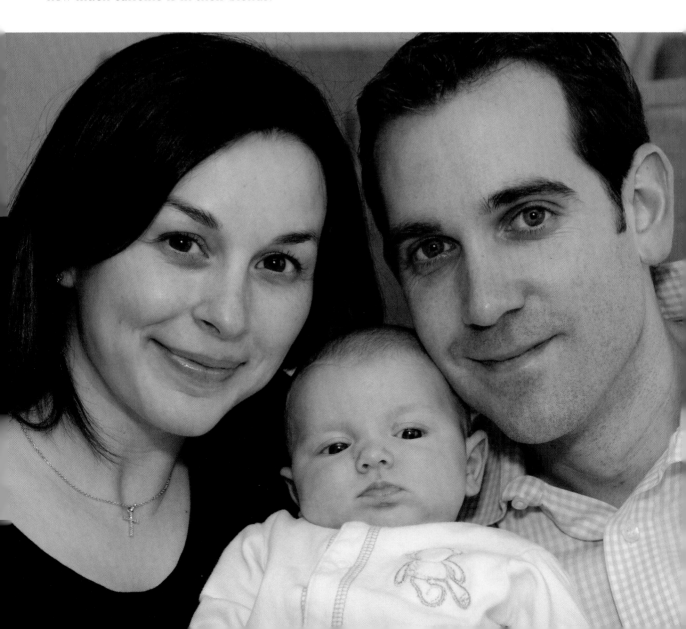

Pregnancy Care Resources

Obstetrics and Gynecology Associations

Up-to-date guidelines and extensive lists of resources for women in specific circumstances (Aboriginal women, disabled women, single parents, abusive situations) and with specific conditions (diabetes, drug dependency problems, cancer), as well as information about maternity and parental leave, parenting and many other concerns.

American College of Obstetricians and Gynecologists
409 12th Street, SW, PO Box 96920
Washington, DC 20090-6920
Tel: 202-638-5577
www.acog.org

The Society of Obstetricians and Gynaecologists of Canada
780 Echo Drive, Ottawa, ON K1S 5R7
Tel: 613-730-4192
www.sogc.org

National health resources

Include up-to-date information about many aspects of pregnancy, including food-borne, environmental, and infectious risks.

Health Canada
www.phac-aspc.gc.ca/hp-gs/index-eng.php

Centers for Disease Control and Prevention (CDC)
www.cdc.gov/reproductivehealth

National Institutes of Health (NIH)
www.nlm.nih.gov/medlineplus/pregnancy

Prenatal education and childbirth classes

International Childbirth Education Association
1500 Sunday Drive, Suite 102
Raleigh, NC 27607
Tel: 919/863-9487
www.icea.org

Lamaze
2025 M Street, NW, Suite 800
Washington, DC 20036-3309
www.lamaze.org

Midwives and Doulas

Canadian Midwives
#442-6555 chemin de la Côte-des-Neiges
Montréal, Québec H3S 2A6
Tel: 514-807-3668
www.canadianmidwives.org

Association of Ontario Midwives
365 Bloor St E, Suite 301
Toronto, ON M4W 3L4
Tel: 416-425-9974
www.aom.on.ca

DONA International
PO Box 626
Jasper, IN 47547
Tel: 888-788-3662
www.dona.org

Teratogen information services

There are a number of teratogen information services that report on current research in this field. The information can be complex, so be sure to discuss it with your health-care providers for a clear understanding of these risks in pregnancy.

European Network Teratogen Information Services (ENTIS)
Serves Europe, Israel, and South America. See the list of ENTIS services at www.entis-org.com

Organization of Teratology Information Services (OTIS)
Serves most states and provinces in the United States and Canada. See the list of OTIS services at www.otispregnancy.org

Motherisk
Based at the Hospital for Sick Children in Toronto, Canada. See the list of Motherisk services at www.motherisk.org

Mental health information

Dalfen A. *When Baby Brings the Blues: Solutions for Postpartum Depression.* Toronto, ON: Wiley, 2009.

The MGH (Massachusetts General Hospital) Center for Women's Mental Health
Perinatal and Reproductive Psychiatry Program
Simches Research Building
185 Cambridge Street, Suite 2200
Boston, MA 02114
www.womensmentalhealth.com

BC Reproductive Mental Health Program
BC Women's Hospital and Health Centre
4500 Oak Street
Vancouver, BC V6H 3N1
Tel: 604-875-2424
www.bcwomens.ca

Perinatal Bereavement Services of Ontario
PO Box 177
Pickering, ON L1V 2R4
Tel: 905-472-1807
www.pbso.ca

Postpartum Support International
www.postpartum.net

Breastfeeding support

Newman Breastfeeding Clinic and Institute
Canadian College of Naturopathic Medicine (CCNM)
1255 Sheppard Avenue East
Toronto, ON M2K 1E2
Tel: 416-498-0002
www.Drjacknewman.com

La Leche League
National Administration
PO Box 700
Winchester, ON K0C 2K0
Tel: 613-774-4900
www.lllc.ca/

International Board of Lactation Consultant Examiners
www.iblce.org

Nutrition

Health Canada
www.hc-sc.gc.ca/fn-an/nutrition/prenatal/index-eng.php

Kalnins D. and Saab J. *Better Food for Pregnancy.* Toronto, ON: Robert Rose, 2006.

Smoking cessation in pregnancy

Pregnets
Tel: (416) 535-8501 ext. 6343
Fax: (416) 599-8265
www.pregnets.org

Baby care
Friedman J. and Saunders N. *The Baby Care Book.* Toronto, ON: Robert Rose, 2007.

468

Acknowledgments

Elephants have a much longer gestation period than humans — 22 months — but still only two parents. This book has had an even longer gestation period, and many, many more contributing parents. We are grateful to so many people for their enthusiasm and participation in this elephantine project.

Our contributing authors: Yoel Abells, Lisa Allen, Marshall Barkin. Elizabeth Brandeis, Laura Crouse, Ariel Dalfen, Eric Goldszmidt, Preeti Jain, Elyse Levinsky, Erin Love, Elliot Lyons, Jesseny Rojas, Jodi Shapiro, Matthuschka Sheedy, Ants Toi, and Beverly Young. This book relies on their specialized knowledge and experience, and without their contributions there would not have been a book.

Our coordinator: Helen Robson was instrumental in shepherding this project to completion by coordinating the authors, the photographers, and the models. Her organizational skills and, particularly, her patience, go beyond the bounds of reason.

Our photographers: John Loper, of J.C. Loper Photography, took most of the beautiful pictures in the book, and his good humor and sensitivity were universally appreciated by the participating families and by us. Bryan Kautz and Keith Oxley, of University Health Network PhotoGraphics, also contributed many beautiful pictures. Ken Meats, of the Department of Graphics and New Media at Mount Sinai Hospital, expertly assisted in the preparation of many photographs and ultrasound images. Gwen Rayner, R.R.T., who always provides photography services along with her usual excellent respiratory therapy care to newborns in the Caesarean section room, provided a few of her photos to grace these pages. Grace Donald, RN, a labor and delivery nurse at Sunnybrook Health Sciences Centre and a photographer, combined her skills to provide a series of wonderfully unique photographs of a spontaneous birth.

Our models! We are grateful to the many women and their families who consented to be photographed for this book. We think you will agree that they look fabulous!

Our publisher: Bob Hilderley, Senior Editor, Health, of Robert Rose Inc., calmly guided us (and the manuscript) from beginning to end with patience and skill. The support of Marian Jarkovich, Bob Dees, and the remainder of the team at Robert Rose has been much appreciated.

Our designer: Andrew Smith and the team at PageWave Graphics were so successful at presenting the text in an interesting, readable, and clear format.

Our hospital: Members of the Department of Communications and Marketing at Mount Sinai Hospital, notably Judith John, the former VP of this division, encouraged us to take on this project, and Lyn Whitham, the current VP of the Department of Communications and Marketing at Mount Sinai Hospital, has continued to support this project.

Our families: And finally, but not least, our families gave us understanding and support when time contributed to this book took us away from them: David, Sebastian, Beatrice, and Grace Dal Bello; R.J., Sam, and Hannah Cusimano; and Barbara Bernstein.

Photo Credits

Principal photographer: John Loper/J.C. Loper Photography.

Subsidiary photography by: Bryan Kautz and Keith Oxley, Medical Photographers, University Health Network PhotoGraphics; Ken Meats, Department of Graphics and New Media, Mount Sinai Hospital; and Gwen Rayner, R.R.T.

Vaginal birth photography by Grace Donald, RN.

Thanks to Lynn Sharples, RN, and Karen Meadwell, RN, for supplying a partogram.

Stock Photography as follows: page 3: © iStockphoto.com/Marie-France Bélanger; 12: © iStockphoto.com/Derek Lotta; 26: © iStockphoto.com/pix deluxe; 32: © iStockphoto.com/johannes norpoth; 39: © iStockphoto.com/RonTech 2000; 43: © iStockphoto.com/Jelani Memory; 52: © iStockphoto.com/gary milner; 56: © iStockphoto.com/Valentin Casarsa; 60: © iStockphoto.com/laartist; 63: © iStockphoto.com/Sara Sanger; 75: © iStockphoto.com/iofoto; 83: © 2009 JupiterImages Corporation; 94: © iStockphoto.com/Nicolette Neish; 102: © iStockphoto.com/Leah-Anne Thompson; 107: © iStockphoto.com/Dean Mitchell; 113: © iStockphoto.com/Suprijono Suharjoto; 116: © iStockphoto.com/Rhienna Cutler; 117: © iStockphoto.com/Elena Schweitzer; 121: © iStockphoto.com/Doxa Digital; 123: © iStockphoto.com/Dan Moore; 124: © iStockphoto.com/kivoart; 126: © iStockphoto.com/Leah-Anne Thompson; 127: © iStockphoto.com/Klaudia Steiner; 131: © iStockphoto.com/jo unruh; 137: © iStockphoto.com/Hannes Eichinger; 141: © iStockphoto.com/forgiss; 144: © iStockphoto.com/1001nights; 149: © iStockphoto.com/Tomasz Markowski; 160: © iStockphoto.com/Kevin Panizza; 161: © iStockphoto.com/Dean Mitchell; 246: © iStockphoto.com/Anthony Rosenberg; 260: © iStockphoto.com/amaxim; 311: © iStockphoto.com/Jacqueline Huntzele; 330: © iStockphoto.com/Joshua Mort; 365: © iStockphoto.com/Sean O'Riordan; 368: © iStockphoto.com/Damir Cudic; 371: © iStockphoto.com/susaro; 373: © iStockphoto.com/Rich Legg; 384: © iStockphoto.com/Marcos Paternoster; 386: © iStockphoto.com/ijoe; 391: © iStockphoto.com/Joshua Mort; 392: © iStockphoto.com/Kati Neudert; 394: © iStockphoto.com/1joe; 397: © iStockphoto.com/gaia moments; 398: © iStockphoto.com/Emre Eldemir; 416: © iStockphoto.com/Brian McEntire; 417: © iStockphoto.com/Brian McEntire; 419: © iStockphoto.com/Rohit Seth.

Library and Archives Canada Cataloguing in Publication

Farrugia, Mary Michèle
    Mount Sinai Hospital : the pregnancy care book / Michèle Farrugia, Jacqueline Thomas, Paul Bernstein.

ISBN 978-0-7788-0226-6

1. Pregnancy—Popular works. I. Thomas, Jacqueline, 1961– II. Bernstein, Paul, 1943–
III. Mount Sinai Hospital (Toronto, Ont.) IV. Title. V. Title: Pregnancy care book.

RG525.F37 2009a   618.2   C2009-904493-5

Farrugia, Mary Michèle
    Canada's pregnancy care book / Michèle Farrugia, Jacqueline Thomas, Paul Bernstein.

At head of title: Mount Sinai Hospital.
ISBN 978-0-7788-0231-0

1. Pregnancy—Popular works. I. Thomas, Jacqueline, 1961– II. Bernstein, Paul, 1943–
III. Mount Sinai Hospital (Toronto, Ont.) IV. Title.

RG525.F37 2009   618.2   C2009-902269-9

Index

formula-feeding, 258, 410
deciding on, 255, 256
friends (as support), 90–91

G

galactogogues, 409
galactosemia, 399
GBS (group B
streptococcus), 289–90,
304, 338
genes, 38, 39
mutations, 41–42
genetic counseling, 72–73
genetics, 38–43
of Rh, 284
genital warts, 445
German measles. *See* rubella
ginger (as nausea remedy),
134–35
gingivitis, 137
glycemic index, 102
gonorrhea, 445
Grave's disease, 438

H

hair
changes in pregnancy,
66, 142
coloring or processing, 142
loss of, 427
hay fever, 450
headaches, 139
from epidural, 266
medication alternatives,
450
health
optimizing, 44, 45
in pregnancy, 61, 130
health-care providers, 68–75
specialists, 71–74
trainees, 75
hearing disorders, 399
heart disease, 433, 434–35
heart rate (fetal), 344

in labor, 339
monitoring, 342–43, 363,
366
non-reassuring, 366
oxytocin and, 363
heart rate (maternal)
in early pregnancy, 66
in exercise, 172
heartburn, 67, 136–37
HELLP syndrome, 322
hematomas, 372
hemophilia, 41, 429, 430
hemorrhage
Caesarean section and,
381, 382
postpartum, 387–89
hemorrhoids, 67, 208,
304
hepatitis B, 445–46
hepatitis C, 440
herbal remedies, 451
to increase milk supply,
409
for nausea, 134–35
herbal teas, 455
heredity, 38, 42. *See also*
genetics
heroin, 452
herpes, 446
HIV (human
immunodeficiency
virus), 447
hormones of pregnancy, 66
hospitals, 82–83, 84
hot tubs, 453
HPV (human papilloma
virus), 445
Huntington's chorea, 41,
429, 430
hydrops, 441
hypertension, 433. *See also*
pre-eclampsia
chronic, 435–36
diabetes and, 229

drugs for, 49, 435
gestational, 291–92, 322
measuring, 436
hyperthyroidism, 433,
438–39
hypnosis (during birth), 80,
262
hypothyroidism
in mother, 433, 438–39
in newborn, 399

I

immunization, 52, 440
in-laws (as support), 90
in vitro fertilization (IVF),
36, 37, 43
infections, 439–43
of breast, 413
Caesarean section and,
380, 381–82, 420
and labor, 338
in newborns, 400, 401
postpartum, 420
during pregnancy, 51, 52
infertility, 33–37
influenza, 440
intrauterine growth
restriction (IUGR),
282–83, 292
iron (dietary), 111–12
breastfeeding and, 410
and constipation, 136
supplemental, 450
and zinc absorption, 113
itching. *See also* rashes
from epidural, 266
IVF (in vitro fertilization),
36, 37, 43

J

jaundice
in newborn, 404
during pregnancy, 210
joints, 168–69, 296